T0200871

Managing Minor Musculoskeletal Injuries and Conditions

David Bradley

Formerly Senior Lecturer in Emergency Care at
Liverpool John Moores University
Liverpool, UK

WILEY Blackwell

This edition first published 2014 © John Wiley & Sons Ltd.

Registered office: John Wiley & Sons, Ltd., The Atrium, Southern Gate, Chichester, West Sussex, PO19 8SQ, UK

Editorial offices: 9600 Garsington Road, Oxford, OX4 2DQ, UK
The Atrium, Southern Gate, Chichester, West Sussex, PO19 8SQ, UK
111 River Street, Hoboken, NJ 07030-5774, USA

For details of our global editorial offices, for customer services and for information about how to apply for permission to reuse the copyright material in this book please see our website at www.wiley.com/wiley-blackwell

Library of Congress Cataloging-in-Publication Data

Bradley, David, 1945– author.
Minor musculoskeletal injuries and conditions / David Bradley.
p. ; cm.
Managing minor musculoskeletal injuries and conditions
Includes bibliographical references and index.
ISBN 978-0-470-67310-2 (pbk. : alk. paper) – ISBN 978-1-118-51282-1 (epub) – ISBN 978-1-118-51283-8 (emobi) –
ISBN 978-1-118-51284-5 (epdf)
I. Title.   II. Title: Managing minor musculoskeletal injuries and conditions.
[DNLM: 1. Musculoskeletal System–injuries.   2. Musculoskeletal Diseases–therapy.   3. Wounds and Injuries–therapy.   WE 140]
RD680
617.4′7044–dc23
2013024792

A catalogue record for this book is available from the British Library.

Wiley also publishes its books in a variety of electronic formats. Some content that appears in print may not be available in electronic books.

Cover image: Photograph, showing a mallet deformity of a finger, taken by the author.
Cover design by Workhaus

Set in 8.5/11 pt Utopia Regular by Toppan Best-set Premedia Limited
Printed and bound in Malaysia by Vivar Printing Sdn Bhd

1   2014

Contents

Dedication

To Jeff Mearns
1944–2012

'I've built some beautiful oil rigs, Bren.'

'He built great structures in the sea
and brought power and light to the world.'

Acknowledgements

Acknowledgements go to:

My wife Bren, who throughout illness has put up with the love triangle with my computer for several years.

Ian Fairclough and Kay Hughes, both senior lecturers in Liverpool John Moores University, for reading drafts, pointing out mistakes and offering suggestions in the development of the book.

Magenta Styles, the Executive Editor at Wiley Blackwell, for initially recognising the worth of my ideas and accepting the book's proposal.

Madeleine Hurd, Catriona Cooper and Andrew Hallam, all editors at Wiley Blackwell who have guided me through the frightening publishing process.

Kathy Syplywczak, Project Manager at PM-Bookpublishing and Anne Able Smith, copyeditor at Abel Communication, they are two of quite the most meticulous people that I have ever worked with, all credit to them.

My many nurse and paramedic students over the years, who, because of their enthusiasm and comments, have moulded my ideas.

About the companion website

To help you with your studies, this book is accompanied by an exciting website containing a range of special features. Check it out here:

www.wiley.com/go/bradley/musculoskeletal

If you have any problems accessing or finding your way through the site, contact Wiley Blackwell at:

nursingeducation@wiley.com

The site may be used either as a stand-alone source of additional information; or the book may be used to point you to relevant sections on the website which will provide you with a variety of more detailed experiences as you progress.

The contents

- **PowerPoint X-rays** that can be freely used by lecturers as base materials for teaching sessions as well as by students working alone. These X-rays are grouped, as in the book's chapters, to test recognition of key signs and visuals and includes enlarged sections to show significant details, plus accompanying comments or questions and answers.
- A range of clinical **photographic tutorials** of patients, plus accompanying comments or questions and answers.
- **Legal scenarios** testing you on management of common problem areas and offering guidance.
- **Clinical notes scenarios** demonstrating examples of good and bad practice and accompanied by key learning points.
- **Patient history scenarios** to test your diagnostic skills.
- Although basic answers to the **multiple choice questions (MCQs)** are provided in the book, more detailed explanation to each answer is given on-line.

A note from the author on how to use this site

This site is of great use to both students of the subject and lecturers.

First, lecturers may find the PowerPoint presentations, especially of the large selection of regional groupings of X-rays, a useful addition to their own collections. All may be enlarged to show minute detail to large groups of students, or of course downloaded to show to students in the clinical sphere.

In these days of ever-increasing workload for university lecturers, all the other scenarios and tutorials may be rapidly adapted to meet specific classroom needs. Therefore, using this work as a foundation will assist in the delivery of quality sessions to students, in reduced time.

For the student, the website is an excellent additional resource to develop the distance learning (DL) process. Just reading is never the optimal way to learn: learning is aided by increasing the variety of forms of presentation that are used. Everything on this website can be worked through by a student on their own, but yet another variety of presentation would be to team up with another student. A prime example of this would be the patient history scenarios; two students could divide the scenarios between them and verbally 'act out' the situations to make them more interesting and fun.

Part 1

The background

How to use this book

Introduction

This book aims to bring together the diverse aspects of the management of minor musculoskeletal injuries and conditions. A number of texts already exist to cover subjects such as:

- anatomy and physiology
- history taking and physical examination
- minor musculoskeletal injuries
- minor musculoskeletal conditions
- patient documentation
- X-ray interpretation
- legalities and ethics.

Here I've brought several of these together into one volume for your convenience. No one can give you everything that you require, but it will provide a firm basis for your initial study and your further development.

The book

The format

The book uses a **distance learning** (DL) approach to study and is written in a friendly, encouraging and **minimally academic** tutorial style. For extra clarity, the text is supported by hundreds of illustrations. There is also a wide variety of 'boxed activities', which will test and deepen your understanding, providing you with added interest.

Associated with the book is a large and informative website, giving you free access to the following:

- Regional PowerPoint presentations of X-rays for interpretation.
- Multiple choice questions (MCQs) with detailed comments on answers.
- Documentation exercises.
- History taking scenarios.
- A clinical photo tutorial.
- Legal and ethical scenarios.

Who is the book designed for?

Senior nurses and paramedics are the main target groups, but A&E nurses, paramedics, school nurses, practice nurses and many physiotherapists will find a wealth of essential information, making the book a valuable resource.

Managing Minor Musculoskeletal Injuries and Conditions, First Edition. David Bradley.
© 2014 John Wiley & Sons, Ltd. Published 2014 by John Wiley & Sons, Ltd.
Companion website: www.wiley.com/go/bradley/musculoskeletal

How the book may be used

There are two ways of using it. Few standard texts are ever read cover to cover, or anything approaching that. So first, just pick and choose: you will find both the illustrations and the explanations clear and mostly at the level you require. If you do not need the boxed activities, just ignore them.

Second, use the book as a guide for independent organised study. To do this, start here and slowly work your way through the remainder of this chapter. Let my experience direct you to an activity, or onto our website, to have a rest or to gain clinical experience as you progress.

This approach is the next best thing to a full university 'face-to-face' programme and is based on my many years of experience running both diploma and degree courses.

You, the student

Organise yourself

To study to the best advantage, you have to make an initial agreement with yourself to try to complete the work in a given time and also to get into a habit of **regular study**.

The study habit can be difficult, because it 'eats' into your time (Figure 1.1).

Making a flexible study plan is one of the better ways to start.

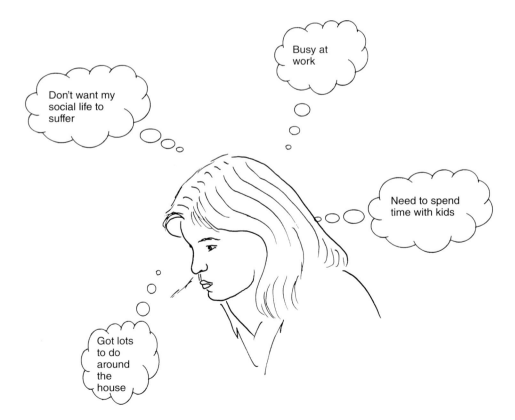

Figure 1.1 Organise your study to fit your life; something has to go.

Each of the book's chapters would take you approximately a week of study. Note, **this is not the time taken to read the book** – anyone can do that in hours: it is the time when you are:

- reading text
- highlighting and making notes
- completing activities
- sampling clinical practice and receiving feedback
- using the book's specific website for tutorials
- reading suggested texts
- looking at suggested YouTube videos.

Try to avoid commencing study at times that are likely to be exceptionally stressful, such as Christmas, during overtime, when you are decorating, or perhaps when there is illness in the family. It will simply spoil your enjoyment.

Although not always practical, it is best to complete the basic examination skills for a particular region of the body before starting the next.

Record clinical accomplishments

In each of the regional chapters, there is a checklist for you to complete, or get your clinical mentor to sign to prove your competencies in this area. These tables are excellent as an aid to your memory, but also your clinical mentor can see at a glance which skills still need to be accomplished and can work towards your continuing professional development (CPD). Further information on CPD for paramedics may be found in Fellows (2008).

Let others know you are studying

Some students do not see the need to tell anyone about their self-directed study. So, if they are noticed 'just' reading this book, others will see no harm in asking them to do something else for them instead. **They cannot understand a student's annoyance if they are not told they are studying**. Studying on your own is **almost impossible without the help of your family and friends**. So let's make a 'golden rule':

GOLDEN RULE

Include others in your study plans, so that they understand what you are trying to achieve.

When to study

No one can tell you the best way to study, or when – there are too many variables. However, I can give you some general rules students have found useful. Give them a trial and keep using them if you find them effective. Most of you don't have the luxury of choosing a time to study. More often than not it is a matter of fitting in with commitments. Try for regularity and what suits you.

Everyone reads and learns at a different rate. But **never rush** – I can skim read an article in minutes to update myself before a lecture, but one of my students could need about an hour.

Have frequent breaks

Whatever is the best time for you, **break your study up into small portions**, never longer than an hour.

Changing the type of study or **having a short break** is also beneficial. Don't feel guilty about having a break. I will remind you occasionally in the text.

Why?

You know that age children reach when all they do is ask you 'why'. Why does the sun rise? Why is the sky blue? What makes it rain? Endless questions.

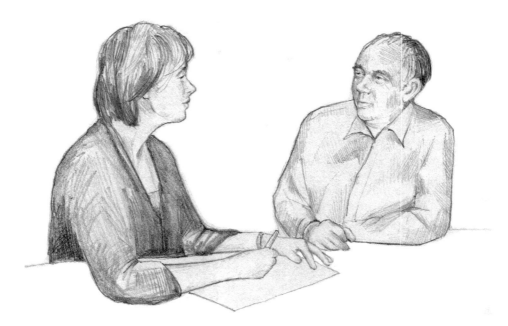

Figure 1.2 Use a mentor to talk through experiences, ask advice and 'bounce' ideas off them (Dustagheer *et al.*, 2005).

In some way, that is how you must act as a student studying with this book. **Question all you see, hear, read and do**. That includes what I write: **there is not a book published without a fault**. The more you ask, the more people will notice your enthusiasm and try to help. Of course, you must choose a time when people are not too busy.

Someone to help you

Embarking on a moderate level of study, such as this book, can be made far easier and more interesting by approaching a work colleague or acquaintance to act as your mentor. No formal contract is necessary: simply talk with them during a break. Say you are studying this book for a few months and ask to 'bounce' ideas off them, talk through experiences and seek advice (Figure 1.2).

Ideally they should be more knowledgeable or experienced than you, but that is not absolutely necessary. Discussing points with a colleague at the same level can make you feel less alone in your study and add interest. Studying on your own is lonely!

Look studious

Now leave this book and go to a mirror. No, don't just read on, it sounds silly but is important: just do as I ask and go to a mirror . . . Ready, look into it, what do you see? That face is exactly the same face as always, you look the same. However, both you and I know you are now studying minor injuries and conditions, but it doesn't show. So, what you have to do is **let people know and keep reminding them that you are studying, if you want any substantial form of support.**

Another small but important point is to tell people that you are **studying**, not just reading, but **studying**. There is a very important difference: you will get no 'Brownie points' for reading, we all read. But, if you are studying, that's a different matter and you tend to get more help.

Having said that, what you tell a busy colleague with a waiting room full of patients or just rushing out to a call will maybe register in their mind for a matter of minutes. You have to **keep on telling them,** again and again, day after day.

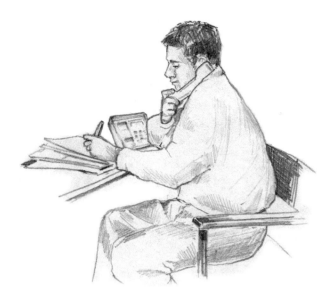

Figure 1.3 Phoning to follow up is often the only way of knowing if you managed your patient correctly (Dustagheer *et al.*, 2005).

Then eventually it clicks and they remember to call you over to discuss something or see an interesting point – success!

Many years ago when studying for a degree with the Open University, I would bring study units, books, papers etc. into A&E with me on a shift. Although it would be rare to get much study done except in breaks, I used this as an opportunity to promote conversation with passing clinicians. In time people got used to the fact that I desperately wanted to learn more and they came to me with stimulation; it helped.

Follow patients through

Following your patients through hospital departments can prove rather difficult. All I can say is you must be persistent. In this context there is no legal problem with patient confidentiality: you are part of the professional team managing them and are just requiring basic diagnosis and early management details. Phoning to follow your patient's progress to find this information is often the only way of knowing if you managed your patient correctly or in some way let them down by your inexperience (Figure 1.3).

Maybe time for another golden rule:

> ## GOLDEN RULE
>
> **Do your best to follow up the definitive diagnosis and management of your patients.**

Note taking

You may ask, 'Do I have to write notes about what I read?' Well no, but, if not, you are unlikely to learn as much as someone who does. Writing includes you more in the learning process, assisting pure memory and helping the pieces of the knowledge 'jigsaw' fit together.

You will find that in many of the activity boxes, you are asked to write comments before continuing to read the page. For this, although you could scribble the occasional word in the margin, it is far better if you have a notebook to write in as well.

Now try this first activity, writing your four brief answers in a notebook.

 Activity 1.1   **Time: 5 minutes**

Without searching the previous text, list three of the major paragraph points that I made in the text you have just read about 'Someone to help you'. Then look back and check what you have written.

Sneaky trick eh!

What I am trying to explain is that, if you read text effectively and understand it, that does not mean that the knowledge is firmly in your brain. However, if while you were reading it you had underlined parts, highlighted them or scribbled notes all over the page, I bet you would have remembered most of them. Notes all over a book are a sign of a busy mind and proof that you are involved in the learning process. Please, **make this the most scribbled-in book you ever study**, unless it's a library book!

Enjoy the frequent breaks in the text to attempt the suggested activities, each with their own (rough) estimate of time for completion. The amount that you learn, even with an interesting topic, will rapidly fall off even after half an hour. This method refreshes you and you will see that because of the more leisurely approach you will learn more.

Questions are sometimes asked in the activities. These are to ensure that you understand rather than just read, and rest assured: the answers are provided for you to check later if necessary.

Your study

Academic level

This is not a standard academic text. **Simple everyday language is purposely used throughout**, so that it **feels just like a tutor is talking with you**, along with the associated occasional humour and stories. However, don't for one moment think that this means that the book is in any way basic: it's primarily intended for diploma and degree levels of university study. Challenging subjects, put over palatably.

At this stage, don't become too involved with the precise academic level that a piece of work like this is aimed at. Knowing the name and function of a ligament, having the ability to perform a specific examination, or writing up case notes doesn't hold a particular academic level. **What your employer wants you to do with a particular knowledge or skill is where the levels vary**.

Let me explain this a little more by discussing a very complex skill – emergency endotracheal intubation – which is surrounded by a complex area of knowledge. Over the years, I have taught the theory and practice of this to both paramedics and senior A&E nurses. What I taught the different groups was exactly the same, because they all had to clearly understand exactly when and under what circumstances to perform the skill and how to get out of trouble if the patient reacted badly. Their background knowledge had to be immense to cover all eventualities without immediate medical back-up. Yet, all **this extremely complex theory, and hours of individual, stressful, simulated practice, came under part of a diploma-level university programme**.

In these days of funding and resource scrutiny, it is often the university **form of assessment** that is the major indicator of an academic level – basically, a student at a lower level only needing to repeat facts, at higher levels needing to be able to analyse and discuss, and finally at Master's and Doctorate levels being able to turn water into wine! It is the **competency to practise** that is important, and that requires different levels of knowledge and understanding, depending on the operator's role.

Referencing

A form of the Harvard referencing system is used throughout, with essential listings at the end of each chapter along with any recommended reading. In major academic works and essays, new thoughts and comments are expected to be referenced exhaustively. However, I have purposely used references sparingly, to improve the flow of the book as in a face-to-face tutorial.

You will find that in many major established texts, especially those centered around anatomy and physical examination, evidence-based references are scarce to non-existent – authors tending to rely more on suggesting further 'backup' reading for you (Douglas, Nicol and Robertson, 2009; Gosling *et al.*, 2008, for example).

The references in this book are important for your study for two reasons. First, you must use them extensively in assignments. You are most unlikely to even gain a pass grade unless you support your opinions and major facts, with adequate referencing. Second, they will assist your reading in more depth around a presented subject. This will be a tremendous help to you and the places to start will be the references or further reading suggestions provided at the end of the chapters.

Beware the subtle trap of becoming too studious at too early a stage. Unless you have a burning desire for a particular answer, leave further specific searches, such as in the excellent Cochrane library, until most of your study of this book is complete. Too many resources can sometimes cause confusion.

A great problem in the management of patients in A&E minors, minor injury units, walk-in centres and the ambulance service is that they deal with a multitude of diverse conditions – many of these comparatively trivial in themselves, not lending themselves to research funding and not 'sexy' enough to encourage research – compared with major conditions such as acute myocardial infarction (AMI).

In a bold attempt to counter this problem, a website was set up and developed a few years ago by the professionals at the Emergency Department of Manchester Royal Infirmary. Called 'Best Evidence Topics', it covers many of the small areas that are in urgent need of firm evidence to lead clinical practice (www.bestbets.org). In many areas, I have made a point of using this site as a valuable and up-to-date source for you. My hope is that you continue to use it, **or even add to it yourself**, as you become a more experienced practitioner.

A study plan

One of the major disadvantages of self-directed study is that you tend to be mostly on your own, without the daily banter and support of other students, or the occasional passing comment of a tutor in the university corridor. To overcome these difficulties, you have to be focused in your approach and set a plan. In the simplest form, you would write out a section of a diary, or calendar on the fridge, with a set time to try to study, but a more thorough approach would list topics and set aims to stage the study through the month.

The whole patient

This book is mostly organised around anatomical regions – for instance, the knee, the shoulder. But one of the most important lessons for you to learn is that **when you deal with a patient, it is wrong to consider them mainly by a body region** (Figure 1.4).

This is partly because of the following:

1. Their presenting pain may be referred from another part of the body.
2. An injuring force may mainly affect one area, but may travel, also damaging another area
3. The presenting pain may be so severe as to mask lesser pain elsewhere.
4. A medical condition may have caused the initial accident.

In a standard book, we would simply go on to the next point, but because this is DL I want you to become involved. So, think of the four points now and try the following activity, either in your mind, or on some paper, whatever suits you.

 Activity 1.2   **Time: 5 minutes**

Cover up my observations on this activity.
Now give an example of each of the four numbered points in your notebook.
Check your answers then with my observations.

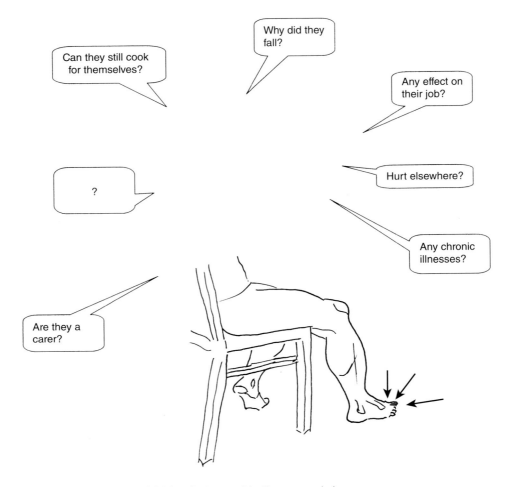

Figure 1.4 Don't manage a semi-'invisible' patient – consider them as a whole.

Observations on Activity 1.2

I thought of the following that I have seen occasionally:

1. Shoulder pain referred from an acute abdomen.
2. Wrist fracture associated with a fractured neck of radius.
3. A painful clavicle fracture 'hiding' abdominal trauma following a road traffic collision (RTC).
4. A transient ischemic attack (TIA) causing a fall.

You will notice how these facts tend to stay in your mind more easily when you have short activities; so, although you may miss them out to get on with the study faster, it's just not advisable.

Maybe now would be the best opportunity to state our first **clinical** golden rule:

GOLDEN RULE

Always consider your patient as a whole, never just the part of the body with the obvious problem.

You will find occasional golden rules scattered throughout; they are designed to act like trusty mentors looking over your shoulder and giving advice.

Aims and outcomes

At the start of each further chapter are listed aims and outcomes to guide you if you are studying this book by directing your own learning. The **aim is the main (overall) reason** for the chapter, whereas the **outcomes are the detail** of exactly what I would like you to have achieved. However, and this is important: I only expect you to have completed the outcomes after thoroughly studying a specific chapter **and the associated activities both in the book and on the website**. Also, that you have had appropriate, **structured clinical practice**. Quite a tall order, isn't it?!

   The aim of this first chapter:

To introduce you to study with this book and the best way of using it.

   Its outcomes:

That by the end of the period of study and experience, you will:

- effectively use the book and website to the best advantage, not just read them
- organise your own individual system of study
- choose at least one effective mentor
- refamiliarise yourself with major study skills
- make increased use of references.

Without further ado, make yourself comfortable and progress with the first chapter of actual clinical study. Do not rush, don't even push yourself to complete a chapter, take it a section at a time at a reasonable rate, so that you can take in the knowledge at your own educational pace and enjoy the experience!

REFERENCES AND SUGGESTED READING

Douglas, G., Nicol, F. and Robertson, C. (eds) (2009) *Macleod's Clinical Examination*, 12th edn, Churchill Livingstone, Oxford.

Dustagheer, A., Harding, J. and McMahon, C. (eds) (2005) *Knowledge to Care: A Handbook for Care Assistants*, 2nd edn, Blackwell, Oxford.

Fellows, B. (2008) Continuing professional development: who needs it?, in *Foundations for Paramedic Practice: A Theoretical Perspective*, 1st edn (ed. A.Y. Blaber), Open University Press, Maidenhead.

Gosling, J., Willan, P.L.T., Whitmore, I, Harris, P.F. (2008) *Human Anatomy: Color Atlas and Text*, 5th edn, Mosby, Edinburgh.

Moore, S., Neville, C., Murphy, M. and Connolly, C. (2010) *The Ultimate Study Skills Handbook*, Open University Press, Maidenhead.

Introduction to Multiple choice questions

At the end of each chapter you will see some MCQs to try. These will allow you to test yourself and get just **a little idea of how effectively you have been studying**, rather than the usual of **just reading** a book. In university when my students have attempted questions like these, the **major fault** they have had is that they have tried to **answer the questions after just quickly reading through the work**. Do not even attempt the questions until you have completed all the chapter **and the associated activities and practical experience**. Now, I know you may not heed this advice, but honestly, it is best if you wait.

Now before you go further, here are just a few points to note. Read the questions carefully – some may even depend on you noticing **deliberate spelling mistakes**, or the **exact meaning** of a word.

Not all the information required for a correct answer will be found in this book. By the time you attempt the questions, you will have been expected to have read around the particular topic, to enrich your experience. To gather the basic concepts of a topic, it is often an advantage to stick with a particular 'reader' such as this book. However, following that, it is very advantageous to read the works of others. That is one of the reasons for lecturers to give you references and tests, to encourage you to study more.

Unlike many collections of MCQ questions, there may be:

- all answers correct
- no correct answers
- any number correct in-between.

Just circle the correct answer/s.

The correct answers will be shown at the end of the book. However, all the questions, answers and detailed comments supporting the answers are to be found on the book's website.

If **all the parts** of your individual question are completely correct, just score yourself one mark.

How to interpret the result

Very important for you to understand is that these MCQs **will not tell you how clever you are** – few tests in this world ever do! What they **will do, if you complete them at the correct stage**, is give you a reasonable idea of how effectively you have studied the chapter.

The number of questions varies with each chapter, so I talk here in percentages.

100% correct. This would be a really excellent score, but difficult to achieve, requiring intense study. Perhaps only one or two of my students a year would be able to put the commitment in to achieve this score.

75% correct. Be very pleased with yourself. A score around this level shows that you either knew a lot already or have understood what is required of you and put the hours of study in. You would only have to top up occasional areas to improve. Very well done.

50% correct. Well, not to be sniffed at; quite a bit has stuck in your brain. What has probably happened is that you have enthusiastically gone through the chapter fairly quickly. Best read through the sections that you went down on; possibly making the occasional note in the margin or highlighting text will help the information to stick in your mind. Don't be downhearted; spending more time with the following chapter will probably work wonders.

15–25% correct. Oh dear! Possibly not one of your best attempts. There are several likely reasons for a low score like this:

- You have rushed the study, not putting the time in. Maybe too busy at home or trying to catch up.
- The area is not one that you particularly enjoy; we all tend to skimp over things we don't like.
- It's just a fluke: you may have misread questions, become distracted or tried to answer them too quickly.
- You have been putting the time into study, but not effectively. Possibly rethink how you study.

Only you will know exactly what happened. Remember I said that these are only a reflection of how well you have studied, **not how clever you are.** Better next time eh!

1% correct. Well, some people just don't do well at tests; consider the bullet points in the previous section; it may just be a one-off. Sometimes your mentor may work through the answers with you, offering advice and explanation.

Another explanation is that sometimes with a group of questions you have got most of the individual answers correct, but maybe just one or two in each set of four were a puzzle to you and that dragged your score down.

DL just does not work well with some people. If very low scores become a trend, perhaps face-to-face learning in a university would be a better option.

Multiple choice questions

1. **As a general rule, studying is most effective:**

   A In one long session so that you are not disturbed
   B Broken up into short sessions
   C Done in the morning, when you are alert
   D If you vary your study activities

2. **Regarding the aims and outcomes in this book:**

   A An aim is an overall statement of what I want you to achieve from the chapter
   B Outcomes are the detail of your individual achievements
   C Aims must be achieved, whereas outcomes are extras for you to attempt if you have time
   D You cannot use this book unless you work through the objectives

3. **It is wrong to think of a patient as having an injury in just one body region; you should always consider the whole patient. This is because:**

   A The presenting pain may be referred
   B The injuring force may travel to a more distant part
   C The presenting pain may be so severe that is masks another
   D A medical condition may have helped cause the injury

4. **Finding and reading up some of the references in this book will:**

   A Encourage you to reference your own university assignments
   B Help you to 'read around' a topic in this book, to consolidate your knowledge
   C Help you to become more familiar with the Harvard system
   D Assist you in future full-time courses

5. **Having a mentor while reading through this book:**

   A Is essential.
   B Will aid discussion of points you find difficult or challenging
   C Will be especially useful to help you through the practice experiences
   D Is quite desirable because they may be used to 'sign off' competencies

6. **The advantages of DL are that:**

   A You have more control of when to study
   B It is generally easier to study this way than in 'face-to-face' education
   C It blends easier into a full-time occupation
   D It is cheaper

 Answers are available at the end of the book. For an explanation of these answers and further resources visit the companion website at:

www.wiley.com/go/bradley/musculoskeletal

2

Taking a patient's history

Aim

To increase your awareness of good communication in healthcare, and to introduce systematic history taking for minor injury patients.

Outcomes

That, by the end of this study, and all the associated activities and clinical experiences, you will be able to:

- discuss communication issues with colleagues as they arise
- communicate effectively with patients, their relatives and other professionals
- use a systematic approach to history taking
- obtain detailed mechanisms of injury.

The greatest challenge you have is to make an accurate assessment of your patient and ultimately arrive at a safe working diagnosis. The very first step along this road is also the most important, yet in the past many inadvertently trivialised its importance by giving it scant mention in textbooks.

Here I try to reverse the trend. This chapter will give you the basics of an approach to history taking, and each chapter in Parts 2 and 3 will have its own comprehensive section detailing specifics for that particular region of the body.

Communication skills

Most of you reading this book will be experienced and working towards becoming some form of advanced practitioner. Because of that, you may feel irritation at my wanting to discuss communication skills. However, please bear with me – there are few in the world who cannot benefit from some revision, and you may be pleasantly surprised. Good communication is, after all, **the single most important skill a caring professional has to achieve**. No doctor, nurse or paramedic can be truly excellent in their role unless their communication skills are also excellent.

As we go about our daily lives we constantly meet new people and for our own safety have to 'weigh them up' in seconds.

Managing Minor Musculoskeletal Injuries and Conditions, First Edition. David Bradley.
© 2014 John Wiley & Sons, Ltd. Published 2014 by John Wiley & Sons, Ltd.
Companion website: www.wiley.com/go/bradley/musculoskeletal

Activity 2.1   Time: **A few minutes' thought only, or as classroom discussion**

At a meeting or social function, how long does it take you to make your mind up if you initially like someone? Write a few brief comments in your notebook. Then read on.

Of course, sometimes we will be wrong and have to change our opinions of them after a few minutes or following several meetings.

 Activity 2.2   Time: **15 minutes**

Cover up my observations on this activity, then read on.
What factors will be rapidly and automatically considered when forming an initial opinion of them?
Write as many as you can think of on some rough paper or in your notebook. Then continue.

Observations on Activity 2.2

I would have listed:

- facial appearance
- body appearance
- what they are doing at the time
- who accompanies, or introduces them
- expression
- clothing, uniform
- mannerisms, gestures
- what they say
- how they said it
- my experiences of others in the past
- my knowledge (or what I have heard of them previously).

Quite a list isn't it? And I'm sure there are others that you have listed and I haven't. So someone's opinion of us (the professional) is a very complex judgement.

If we want accurate and detailed information from them, we have to ensure that all these points are considered. If you are mentoring any students at the moment, working up a discussion with them around this topic can be really helpful to their future approaches.

Of course, some have a 'foot in the door' in the instant acceptance stakes: they look like one of what I call the 'beautiful people' that you see on TV, all good looks and perfect teeth. The remainder of us 'ordinary people' have to battle for acceptance from the first glance.

If you look around at friends and colleagues, you will know many who are very accomplished communicators and also a few who are lacking, especially under specific circumstances. However, what about you – do you know how good you are at communicating, or do you just **think** you know? Give yourself a quick score for **face-to-face communication in general**, with 1 being terrible and 10 fantastic. Then ask a friend to tell you the truth. Of course, if your score is low, you are just a natural Victor Meldrew – but don't worry, several aspects of communication can be improved with a little insight and practice.

We mostly change the way we approach a situation by reflecting on our past experiences. This is a valuable tool when mentoring students, but although it is a little more difficult you can do it yourself. Here is a true example of an incident that made me change the way I handled situations with students.

The situation occurred years ago, with me in charge of an A&E department. A close member of staff died in the department, cardiac arrest, tragic circumstances. A young student and I were the main participators in the resuscitation.

Post-arrest, very, very busy.

The student comes to me, 'Mr Bradley, can I have a word with you, please?'

I reply, 'I can't, I'm busy at the moment, sorry.'

All was then forgotten and the shift ended.

The next day I found out that she was severely disturbed by the incident, crying and trying to come to terms with it, feeling that she had 'let the patient down' by her lack of knowledge and skill.

I was mortified. Her immediate need was of far more importance, **at that time**, than that of any of the other patients in the department. I just did not realise it when she approached me.

 Activity 2.3 **Time: About 10 minutes**

How could I have handled the situation better?

Can you now think of a situation when you have realised the need to communicate differently?

Observations on Activity 2.3

Usually even if very busy, I now **ask what the person wants me for** and give them an approximate time that I can listen to them. I then have a better chance of not making the same mistake again.

Non-verbal communication

Perhaps 20 years ago I read a book about body language by Allan Pease, a salesman. He has gone on to write more over the years and just one of his latest, *The Definitive Book of Body Language* (Pease, 2005), is well worth a read (it could help your social life as well).

Alternatives are available, although few are as interesting. The internet is another powerful source of information, simply bulging with examples.

 Activity 2.4 **Time: 15 minutes**

In the management of minor injuries there's you, the practitioner, meeting members of the public with their problems. Can you think of a few circumstances that would have a negative effect on your communication?

Write them in your notebook now before you read on.

Observations on Activity 2.4

I thought of the following complicating factors:

- Just a few years ago everyone with a minor injury would have gone to an A&E. Patients may now be worried in case they have come to the wrong type of department.
- Is their idea of 'minor' the same as yours?
- Elderly people are more used to being seen by a doctor and may not understand why they are seeing another kind of professional.

- A possible thought: 'Because this is a minor injury unit, I had better not mention that I'm worried about my diabetes.'

So you see, quite a few points may be working against you before you even meet the patient.

The initial meeting

The first contact with your patient is a critical time: you are constantly weighing up incoming information about them, and automatically adjusting what you say and do depending on their words and actions. I wonder, can you remember most of the factors listed in my observations on Activity 2.2? They will have had an impact on how you initially judged the patient.

Your aim now is to **make the patient feel comfortable with you in their new surroundings, so that you can gain an accurate history.**

Points that would usually have a positive effect on your relationship with them in a minor injury situation could be:

- having an unrushed approach
- using their correct name and style
- going to the patient, rather than calling them in to see you
- giving a smile, or, if not appropriate, showing a caring expression
- looking smart
- introducing yourself and your role
- inviting someone accompanying them to be present, if that is what the patient wants
- ensuring privacy.

I have mostly noticed staff managing this list very well in difficult circumstances; but there is no room for complacency.

Just an accurate history?

 Activity 2.5   **Time: A quick question**

Do you think that your conversation with the patient should be just to get an accurate history?
Write a brief answer in your notebook, then read on.

Observations on Activity 2.5

The answer here must be both yes and no. Yes, because that it is our **primary aim**, the one thing that we must obtain. No, because the whole process should be **a two-way conversation**, when the patient has the opportunity not only to say what has happened, but also to talk about themselves and ask questions about their present problem and other health worries.

The importance of detailed questioning

In the past your questioning of patients has of necessity been superficial. Now, however, when you are learning to become an autonomous practitioner, obtaining a history is a major part of your role and has to be approached systematically.

The major history taking problem with nurses and paramedics, early on in their university programme, is that **they do not ask enough detail**.

When listening to your patient's history, you must ask enough detail of what happened to be able to visualise the situation yourself. Only then will you be able to form a clear idea of the injury sustained or the build-up to a condition.

Consider the following short scenario as a paramedic approaches an incident in a local park, or a nurse is talking to a patient in A&E:

Practitioner (P): 'Hi, what's happened to you?'
Teenager (T):   'I fell.'
P: 'What were you doing?'
T: 'Playing football. I had the ball and got tackled.'

This conversation could have been satisfactory for the non-specialist; however, if you want to even start to form a diagnosis, far more is required.

Extracting more information

Occasionally you will come across 'poor historians', meaning that to get more accurate and useful information out of them will be difficult or impossible. However, sometimes an accident happens so quickly that it would be difficult even for the most articulate among us to assist you more.

Let me take the conversation in the earlier scenario a little further now and show you how increased questioning by the practitioner can open up possibilities:

P: 'Fine, but are you able to describe **exactly** how it happened?'
T: 'Yeh! Someone tackled me from the right side as I was running. I twisted to the left, I think my right foot stuck in the ground and I felt this sudden pain in the knee.'
P: 'Anything else? For instance, did you hear anything?'
T: 'Funny you should say that; I think I heard it sort of 'pop', but it was just immediately so painful.'
P: 'Nothing else?'
T: 'I couldn't continue with the game.'

With coaxing, you have far more information and are well on the way to the formation of a shortlist of possible diagnoses (differential diagnoses). Or, perhaps I should say that, after you have read Chapter 10 about knee injuries, several should be in your mind.

This brief glimpse of part of a useful history taking is just one aspect of a 'history conversation' that you have to develop with all your patients. No more quick few words, but rather:

- **get to know your patient properly**
- **get them talking in detail** about their condition, or their accident
- **get them talking about themselves**.

Only then will you become a truly effective professional. Of course, an added bonus will be that they will rather like you taking such an interest in them.

Often I give my students some scenarios to get points over to them about taking a history (and possibly catch them out); why not try this next activity and see how you manage?

 Activity 2.6   **Time: 10 minutes**

What do you think may be wrong with this patient?

- Male aged 65 years.
- Complaining of (c/o) pain in right knee.
- Limping slightly.

Practitioner (P):   'Hello', and preliminary chat. 'What has happened to your knee?'
Male patient (MP): 'I'm not sure really; it's been very painful for a while now (rubbing the side of his knee). Foolishly I tried gently kicking a football with the grandson in the garden yesterday evening; it seems to have made it worse.'

On examination (OE), the knee looks fairly normal for the patient's age and is visually comparable to the left side. There are no areas of tenderness and it has almost a full range of movement, although he doesn't particularly like you moving his leg. He has no relevant past medical history.

What are your initial thoughts? Write some down, along with how you would progress from here.

Observations on Activity 2.6

Well, obviously I have not told you everything; this scenario could be the most that some would question the patient and, if so, could lead to disaster.

The practitioner has failed because of four points:

1. Lack of depth in general conversation about the patient.
2. Failure to reveal a limitation of walking activity over the past years leading to an early retirement.
3. Lack of specific knowledge of referred pain – in this instance, pain from a condition in the hip is commonly felt in or around the knee.
4. Only examining the obvious part that was injured.

Our patient quite simply has had steadily worsening osteoarthritis of the right hip, with increasingly limited movement and ability.

The patient didn't like you examining the knee, because examining the knee also moved the problem hip.

If your answer to the activity question was anything like, 'to consider the patient as a whole, ask more questions and look elsewhere', very well done.

 Activity 2.7   **Time: 30 minutes**

References sound a little 'dry', but just bear with me. Earlier I told you about a rather unusual presentation.

As a student, it is the ideal for you to get used to reading around a subject. Just to read this book will not make you the most knowledgeable paramedic or nurse in the world, but, if it encourages you to take every opportunity to read and ask further questions, it will have done a good job.

I am now citing a reference to a piece of work written by a doctor in Liverpool who met a patient with a similar problem (Emms, 2002). If you follow this up in the reference list at the end of this chapter, all the information required to find it is there. I was even able to download it from the internet; it makes fascinating reading.

You have now to get into the habit of a systematic approach even with minor injuries, so that nothing is missed.

Before going further, let us have some thought about factors that may have a bearing on what damage could occur to any of our patients.

 Activity 2.8   **Time: 10 minutes**

First, cover up the observations on this activity.

A set force is applied to a patient. What factors surrounding the incident have any influence on what damage is done? List those you can think of.

Observations on Activity 2.8

I thought of the following:

- Direction of force, the angle.
- Duration of force.
- Strength of patient's tissues.
- Any illnesses to complicate matters?
- Patient wearing any protection?
- Surface soft or hard?

I'm sure that there are others. Each of them could make differences to the end result. Each should be in your mind as you are asking the questions.

Variety of presenting problems

The overuse (accumulative) injury

So far we have considered 'straightforward' forces applied to a body. These have been known about by the patient or witnessed by an onlooker. However, history taking is not always as simple as that.

The understanding and acceptance into your daily patient management of the concept that I am to explain now will be a 'cornerstone' of your effective patient management in the future – it's simply as important as that.

Most of you reading this text will be comparatively young to middle-aged. Your body cells, especially in the musculoskeletal system, will be fully functional, able to cope with most that you ask of them and, if not, will repair quickly. Lifting a heavy patient, chasing your children up a steep hill, painting a ceiling or gardening all day will all be within your grasp.

Contrast this with a more elderly person (see Figure 2.1). Presume that I spend hours running around a football field with my grandchildren. My less able cells will be overused, not by a massive single trauma but by prolonged small incidents of trauma **accumulatively** causing injury that I did not realise was happening.

Microscopic haemorrhages into your soft tissues may make you ache the next day and the occasional cell may be unable to recover, but on the whole you will be unaware of any problem.

Now, my ageing cells are more used to a gentle walk to the train station; football would make them quiver in fear. They will have more haemorrhages, tiny fibres will be actually torn, quite a few will have their cell walls damaged or will have died. Irritating substances will have leaked out, a degree of inflammatory response may set up. Not a pretty sight and I will know about it in no uncertain way: stiff, aching, swollen, painful, limbs, unable to move as they could before.

Now apply this to your patients. If you ask them, '. . . what has happened?' or '. . . have you injured your knee?', their answer may quite simply be 'no'. They may not connect the overuse trauma with what they are presenting you with. You have to think ahead of these possibilities for them by excellent, detailed history taking. Perhaps it's time for another activity.

 Activity 2.9   **Time: 5 minutes**

Cover up the observations on this activity.
   Let's try another scenario.

- It's one of those Monday mornings . . .
- Woman, 65 years, looks healthy, walks in to you with a limp.
- Complaining of pain near the patella when she walks.
- Has had it only since she got up today, finding it difficult to get around the house.

What history questions would you ask her? Write your ideas in your notebook and then read on.

Observations on Activity 2.9

I wonder if you have been able to do well here. Remember this is not about examining the patient just yet, it is about your questioning them. Most importantly, I wanted you to ask about interests, hobbies, what's happening in their life, what they did over the weekend, etc.

Quite unknown to the patient, their present condition is because of their past. She went walking for a couple of days over the weekend (remember I said that this was a Monday morning). The soft tissues of her knee were not used to this type of accumulative trauma and are now complaining. If you had taken a good history, you would be approaching the examination with something like a possible patella tendonitis in your mind. Not set on that diagnosis, but firmly among the possibilities.

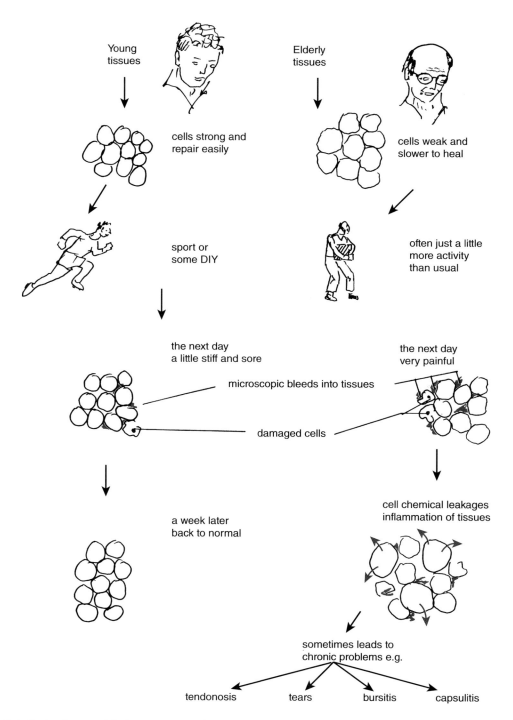

Figure 2.1 Contrasting possible tissue responses between young and elderly people.

Other illness presentations and patterns of disease

Illnesses will mostly present to you in a uniform way, but the body may demonstrate tremendous variety. For safety, it is wise to consider the mix of local plus general features that may occur, with one or the other being more obvious when the patient presents to you. Let me give you an example.

One is the uncommon condition called **sarcoidosis**. This is a tremendously variable autoimmune disease, commonly affecting young adults. Among the many tissues of the body that can be affected are the joints, giving the patient severe pains, but also they feel unwell, often with severe breathing problems.

Just to focus on the area that they tell you about – for instance, shoulder pains – and not to ask about general feelings will lead you astray in this history 'puzzle'. Always give yourself the best possible chance by **considering the patient as a whole** and asking about other problems, examining as necessary.

 Activity 2.10   **Time: 10 minutes**

Before you leave this section, think about my mentioning of sarcoidosis earlier. You are now a student and studying this book as DL material. If you come across such a condition, which you are not too familiar with, take the opportunity to review it to get the basics clear in your mind. Just a few minutes, nothing in depth.

Elderly people and falls

An important example of your consideration of the whole patient rather than just the obvious site of injury, is that elderly people have proven risk factors for the practitioner to recognise the future likelihood of a fall (Close *et al.*, 2003).

 Activity 2.11   **Time: 30 minutes**

From your own clinical experience, are you aware of these risk factors? **If you are inexperienced or unsure**, take about 5 minutes now to consider possible risk factors, writing your ideas down in your notebook.

Once completed, I want to do something a little unusual. Here, rather than at the end of the chapter, you will find a reference for an article: Anderson, K.E. (2008) Falls in the elderly. *Journal of the Royal College of Physicians of Edinburgh*, 38, 138–143, www.rcpe.ac.uk/journal/issue/journal_38_2/anderson.pdf

So many students rush study in their enthusiasm, ignoring references, but I would really like you to see the benefit of this article. It is easily accessed on the web: just 'Google' it.

As stated in the NICE guideline, *Falls: The Assessment and Prevention of Falls in Older People* (National Institute for Health and Care Excellence, 2004, p. 8): 'Older people in contact with healthcare professionals should be asked routinely whether they have fallen in the past year and asked about the frequency, context and characteristics of the fall/s.' If they then meet the criteria, the carrying out of a 'multifactorial falls risk assessment' is the gold standard for management.

Of course, if you don't do this, or don't refer your patient to someone who has the skill, you will never know of the opportunity that has been lost. You may never know of how a particular intervention might have prevented a further fall and possibly early dependency or death.

This applies to many of our, broadly speaking, 'accident prevention strategies'; at the working end, we get little feedback and never know what might have been.

Questioning your patient

What should I ask first? Possibly 'What has happened?' is reasonable, to find out if the problem is the result of an injury or a condition. This is not always as obvious as you would imagine. A common example would be a stress fracture of a metatarsal. No obvious injury as such, but the patient will get a rapid onset of pain while running or walking.

Another example could be a torn extensor pollicis longus tendon at the base of the thumb; this is a complication of a Colles fracture, occurring weeks later when the fracture is all but forgotten.

Time for a golden rule I think.

GOLDEN RULE

The patient's presenting problem is not always what they primarily want to see you about.

The patient may indeed have something like a sore heel, but sometimes a certain expression or the 'May I ask you about my . . .' is very important to them. Try to be open to the possibility.

What you do about it is up to you. Maybe in your new role you will be able to **make the time** to listen to the patient.

How much depth in questioning?

No one in this world can tell you that your interview must cover ABCDE . . ., etc. The process must be fluid: a great deal of depth perhaps when you think you may have met a major condition, reasonably superficial when dealing with one straightforward common entity. To stress this point, here are three examples:

1. A 30-year-old woman asks you about stiff, painful joints on her fingers. You immediately consider rheumatoid arthritis (RA) and ask her many general questions.
2. A 30-year-old woman shows you a mallet deformity of her finger. You ask mechanism of injury (MOI) questions and briefly ask about lifestyle, help and further problems.
3. A 30-year-old woman shows you a mallet deformity of her finger; she also seems very 'on edge', with a fine tremor of her hands, hardly answers you and tries not to allow eye contact. You talk at length until you have either understood the reasons for the behaviour or are sure that there is no need for referral.

When did the injury occur?

Never presume; I can think of conversations when I have been listening for minutes before I realised that my patient was talking about a week-old injury.

Even hours can make a difference; consider the amount of swelling into a joint cavity. If you know the time that an injury occurred, it allows you to make a judgement as to whether it is a slow-growing effusion or a rapidly filling haemarthrosis.

The likely contamination of a wound is also time dependent.

When did the problem first start?

Try not to let a patient come into a conversation halfway through their problem. Ask when the problem first started so that you get a 'clear picture'.

In recent years, statins have been implicated by some in the development of joint and muscle pains. This is an example of how your general questioning can be of great significance.

What is the pain like?

Some or all of the following 10 questions may be asked as part of your routine:

1. What were you doing just before the pain started?
2. When did it start?
3. Is it continuous?
4. How severe is it?
5. Where is it?
6. Does it travel?

7. What's its character?
8. Does anything worsen or ease it?
9. Have you ever had it before?
10. Have you taken anything for it?

How old are they?

Confirm the age of the patient, especially if they do not look their age.

Any allergies?

Always ask, no matter what the presentation. Also, the use of the word 'allergy' is not completely understood by everyone. Enquire also about 'bad effects' following tablets or creams, etc. Try to jog memories about past courses of antibiotics, or changes of treatments that were necessary.

Do they have any major illnesses?

Ask specifically about diabetes. If your diabetic patient gets a minor soft tissue infection, it could run out of control. Asthma is another example of a condition that the patient often doesn't think of as important or major, because they simply live with it.

As you know, epilepsy, heart disease and high blood pressure can all lead to falls, so your judicious questioning may uncover instability of the condition.

Any medicines?

This could have a bearing on what you prescribe.

Some people do not think of insulin or inhalers as medicines. Also, a given drug (or lack of it) may have been the cause of the accident that injured them. Find out if any of their drugs are causing problems.

Steroids would certainly affect your management of a leg laceration, for instance, so it is vital to know of them, or if the patient has had courses of them in the past.

Any previous injuries or operations?

Previous operations can hint at conditions behind the patient's present visit to you – for example, a hip replacement pointing to possible arthritis elsewhere.

Do they smoke?

Smoking seems to be the basic cause of 50% of the world's ills, so this is an essential question. Consider the terrible calf pain of intermittent claudication; also circulation problems to the fingers.

Do they drink?

Drink seems to be the cause of the other 50%; any evening in an A&E department will prove that to you. It is a major contribution to much trauma and general unhappiness, both to the individual, their families and complete unfortunate strangers. If appropriate, always ask.

Job and hobbies?

Think of repetitive strain injury, vibration injury, amateur athletics, welder's flash or gardening. The list of 'hidden' activities is vast.

Hand dominance?

This question certainly has its place; but I can think of few instances from my experience, where it had a direct bearing on how I managed my patient.

Can you think of anything else?

Home conditions, psychiatric and social history are sometimes important, but you may have to invent creative ways of asking questions about these so as not to give offence or form barriers.

General points of style

If you come to realise that a patient has a condition their doctor is unaware of, it is important that you give them the relevant advice. Although you may be working in a specific 'minors' access point to the NHS, you must always treat the whole patient.

Consider their vocabulary; never presume that they will be familiar with your words. TV has brought many medical terms to the general public, but their exact meaning can be lost. Below are some examples that may confuse intelligent members of the public:

- Emergency nurse practitioner (ENP).
- Emergency care practitioner (ECP).
- Paramedic practitioner.
- Advanced practitioner.
- Nurse consultant.
- Triage nurse.

I'm sure that you can add many medical words to this as well.

You must routinely put the generally inarticulate at their ease with thoughtful questioning. You will have done this in the past with a junior colleague in someone's home or, if a nurse, when accompanying a junior doctor. It will have been as though they were talking different languages and you had to intervene so that the patient understood. It's even more obvious with those who are hard of hearing.

Never underestimate the worth of a patient's accompanying friend or relative. Include them in the conversation at some stage (if privacy permits); they may be waiting for a prompt from you before they offer the key to the diagnosis.

 Activity 2.12　　　　　　　　　　　　　　　　　　　　　　**Time: 10 minutes**

What are your feelings about **when** to start writing information down in a patient's notes? Write your thoughts briefly in your notebook and then read on.

Observations on Activity 2.12

This may sometimes be rather awkward – writing while a patient is talking to you tends to say, 'I'm not listening.' But, if you leave writing down information too long, you may forget and have to ask them again, which also doesn't send a very good message.

One answer could be to jot down the occasional note so that you can write them up properly later. But probably better is to explain that you have to write sometimes and that you are still listening to them. Your later reflections can reinforce that you have listened.

Activity 2.13

Time: About an hour as a university discussion group, or 20 minutes' jotting down the occasional comment by yourself

Your approach with patients will vary, but with the following groups of patients there may be considerable differences:

- School children.
- Elderly people.
- People with hearing impairment.
- Busy mothers.
- 'Posh' businessmen.
- People with a language difficulty.
- Timid patients.
- Those afraid of hospitals or departments.
- Chatterboxes.
- Teenagers.
- The alcohol impaired!
- Friends or relatives.
- Other health professionals.

Try making some pertinent points for each of these groups now.

Observations on Activity 2.13

Discussion with work colleagues may bring up excellent points, but, using **teenagers** just as an example, I have given pointers to the amount of detail that I would like discussed:

- Teenagers can be a large, and often artificial, grouping.
- Some will still want their parents there as support; others will wish to be considered on their own.
- Some only **appear** to be 'cool' about something, when they are actually quite worried.
- At specific times of the year the timings of college examinations can be a big worry.
- Accompanying 'friends' sometimes need to be controlled.
- Ill-advised experimentation with alcohol can easily catch them out, making them act out of character.
- Body image can be very important to them.

Leading questions

Avoid subconsciously leading your patient into giving you the answer that you want.

An example of this would be walking up to an elderly patient in the waiting room and saying, 'Hello, Mr Smith?' A perplexed, deaf Mr Jones, not wanting to appear deaf, says, 'Yes', and you both walk into the consultation area. Accidents so easily happen!

Dealing with interruptions

Interruptions by people in person or on the telephone can always occur. Give them the same courtesy you would if it were your mother sitting there: cut the interruption short, ask to call them back and then apologise.

A friendly chat!

History interviews have their specific aim: a two-way conversation with both parties learning from one another, and even the talk itself can be therapeutic. The comparatively insignificant physical help you have given the patient for their presenting condition is sometimes overshadowed by **the psychological boost you have given them by simply talking** about their condition or just showing an interest.

Those with chronic conditions highlight this point very well. I can vividly remember an overweight, middle-aged woman with severe chronic asthma. Just attending the clinic with a finger injury had been quite a struggle for her on a very hot, pollen-laden day. The fact that I took a couple of minutes to let her know that I understood her difficulties of transport, feeling tired and being a little breathless seemed to mean a lot to her.

Helpful words or grunts!

Sometimes your patient will have difficulty in knowing exactly what to say or how much detail to give, or they may freeze with embarrassment. In these situations, they will often benefit from a well-timed prompt from you. Some examples could be:

- 'Yes, I see.'
- 'Hmmm . . .' with a nod of the head.
- 'Go on, good.'
- 'How terrible for you.'
- 'I'll just make a note of that, but carry on; I am listening.'
- Echoing what they say: 'The pain was very sharp!'

All the above act as reinforcement, encouraging continuation.

The cut-off

What if, rather than encouraging the patient, we need to halt a drift of the conversation without causing them distress. This is far more difficult and I'm sure that all of you have prayed for something like a TV sound control to control humans.

Basically, if all polite methods fail, you have to be strong: interrupt firmly and re-establish your agenda. If you don't, your other patients will suffer; you don't have infinite time. Often you will find those who behave this way are well used to being cut off and will not be offended.

Sifting through the features

At some stage towards the end of the interview, you need to ensure that you have understood what the patient wants out of the visit.

Ask yourself, 'Do I understand their main problem?' Is it their arthritis pain in their hip; or are they used to it, but concerned that they have been forgotten on the operation waiting list?

So, you could either give effective painkillers, resulting in tragedy for the patient, or you can confirm their 'lost' appointment; everyone is happy.

Before goodbye!

Finally, ask, 'Do you have any questions you would like to ask me, or is there anything you would like me to repeat?'

Practice, practice and more practice

From now on, get as much practice of history taking as you can: talk to doctors, ambulance mentors, ENPs, etc. about their experiences and styles. **Develop a system of your own** to work through, or choose an existing system and adapt it to your personal needs and likes – just so long as it does its job.

Reflection

Reflection is being used increasingly in health education for self-development by using past experiences. Although there is far more to it than seen here, try this small reflective exercise, Activity 2.14.

Activity 2.14   **Time: 30 minutes**

Read again the earlier text under the heading 'A friendly chat!' Consider a recent elderly patient you have dealt with and your conversation with them, asking yourself:

- Did I engage with them enough to gain an accurate impression of their lifestyle and interests?
- Could the altering of my style, or method of questioning, have helped?
- What else could I have spoken to them about that would have increased both their pleasure of the experience and the amount of potentially useful information gained by me?

Writing brief notes about this will assist your retention – or possibly just highlighting the text if that is more your style.

Reflection may be done simply by means of thinking a situation through yourself at the end of a shift; but it is far more effective if done with the help of a clinical mentor (not necessarily someone official, but one of your own choosing) who is willing to give you an occasional few minutes' conversation.

On this book's website, you will find some history taking exercises that will help you to keep an open mind when taking a history. Why not skim over this chapter fairly quickly again, highlighting what you feel are the most important points, and then try the website.

REFERENCES AND SUGGESTED READING

Close, J., Hooper, R., Glucksman, E., Jackson, S. *et al.* (2003) Predictors of falls in a high risk population: results from the prevention of falls in the elderly trial (PROFET). *Emergency Medicine Journal*, 20 (5), 421–425.

Douglas, G., Nicol, F. and Robertson, C. (eds) (2009) *Macleod's Clinical Examination*, 12th edn, Churchill Livingstone, Oxford.

Emms, N.W. (2002) Hip pathology can masquerade as knee pain in adults. *Age and Ageing*, 31: 67–69.

Marsh, A. (2004) *Crash Course: History and Examination*, 2nd edn, Mosby, Oxford.

National Institute for Health and Care Excellence (NICE) (2004) *Falls: The Assessment and Prevention of Falls in Older People*. NICE clinical guideline 21 (updated June 2013), www.nice.org.uk (accessed 24 May 2013).

Pease, A. (2005) *The Definitive Book of Body Language*, Orion Publishing, London.

Welsby, P.D. (2002) *Clinical History Taking and Examination: An Illustrated Colour Text*, 2nd edn, Churchill Livingstone, Oxford.

Multiple choice questions

Before you start, take in the reasoning behind these MCQs, how to answer them and how to interpret the results, from the section at the end of Chapter 1.

1. Which of the following are possible indicators that someone is not liking or agreeing with what you have said to them:

    A   Arms are folded
    B   Fists clenched
    C   Legs are crossed
    D   Eye contact with you

2. A handshake with a patient is:

    A   Always good on a first meeting
    B   Sometimes best as you say goodbye
    C   Sometimes quite inappropriate to use
    D   Something you should never do while wearing latex gloves

3. Touching a patient is:

    A   Something to avoid until you have built up a relationship with them
    B   Often very therapeutic for them
    C   Not advisable if they have eczema
    D   Occasionally 'off-putting' for the patient, so best avoided

4. Which of the following is/are the best way/s of finding out the type of pain a patient has?

    A   Tell me about your pain
    B   Is your pain sharp?
    C   What is your pain like?
    D   Is your pain there all the time?

5. Which of the following are factors to be considered when looking into the history of a patient's fall?

    A   The type of surface they fell onto
    B   The direction of the force when they fell
    C   What made them fall
    D   If they have fallen before recently

6. Which of the following history features would be suggestive of RA?

    A   One-sided distribution
    B   Male patient
    C   Patient in their twenties
    D   DIP joint involvement

7. Which of the following history/MOI features could be suggestive of a fracture?

    A   Insulin-dependent diabetes
    B   Known osteoporosis
    C   Previous CVA
    D   Previous fracture in the same location as a child

8. Your patient, an overweight 13-year-old girl with no previous illnesses, complains of sudden onset of pain in the groin and knee. She doesn't remember any injury. Which of the following should be considered the most likely cause/es?

   A   Dislocation of the patella that has slipped back into place
   B   Fractured neck of femur
   C   Slipped femoral capital epiphysis
   D   Perthe's disease

9. Which of the following may have implications for the diagnosis of a patient presenting to you with leg pain?

   A   Pregnancy
   B   Smoking
   C   Previous injuries
   D   Hobbies

10. A history of taking which of the following drugs may lead to damage of your patient's Achilles tendon?

   A   Steroids
   B   Group of antibiotics
   C   Vitamin C group
   D   Glucosamine

Answers are available at the end of the book. For an explanation of these answers and further resources visit the companion website at:

www.wiley.com/go/bradley/musculoskeletal

3

An introduction to examining your patient

Aim

To guide you towards a systematic form of patient examination.

Outcomes

That by the end of this study, and all the associated activities and clinical experiences, you will be able to:

- analyse the background to the physical examination of your patients, applying theory to the clinical situation
- effectively examine patients with minor injuries and conditions.

In this chapter we start with some general information about examining patients, then in later chapters we detail the specifics for a particular region of the body.

The background to physical examination

It will be useful to start with an activity.

 Activity 3.1   **Time: 15 minutes**

If you **are not** already a practising advanced practitioner, this should be quite useful for you.

If **you are** an advanced practitioner, why not read quickly through to use the activity as a tool for teaching others.

As an absolute expert at something, having seen and done it all for years, a mistake will be a rarity. However, most of you reading this book will be building towards that state and be vulnerable to errors of judgement. To minimise this, approach all examinations of your patients using a system. There's not just one system – rather, look with care into all that you find and either choose one that suits you best, or develop one of your own. Whatever you use must meet basic criteria. What do you think these could be? List some and then check with the observations on this activity.

Managing Minor Musculoskeletal Injuries and Conditions, First Edition. David Bradley.
© 2014 John Wiley & Sons, Ltd. Published 2014 by John Wiley & Sons, Ltd.
Companion website: www.wiley.com/go/bradley/musculoskeletal

Observations on Activity 3.1

Your examination system criteria should include the following:

- Be straightforward and logical.
- Be easy to remember.
- Greeting, comforting and explaining to your patient.
- Encouraging a dialogue.
- Considering your patient as a whole.
- Considering major problems a possibility.
- Detailing MOI or progression of a condition
- Considering the needs of your employing Trust.

Your wording may not be identical, but just so long as you understand the points.

Standard medical clerking system

This is the routine documentation of information that generations of doctors have had to learn. There are slight variations in practice, but all are very similar to this list:

- PC (presenting complaint).
- MOI (mechanism of injury).
- PMH (previous medical history).
- Drugs.
- OE (on examination).
- Investigations.
- Diagnosis.
- Treatment.

It is systematic, logical, well tried and fits most situations.

 Activity 3.2   **Time: A few moments**

In most situations, yes, this statement is true; but in what major area does such a system 'fall down'?

Observations on Activity 3.2

I hope that you would have immediately thought of emergencies; systems have been developed and introduced around the world to help in these situations.

Advanced Trauma Life Support (ATLS)

This is a worldwide system for the immediate assessment and management of patients with major trauma; it's very widely accepted. It suggests a routine order for the examination of all such patients.

It would also not go amiss to look at the variations of assessment used in specialised critical circumstances, such as Advanced Life Support (ALS), Advanced Cardiac Life Support (ACLS) and Advanced Paediatric Life Support (APLS).

Some other examination systems and prompts

I now list some of the other ideas that I would like you to become familiar with. Notice I don't say 'learn' – I only want you to get a feel for the different systems used.

Who, what, when, where, why system

These are good questions and I have no problem with your using them, but personally I just ask, 'How can I help you?', 'What has happened?' and take it from there. The depth and extent of questioning will vary considerably with each patient.

Some common physical examination mnemonics

Some people find these very helpful and use them all the time; others will never use them. Do what you find is best for you; we are all different.

SAMPLE

This is a quick system for remembering aspects of history:

- Signs and symptoms.
- Allergies.
- Medications.
- Pertinent history.
- Last oral intake.
- Events preceding the incident.

OPQRSTU

A system to remember the questions to ask about pain:

- Onset.
- Palliative factors.
- Quality.
- Region.
- Severity.
- Timing.
- U How does it affect **you**?

BLISS

The stages of a consultation:

- Beginning.
- Listening.
- Information gathering.
- Sharing information.
- Setting goals.

Spend some more time looking at these ideas before you attempt the Activity 3.3.

 Activity 3.3   **Time: 30 minutes**

Try listing the components of your own basic system for examining a patient with a minor injury or condition. Imagine managing a patient at home if you're a paramedic, or in an MIU situation if you're a nurse.

When you've finished, compare your list with the major features in my observations. Don't be concerned if the wording varies, so long as your basic thoughts are similar.

Observations on Activity 3.3

- Greet your patient to start forming the relationship.
- Tell them what you want to do.

- Ask how you can help or what happened (find the PC).
- Detail the MOI or PMH.
- Examine:
  - the part in question
  - the remaining systems.
- Investigations.
- Provisional diagnosis.
- Management.

Once your own basic system is clear in your mind, you should develop it with further thoughts. Remember this is all a negotiated arrangement.

Vital connections

A patient's condition does not always divide itself up into recognised anatomical areas. For example, it is common sense to consider the head and neck together with trauma, so that, if one presents, you always look into the possibility of injury to the other. A golden rule perhaps:

> ## GOLDEN RULE
>
> **Head injury: always consider the neck. Neck injury: always consider the head.**

With non-trauma conditions as well, the two areas often 'share' problems. An excellent example of this is a headache caused by muscular spasms in the neck.

 Activity 3.4   **Time: A few moments**

Can you think of other anatomical areas that should often be considered together, to avoid missing a diagnosis?

Observations on Activity 3.4

Especially with DL, you should do all you can to have repetition of important points to aid memory and, associated with this, to hang new pieces of information on existing 'hooks' of knowledge. You have already learnt, in Chapter 2, of this idea of a condition crossing boundaries. Remember the man with the painful knee caused by OA of his hip?

Most of you will be used to the initial assessment of a range of patients, with a reasonable range of conditions or injuries. So, the more detailed examination of a patient required for the full management of minor injuries should be achieved fairly quickly.

Take this extensive prior knowledge and experience as a baseline, adding to it the detail in this book. In so doing you will find that, with practice, examination of your patient will become fairly easy and you will fall into a safe routine.

Masterly inactivity

Careful decisions have to be made regarding the examination of your patient. You must be selective in what you do and 'masterly inactivity' (a phrase often used by the wise) is sometimes the best option. Just because a particular examination technique has been learnt, doesn't mean that it is best to use it on all occasions. Sometimes effective patient management decisions can be made without the use of (often painful) examination techniques that you read of in texts designed mostly for hospital doctors. Cut your patient disturbance to the minimum, especially if the test is to be painful or tiring.

The whole patient

One of the major points for me to stress, if not **the most important point for you to remember from the whole of this book**, is never simply consider the part that presents in isolation, like a blinkered horse.

Always consider the detail of the MOI, and/or the history of the patient and their condition. This could be summed up in another golden rule:

GOLDEN RULE

What you do not look for, you will not find.

How much to examine?

'How exhaustive an examination should I make?' is a question that students ask time and time again. It does not have a specific answer, because all patients will be so different and the examination develops from the information that you receive, taking you in a slightly different direction every time.

Perhaps I should say that our initial objective is to effectively manage the injury or condition that the patient presents with. At first glance this sounds reasonable, but it would be a sad state of affairs if it stopped there. You have to consider that your patient either may not know of an underlying condition or, strangely, is not too happy about your finding one.

A brief diversion here, the excitement surrounding the London 2012 Olympics brings to my mind that many amateurs may resort to the inappropriate use of anabolic steroids and other performance-enhancing drugs, to emulate their heroes. If because of features you find during examination, you are suspicious of the use of these, you must bring the subject up. The opening conversation could possibly be wrapped up in advice on side effects and the help available from the patient's GP, but to be suspicious of the use of such drugs and simply do nothing is a disservice to your patient.

Every patient contact should be thought of as an opportunity for advice and education. We have to be realistic and realise we cannot hope to perform a general advice and GP service, but focusing completely on the patient's presentation is also wrong. Let me give you some pointers.

 Activity 3.5   **Time: 5 minutes**

With increasing age, it becomes more likely for your patient to have more than one injury, more than one condition and combinations of the two.

Write an example in your notebook. Then check with my observations.

Observations on Activity 3.5

Just two possible examples:

1. The osteoporotic bones of an elderly woman may lead to a wrist fracture and an associated fracture of the radius in the elbow on the same side.
2. A patient with established OA of the hip trips and falls heavily, causing a fractured lateral malleolus, plus a worsening of the OA.

Chronic normality

Chronic conditions become the patients' 'norm'. This makes it easy for them to temporarily forget that they have them, or not to bother mentioning them to you. As examples of this, consider the following:

- A patient who has type 2 diabetes for years and is well controlled doesn't think it is important to tell you when they present with an infected cyst on their neck.
- A patient has 'mild' RA and doesn't think it important to tell you following their whiplash injury.

The excuse

Occasionally a patient will use a completely unrelated trivial condition as an excuse to come and ask you about something else that is worrying them. Another version of this is, 'While I'm here, may I ask you about . . .?' Some practitioners find this approach irritating, but I feel it is in part due to our system of health care, where the patient has many **confusing options for initial entry to our services**, and with often less than ideal access.

   Basically, you have a great honour in being able to put a mind at rest or refer a patient for further advice. Never refuse outright to consider other than the patient's presenting condition, no matter what difficult guidelines you work under; this could be the first opportunity to discover a malignancy! It only takes seconds to listen and guide.

How much of the patient to examine?

Maybe a final activity for the specifics may help. We don't want to undress our patient with a splinter in their finger, but neither do we want our patient with a sprained ankle not to have their sock taken off.

 Activity 3.6   **Time: 15 minutes**

There are no exact right or wrong answers to this activity but, roughly, what would be the extent of your examination of a patient presenting with the following? Write your answers in your notebook. Any format will be fine.

1. A teenager awoke in the morning with a stiff, sore neck for the first time. He walked into clinic.
2. An adult with minor whiplash mechanism the previous day, now with a severe ache, walks in to see you.
3. An adult male, blow to head fighting last night, feels unwell.

Observations on Activity 3.6

The following are reasonable suggestions, but even these will vary with the history detail and presentation.

   Following a detailed history and MOI, all these patients should have what could be termed a routine basic examination of the neck for:

- swellings, bruises, redness
- pain, tenderness on palpation
- the range of joint movements, sensations and paraesthesiae.

Note the following too:

1. Ask about other problems, especially throat, mouth infections, lumps, etc. Possibly take temperature.
2. Question regarding possible injuries elsewhere that may also have just appeared. Did they bang their head? Also, the range of joint movements, sensations and paraesthesiae to all limbs.
3. Always consider all minor blows to the head as head injuries at first and work from there eliminating possibilities. That is the only way to sleep soundly at night and avoid making a tragic mistake one day. Anything that you may consider a head injury also needs that basic examination of the neck. Almost always you will find no features of neck injury, but that doesn't mean that the examination is wasted. What you do not look for you will not find.

Eliminate the major

The main aim of this book is to assist you in learning about and managing patients with minor musculoskeletal injuries and problems. But, to look at this from that single viewpoint will not make you an excellent practitioner. To reach a diagnosis that 'only' a particular minor injury exists, you sometimes have to eliminate more major injuries or conditions in an unrelated body system.

How to start your examination

You do **not** start by observing the presenting injury: you must remember that you are caring for a whole patient, not an injured limb. So, start by observing your patient as a whole when your eyes first meet, and continue throughout (Douglas, Nicol and Robertson, 2009). As you first walk up to them in their own home, or ask them to come through to the consulting room of a clinic, you should note their:

- **build**
- **mode of dress**
- **demeanour**

and ask yourself the following questions:

- Are they **attentive**?
- Can they **hear** you easily?
- Do they **smell**?
- Is their **gait** normal?
- Do they need to **hold onto you**?
- Are they **apprehensive**?
- How are they **holding the** injured or painful **part**?

From this observation, which will shortly become second nature and completed in seconds, you will gain an instantaneous profile of your patient, so that the flow of the consultation will be smooth.

Clothes and cleanliness

Clothing can be a terrible barrier for the inexperienced, especially with some elderly people who may have many protective 'onion skins' for warmth and comfort. A gentle warning: never be in a rush with your examination and, for the sake of a few minutes of sometimes painful exposure of a limb, miss an important feature. Subtle changes in the position of a limb can so easily be missed if they are not undressed sufficiently. So many times over the years, I have seen inexperienced doctors, nurses and paramedics failing to undress patients adequately. Remember our rule: what you do not look for, you will not find.

A stronger barrier to effective examination is that the patient has hygiene problems, either out of choice or circumstance. Although not too pleasant for us, it is not our place to judge and an examination should never be minimised because of it.

The progress

The examination usually progresses from looking, to palpation, then ranges of movement and finally to other abnormal findings.

In all these, the observation of the patient is the one that I find is most often given 'lip service'; yet it is the one that will give the examiner an enormous amount of information if done well.

What should you look for when you examine?

If I always just provide you with the answer, your learning will not be as effective as when you have been involved in some way. With this in mind, try Activity 3.7.

Activity 3.7   Time: **30 minutes**

Cover up the list in my observations of this activity and then try making an exhaustive list in your notebook of all that you would **look** for, with both injuries and conditions of a limb.

Afterwards, compare with my list. If you are already experienced, you should be able to get approximately 75% of these correct.

Observations on Activity 3.7

Routine external observations to be made on a limb:

- **Colour**
  - Pink
  - White/pale
  - Blue
  - Congested/red
  - Black (necrosis)
  - Dirty/clean
  - Pigmentation
  - Mottled
- **Quality**
  - Rashes
  - Thick/thin
  - Hairy
  - Callous
  - Blisters
  - Nail variations
  - Scars
- **Swellings**
  - Effusion
  - Oedema (diffuse or localised)

- **Wounds**
  - Lacerations
  - Incisions
  - Punctures
    - Bites
    - Stings
  - Grazes
  - Burns/scalds
  - Flaps
  - Foreign bodies
  - Bruises
    - Haematoma
    - Ecchymosis
    - Petichiae
- **Muscle wasting**
- **Deformity**
- **Shortening**.

Always comparing both sides will often show up subtle differences that otherwise would not be noticed (*see* Figure 3.1). The patient should be your guide here for the norm.

As you progress through the chapters, we will mention all these points in more detail to develop their significance, but now is an excellent time to start to memorise them.

One simple way is to try writing the list down, or highlighting those points you could not remember and revising them again in a few hours.

Another good habit for your development is to write a word in the margin or highlight it if you are unsure of its meaning. Examples of this are 'ecchymosis' and 'petichiae'. If your dictionary is not available, it only takes seconds on your computer to type 'define' followed by the word, into Google or another search engine of your choice.

In your status as a student, never let a word pass by if the meaning is not understood.

Palpation

You must be sure that you instil confidence in your patients, because gentle palpation can make or destroy a patient's trust in you. Also when acting as a mentor, pass your thoughts on to the next generation of practitioners.

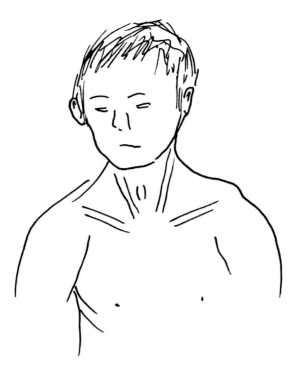

Figure 3.1 Always try to compare the left and right sides. The subtle swelling over the patient's left AC joint may not have been noticed without comparing both joints.

The speed of your palpation also has to be in keeping with the circumstances.

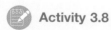 **Activity 3.8** **Time: 10 minutes**

What do you think I mean by, 'The speed of your palpation also has to be in keeping with the circumstances'? Write some comments in rough note format and then read my observations.

Observations on Activity 3.8

With a nervous or anxious patient, you may find that a slow approach may 'settle them down'. Elderly people in particular can often feel uncomfortable with speed, needing time to get used to the character and 'ways' of the individual professional.

With an infant or child, you may find that some form of play helps the situation, allowing them to become accustomed to you. Props such as balloons or drawing paper can be a tremendous help, and the smile of a child is a fantastic reward.

Conversely, a patient may feel that you are inexperienced if you are slow with palpation, or the examination in general; you alone may judge the situation.

Touch has very positive, if not healing, properties. It has been used for thousands of years with the 'laying on of hands' by the clergy. It instils confidence in you and shows that you are interested in the patient and what they say. Some patients will not feel as though they have been managed professionally unless you have palpated their injury thoroughly. Never forget the power of touch (*see* Figure 3.2).

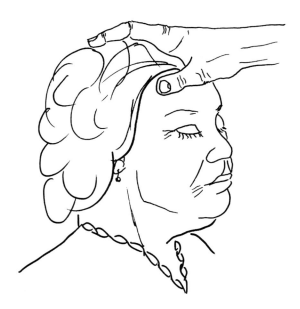

Figure 3.2 Just as the touch of a priest may give great comfort, so your touch of palpation indicates to the patient your interest in what they say.

Explanation

Always explain to your patient what you are going to do. I get this point over to students in the lecture room by singling one out by name and sternly walking up to them. By the time I reach their seat they are anxious and wondering what they have done wrong. Then I explain and they relax, back to sleep! It's exactly the same with your patients. Adequate explanation is of importance so that the patient can give their consent.

As a general rule it is good practice to palpate the 'good' side first, so that the patient's confidence can build up. However, be sure that they understand your reasoning here: it is easy for them to think that you are 'just a little strange' examining the limb with nothing wrong; use your judgement.

Hurting your patient

A final pointer regarding palpation: **sometimes** you have to hurt. A common trend in my students in the early stages of an ENP or ECP course is that they palpate, but they are afraid to apply pressure that causes discomfort or pain. It is important that you don't misunderstand me here: I'm not suggesting screams carrying down the corridors, but, **with prior warning to the patient**, the palpation sometimes has to be firm and deep in order to elicit tenderness. With supervised practice, the amount of pressure will become second nature; best to watch and be guided by a mentor.

What to feel for?

The most logical system for palpation is that you trace the normal surface anatomy of the bones in the first instance. Sometimes if I'm not looking at the patient's face for hints of tenderness, I close my eyes while palpating, getting a mental image of the structures. This would seem to fit better with a clinic environment than for a paramedic on a football field; you find what is best for your circumstances.

Once you have gained confidence and 'found your way' around the bony prominences of a joint, try the far more difficult soft tissues. I will remind you again as we continue through the regions of the body, but, when you are learning to examine these structures particularly, choose a **thin** friend or colleague (*see* Figure 3.3). It is so easy to become 'lost' trying to palpate a joint through significant layers of fat.

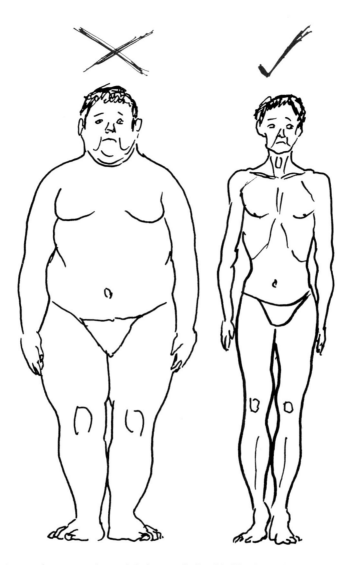

Figure 3.3 In the early stages of your experience, it is best to find a thin friend on whom to practise your palpation techniques!

 Activity 3.9   **Time: Ongoing at work**

Although you will be given specific guidance in the regional chapters, as a general rule try not to examine too many features of a joint too soon. Become familiar with major bony landmarks of a particular joint on a variety of individuals before you progress to the soft tissues.

Checklist 3.1 contains some common examination features that you should try to experience. You may want to add your own extras to the list. Keep a record a good few months into the future and remember what you have yet to accomplish.

Checklist 3.1 Common examination features you should try to experience.

Cysts	☐
Lymph nodes	☐
Fluctuation	☐
Induration	☐
Joint effusions/haemarthrosis	☐
Oedema	☐
Abnormal joint movement	☐
Haematoma	☐
Bony crepitus	☐
Surgical emphysema	☐
Excessive heat/cold	☐
Rigid abdomen	☐
Abdominal tenderness/rebound tenderness/mass	☐
Variations of breath sounds	☐
Neurological variations	☐

© 2014 John Wiley & Sons, Ltd.

Placing joints through a range of movements

This is the final introductory aspect regarding your patient's examination.

There are two forms of joint movement. The first are those that the patient can do by themselves, called '**active**', although sometimes you need to hold their limb and to some extent assist because they are frightened of pain.

Second, there are those that you do for the patient, called '**passive**'. Their muscles will be stretched, but do not actively contract to make the movement; more of this in Chapter 6.

Emergency triage

I would like you to spend just a little time now considering some aspects of emergency triage.

This is a specialised form of examination, which is highly structured and designed to rapidly sort patients into the following categories according to their need:

- Immediate.
- Very urgent.
- Urgent.

- Standard.
- Non-urgent.

Here the practitioner does not have to reach a diagnosis, but rather to decide on priority in management.

 Activity 3.10   Time: **1–2 hours**

The UK leaders in this sphere are the Manchester Triage Group. Their published work, *Emergency Triage*, will give you an interesting insight if you skim read it. Details are in the section on suggested reading at the end of this chapter (Mackway-Jones, Marsden and Windle, 2006).

REFERENCES AND SUGGESTED READING

American College of Surgeons (2008) *Advanced Trauma Life Support Manual*, 8th edn, American College of Surgeons, Chicago, IL.

Douglas, G., Nicol, E.F. and Robertson, C.E. (eds) (2009) *Macleod's Clinical Examination*, 12th edn, Churchill Livingstone, Oxford.

Gross, J., Fetto, J. and Rosen, E. (2009) *Musculoskeletal Examination*, 3rd edn, Wiley Blackwell, Oxford.

Mackway-Jones, K., Marsden, J. and Windle, J. (2006) *Emergency Triage*, 2nd edn, Blackwell Publishing Ltd., Oxford.

McRae, R. (1998) *Clinical Orthopaedic Examination*, 4th edn, Churchill Livingstone, Oxford.

Multiple choice questions

Before you start, take in the reasoning behind these MCQs, how to answer them and how to interpret the results, from the section at the end of Chapter 1.

1. **Induration of the soft tissues means:**

   A A swelling
   B A hardening
   C A fluctulant feeling
   D A crackling feeling

2. **For a patient presenting to you with an ankle injury following a fall, which of the following would be important for you to always examine?**

   A The Achilles tendon
   B The full length of the fibula
   C The hip on the same side
   D The hands

3. **Which of the following would you be particularly looking for while examining the foot of a diabetic patient?**

   A Petichiae
   B Ecchymosis
   C Ingrowing toenails
   D Infections

4. **Which of the following would be most useful when examining a patient's joint?**

    A   Tape measure
    B   Marker pen
    C   Goniometer
    D   Needle and cotton wool

5. **Which (if any) of the following statements are true?**

    A   If the patient has a full range of active joint movements, passive movements will not be required
    B   Full ATLS principles still need to be applied with all minor injury patients
    C   If a part is injured on one side of the body, you should always look at the opposite side for comparison
    D   If a part on one side of the body is injured (unless something like a simple laceration, you should always try to look at the opposite side for comparison

6. **Applying a valgus stress to a joint:**

    A   Means moving the part of the limb distal to the joint, away from the midline of the body
    B   Changes direction depending on the position you find the joint in
    C   Cannot be done to the PIP joints of the fingers
    D   Should not be done if there is any likelihood of its causing pain

7. **Palpation of the joint tissues is a very powerful examination technique. Which (if any) of the following are true?**

    A   Palpation should be avoided if a fracture is suspected
    B   Palpation may be omitted under some circumstances
    C   Palpation is done before, not at the same time as, joint movement
    D   It is best to look at an injured part while you palpate

8. **When examining children in particular:**

    A   It is sometimes best to attend to the 'good' side first
    B   Warning them of your intended actions is very important
    C   It is usually best to build up a relationship first, before attending to the part in question
    D   Their parents, or whoever is with them, should always stay with them during the examination

9. **Which of the following represent some of the items in the physical examination mnemonic 'SAMPLE'?**

    A   **S**igns and symptoms
    B   **L**ast oral intake
    C   **A**BCs
    D   **E**valuation

10. **With the body in the anatomical position:**

    A   The legs are inverted
    B   The sole of the foot is seen in the posterior view
    C   The palms of the hands face forwards
    D   The shoulders and hips are in slight abduction

 Answers are available at the end of the book. For an explanation of these answers and further resources visit the companion website at:

www.wiley.com/go/bradley/musculoskeletal

Patient documentation for minor injuries

Watching a skilled doctor writing up page after page of clinical notes makes it all seem so easy. But it is far from easy, requiring a great deal of thought and practice with a variety of patients.

When you decided to become an autonomous practitioner, I think that documentation would have been the furthest from your mind of skills that you would be looking forward to learning. However, it is right up near the top of the list of importance, when you consider how others will think of you, and **at the very top in protecting you from litigation**. Documentation is too often thought of as a chore, rather than a critical professional skill.

The quality of your documentation is a lasting reflection on you and your level of clinical practice. Quite something to think about, isn't it? If good, it will pay dividends. However, if poor, it will make things difficult for both you (and others), sooner or later landing you in serious trouble.

Activity 4.1   Time: **15 minutes**

A rather basic question and I apologise for any very senior students, but why do we write patient notes?
Cover up the observations on this activity and jot down some notes in your book.

Managing Minor Musculoskeletal Injuries and Conditions, First Edition. David Bradley.
© 2014 John Wiley & Sons, Ltd. Published 2014 by John Wiley & Sons, Ltd.
Companion website: www.wiley.com/go/bradley/musculoskeletal

Observations on Activity 4.1

I thought of the following:

- Protect patients.
- Create a record of a patient and what happened to them.
- Let others know what we found and did.
- Assist with NHS research and audit.
- Act as a formal legal document for:
    - the police
    - insurance
    - the courts.

I'm pleased if you got most of those; maybe the research and audit function was not quite as obvious.

If a number of practitioners were asked to examine the same patient and make notes, each person's notes would be different, but all should in general conform to a set of rules (the medical model of clinical note keeping).

There is no one way of documenting clinical notes. Professions with similar advanced roles will obviously differ. As an example, the notes of a paramedic managing a minor condition in the patient's own home (with few facilities) will vary from a hospital-based ENP (with X-ray facilities, specialist clinics nearby, etc.). But even among the same professions, systems will vary. Some sites use computerised notes, others paper; some ambulance services use wireless portable computer systems, others just A4 duplicated sheets.

With such variety, I have to be flexible in my guidance as to which you apply to your own circumstances.

Remembering that **the best way to learn is not just to read about something, but to become involved**, let's have another activity.

Activity 4.2   Time: **20 minutes**

No matter what system you have to use with your Trust, it is best that you also have a design 'template' in your mind of the essentials.

List on separate paper the items that **you** feel should be documented, and then read on.

Do not hurry this. Note that I have suggested about 20 minutes as an average to think it through properly.

Clinical notes

My record of the essentials are laid out here and you will find that it is very similar to many that you will have seen before.

Clinical notes

Patient details:
  Age, date of birth
  Address
  GP
  Occupation (previous or multiple often useful)

Date and time:

Presenting complaint (PC):

Past medical history (PMH):
  Mechanisms of injury (MOI)
  Medical history
  Allergies/drugs, etc.

On examination (OE):

Investigations:
   X-ray

Provisional diagnosis:

Management:
   Drugs
   Treatments
   Advice
   Disposal
   Follow-up

Signature:
Name:
Time:

I have no hard and fast rules about the general way in which you lay out your notes. You must get into your own way of presenting things **so long as it works**. Forms and styles may also be dictated by your Trust and the type of condition that your patient presents with.

   I now want to detail some of the points in 'Clinical notes'.

Patient identification

You must document the patient's full name, address, date of birth and, if appropriate, a department number. Shortcuts on any of these points can lead to disaster. It's not uncommon for a parent and child to have exactly the same name. Although a second given name usually identifies, the date of birth or department number are sometimes required for confirmation. Oh, wouldn't it be nice to be able to barcode patients (*see* Figure 4.1).

Date of entries

The danger here is with midnight or New Year looming. It is easy to forget, causing confusion for others in the future trying to trace notes.

Timings

When you first meet a patient is obvious; but at least having that stated means you cannot be blamed for anything before that time!

   Some departments or ambulance trusts require other timings for research or audit, but as a base minimum the time when you last see the patient is satisfactory, with intermediate entries for instances of long delay. The timings of phone calls or direct requests for opinions are also useful.

Omission

Perhaps **the most important thing to remember in the whole of this chapter** is the following golden rule:

GOLDEN RULE

If something is not documented, it is presumed that it has not been done.

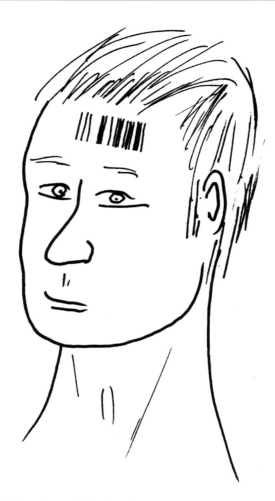

Figure 4.1 Wouldn't it be great to have barcoded patients!

There is no agreed implication that a systematic examination including A through to Z has taken place: **you have to document it**. This whole idea is perhaps **the major mistake made by those new to note taking** (Porter *et al.*, 2008).

Negatives can be important too, if relevant to the situation. To state that you did **not** find something (i.e. no swelling or tenderness) is vital. So, another golden rule in quick succession:

GOLDEN RULE

Also state what you did not find.

For nurses among you, this is an extension of an already familiar area. Think back to drugs and treatments ordered by a doctor in a patient's notes. The nurse who completes the care signs the notes but omits a separate signature for the drug. We all know she **probably** gave it, but unless there is a signature we cannot be sure.

A final point. Imagine that something has gone wrong with a patient and don't let me hear you say, 'It won't happen to me, I'll be very careful' because **all of us fall into a trap sometimes**. Now, if your notes state that you examined this and that systematically, it makes it difficult for someone to say you were **negligent**, although you may still have made an **error of clinical judgement**. So, being meticulous about your notes may save you lots of future worry.

Alterations

Any mistake you have made in the notes at the time of writing can simply have a line drawn through and a correction inserted followed by an initial. There is no need to completely obliterate the original: the inference could be that you are trying to hide what was written.

What you must not do is go back to the notes at a different time or date and make it look like you wrote something at the original time. A separate timed and dated entry should be made, followed by your signature.

What you must always ask is: is there a clear and accurate account of the sequence of events?

Spelling and syntax

At first, you may make many simple writing errors – for instance, spellings. All that it required here is a basic alteration, as you would in a letter or essay.

Offence

Since the early 1960s when I first came into the NHS, I can remember many terrible statements that inexperienced doctors had written about patients in notes. The writings varied from accusations of malingering, vagrancy and being devoid of any mental capacity, to statements that people who subsequently died of cancer could not possibly have the disease.

So, another golden rule:

GOLDEN RULE

You must never write down anything about a patient that you would not like reading either to them or a court.

Three golden rules in a few pages! This should be an indication to you of how important this section is.

Neatness

I have notoriously poor handwriting (*see* Figure 4.2), so I have to concentrate very hard to improve when I am writing longhand. Even then, I often go into a form of semi-capitalisation of the letters. Shopping lists are a nightmare; the coming of the computer age changed my life.

The text in Figure 4.2 says:

> If you can read what I have quickly written down here, you have incredible eyesight, well done. However, don't write like this in a patient's notes, or it could land you in trouble.

If you write patient notes and they are unclear, you may be held in part responsible if things go wrong because of it. Also, use pen, never pencil.

Abbreviations

These are a tremendous help in everyday life and there is most certainly a place for them in your patient documentation. I think everyone has 'pet hates' and mine is the use of the hurriedly written letters 'R & L' instead of the full words 'right and left'. My reason for this is in shown in Figure 4.3.

Activity 4.3   Time: **10 minutes**

Cover up my observations on this activity. I have listed here a few abbreviations that may be used in your documentation. Write your interpretation alongside. Are there any that you would **not** like to use?

T, P, R, BP,
mg, ml, mcg,
FOOSH, MOI, GA, GP,
Mvts, Circ, Sens,
BM, COPD, MI,
BS, PN,
RS, CVS, GIS, GUS, CNS,
LLPOP, BKPOP, WB, NWB,
BAS, C&C

Observations on Activity 4.3

To be honest I have tried to trick you here. I have hidden just one among a variety of quite common and acceptable abbreviations. The one I have a problem with is the use of 'mcg' instead of writing out microgram in full. Why? Because this is usually used in paediatric doses of drugs and it is so very easy to make a 10 times mistake in a drug dosage if that tiny letter 'c' isn't noticed.

Signature

Patient case notes may be required for reference years into the future when you have long since left your present Trust and few if any can remember you. A fine sprawling, exotic signature, like mine (see Figure 4.2) is fine and adds character if not fun to notes, **so long as you print your name clearly underneath**.

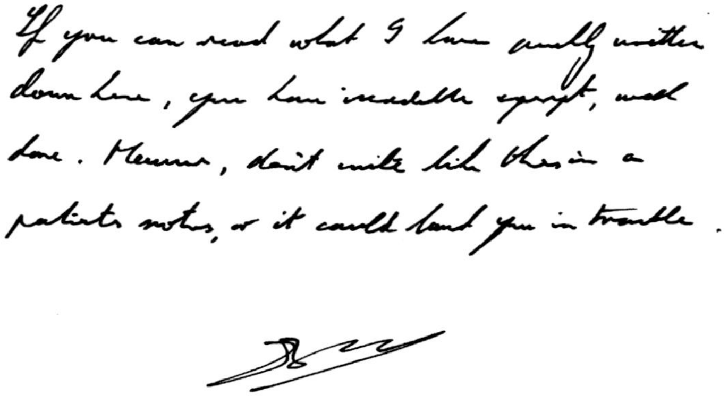

Figure 4.2 An example of my writing and signature; can you read it?

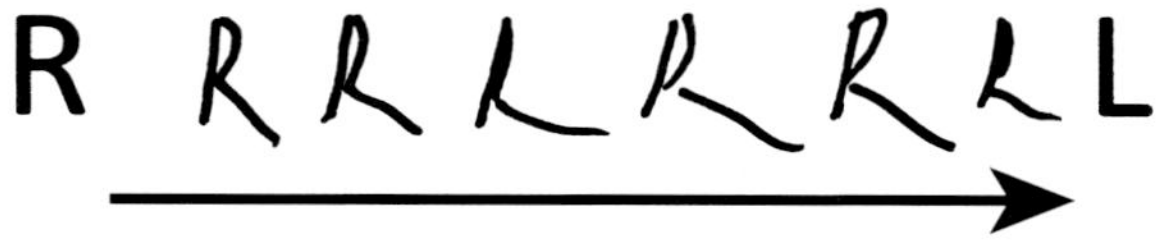

R R R L R R L L

Figure 4.3 How a scribbled 'R' may start looking like an 'L' leading to a mistake.

It's all in the detail

Don't be intimidated by your junior medical colleagues who may scoff at the detail of your notes. Not all doctors provide the 'gold standard' in terms of the correct method of note keeping. Stick to what you know is safe for the patient and it will keep you out of trouble.

Here are two short examples of clinical notes for you to work through. Note that I have not given any background to either of them. When you read good notes, you should be able to get a reasonable mental picture of the patient and everything relevant that has happened to them. Read my comments through after you have read both.

Scenario 1

Mr Peter Dunn
45a Sloane Street
Stockport, SP2 4DT
DOB 15/07/85
GP. Dr Harvest, Seal Rd. health centre.
Police officer, single.
0930hrs 27th Aug ****

P/C
Injury left ankle

PMH
Jumped off a 4ft wall last night while working and twisted left ankle? inversion injury. Sleepless night. Limping since. Brought in by family car.
Says not hurt elsewhere.
No relevant medical history.
No allergies
No drugs

O/E
Throbbing left ankle
Lateral swelling & bruising ++
Tender ++ lateral malleolus
No further tenderness on palpation of fibula up to knee.
Ankle movement severely limited
Circ & sens satis.
NWB
Medial ankle and remainder of left leg nil found
Arms and right leg nil found

Prov Diag.
Fracture lateral malleolus
Ottawa rules, sent for ankle X-ray
See later
X-ray shows undisplaced fracture lateral malleolus, mortise intact, no other injuries.

Management:
BKPOP
Crutches NWB
Raise limb
Analgesia, has at home.
Circulation, mvmts & sens intact.
See fracture clinic in morning 28th Aug
Advice and POP instructions given
See SOS if problems.
Signed D Bradley
1200hrs

Scenario 2

Mrs Pamela S Palmer
20 Laburnum Ave
Peterborough PT6 3HK
DOB 30/02/45
GP. Dr Brewer, Anderson Street surgery.
Retd. Widow.
1304hrs 27th Aug ****
P/C
Pain right shoulder.
PMH
Brought by friend
Increasing, intermittent pain in right shoulder for the past week.
No history of any injury recently or excessive activity.
Enjoys gardening
No significant PMH
No, diabetes, IHD, hypertension or arthritis
Allergic to penicillin
Drugs: occasional analgesics only.
Is overweight
O/E
Looks normal R=L, no swelling
Deep aching pain, not affected by movement
Almost full active ROM
No tenderness
Movt, sens, & circ satis
CVS nil, P86, BP 160/90
No sweating
RS, nil, R18
GIS, c/o some nausea
Tender right upper quadrant abdo.
Investigations:
T 37C
ECG nil
Refer
While on hospital site; discuss with surgeon on call.
Provisional diagnosis:
Cholecystitis with referred pain
Signed D Bradley
Time 1400hrs

My comments

Scenario 1 – Peter Dunn

On the whole quite a good attempt. Just by reading them you are able to get a clear picture of how the injury was obtained, how Peter presented, what was looked and felt for in the examination and finally what was done for him.

There are several points that I would like to stress. All important aspects of the examination are mentioned, so you know exactly where the pain is and where is tender.

You also know where the examiner looked for other injuries and did not find anything.

Finally, note the 'See SOS if problems'. ('SOS' stands for 'si opus sit', 'if needed'.) **This is one of the most important aspects of the whole set of notes. It means that you have told the patient that sometimes things go wrong, even in the best of circumstances, so they should come back to you or telephone at any time of the day or night if they have a worrying problem.**

If you get into a routine of explaining this to every patient you ever see and writing it down clearly, it helps you sleep at night. You have done your best for them and covered every eventuality.

Scenario 2 – Pamela Palmer

First, note that the allergy isn't just mentioned, it is thrown in your face: it should stand out above all else for everyone to see.

Pamela is a prime example of someone who walks into an MIU with something that possibly isn't minor. This type of thing is something that you will always have to be on your guard for. **Never presume that a patient in minors has a minor condition**.

The notes are of course incomplete, just up to the stage of discussion with another.

See how the examiner first examined the shoulder, found nothing, so looked elsewhere for an answer. This is a common sequence. From the patient's history you have a set of main possibilities. You then examine for features to confirm one of these and, if you do not find them, you have to revise your thoughts, ask more questions and look elsewhere.

Note that one of the major steps in the elimination process was the taking of an ECG: it's so easy to miss a 'silent' myocardial infarction (MI).

If you go to the website for this book, you will find a selection of note taking that you can read through and comment on as exercises.

Now for a final run through: detailing important aspects that have either not been covered so far, but are nevertheless important to digest, or deserve reinforcement.

Consent

There are three aspects of consent for you to consider when writing notes:

1. Age and competence.
2. Consent to perform a treatment, be it written or by word of mouth.
3. Consent to tell parents.

Confidentiality

- If your notes are on a computer, log out as routine so others do not have access.
- Don't leave paperwork lying around.
- Reassure patients regarding safety of their details.

Negligence

If you are inexperienced and had to ask for senior advice, document details of this to help avoid claims of negligence.

Reasons

Documenting the reasoning why you made a decision is often useful – for instance, not X-raying a limb because of the Ottawa rules.

Include the patient and relatives

For example, stating that a patient's partner was unhappy with a decision, but you explained the possibilities to them. These are never notes just for you and your thoughts: you must include pertinent others.

Child protection

Be particular about only writing facts about what you see, not what you think you see. For example, have a look at 'Mongolian blue spots' in Google Images. Would you have mistaken them for bruises?

With suspicions of non-accidental injury (NAI) in particular, there is no shame in getting senior advice on wording **before** documenting.

REFERENCES AND SUGGESTED READING

Douglas, G. Nicol, F. and Robertson, C. (eds) (2009) *Macleod's Clinical Examination*, 12th edn, Churchill Livingstone, Oxford.

Porter, A., Snooks, H., Youren, A. *et al.* (2008) 'Covering our backs', ambulance crews' attitudes towards clinical documentation when emergency (999) patients are not conveyed to hospital. *Emergency Medical Journal*, 25, 292–295.

Welsby, P.D. (2002) *Clinical History Taking and Examination: An Illustrated Colour Text*, 2nd edn, Churchill Livingstone, Oxford.

Multiple choice questions

Before you start, take in the reasoning behind these MCQs, how to answer them and how to interpret the results, from the section at the end of Chapter 1.

1. Which of the following are valid reasons for documenting patients?

    A   To gain information for future research
    B   The 10-year national census
    C   To form a legal document
    D   To act as protection for the clinician

2. Which of the following abbreviations are acceptable to write in a patient's notes?

    A   Pupils =& RTL
    B   'o' (as a prefix meaning 'no')
    C   CNs 1-12 intact
    D   PEARL

3. Which of the following statements are true?

    A   For the notes of minor injury and condition patients, to write down everything that was examined would make the notes too extensive
    B   For something so common that everyone would do it, such as to check the circulation to a limb, it is presumed that it was done if not actually written down.
    C   If an item is not documented, it is presumed that it was not done
    D   In practice, to simply write that 'a limb was checked' would imply that the circulation had been checked; the full detail would not be necessary

4. For a patient with a limb injury following a fall from a bike, which of the following would be relevant negatives requiring documentation?

    A   Appetite normal.
    B   No injury to other limbs

C   No LOC
D   No drugs or alcohol

5. **Which of the following apply?**

    A   It is inappropriate to use drawings in clinical notes
    B   Only drawings printed onto the paper should be used
    C   The statement 'no known allergies' is open to differing interpretations, so should not be used
    D   A paramedic comes to you later the same day saying that they brought the patient in and requesting some information from the clinical notes; you apologise, but say that you cannot betray the patient's confidentiality.

6. **Which of the following give a patient the right to see and receive a copy of their written clinical documentation?**

    A   The Data Protection Act (1998)
    B   The Health Records Act (1990)
    C   The Children Act (2004)
    D   Individual local trust guidelines

7. **Which (if any) of the options listed are satisfactory and unambiguous ways of documenting?**

    A   mcg
    B   microgram
    C   μg
    D   mic. gram

8. **You think that your minor injury patient is also drunk. Which (if any) of the following are suitable to enter in the notes?**

    A   Make no comment about it at all
    B   Too much C_2H_5OH
    C   Obviously had a little too much
    D   Smell of alcohol on the breath, but denies taken any

9. **Regarding the time and place of the incident, which of the following are most suitable?**

    A   Patient slipped on the factory floor yesterday afternoon
    B   Patient states that they slipped on the factory floor yesterday afternoon
    C   Patient slipped indoors yesterday afternoon
    D   Patient slipped in Liverpool yesterday afternoon

10. **Your patient has a complete POP applied today (26th). Regarding their follow-up, which of the following are the most suitable to use?**

    A   Returning to # clinic tomorrow
    B   Returning to # clinic Wed 27th 0930hrs
    C   Returning to # clinic Wed 27th 0930hrs & told to contact SOS
    D   Returning to fracture clinic Wed 0930hrs, & attend SOS

 Answers are available at the end of the book. For an explanation of these answers and further resources visit the companion website at:

www.wiley.com/go/bradley/musculoskeletal

Part 2

The upper body

5

The neck

Introduction to Part 2

Following on from the first four chapters that gave you the background knowledge that you require, this is the first chapter showing you how to approach study in a specific region.

For clarity, each of these regional chapters will be divided into the following five sections:

1. Applied anatomy and physiology.
2. History and mechanisms of injury.
3. Patient examination.
4. Minor musculoskeletal injuries.
5. Minor musculoskeletal conditions.

At the end of each chapter will be multiple choice questions and answers.

Aim

To develop an in-depth understanding of the anatomy and physiology, history, examination and early management of minor musculoskeletal injuries and conditions of and around the neck.

Outcomes

That by the end of this study, and all the associated activities and clinical experiences, you will be able to:

- demonstrate an in-depth knowledge of the anatomy and physiology of musculoskeletal structures of the neck
- take an effective history and examine patients presenting with neck problems, forming a differential diagnosis
- demonstrate an in-depth knowledge of minor musculoskeletal injuries and conditions of the neck
- apply these skills to the early management of patients, recognising any need for referral.

Managing Minor Musculoskeletal Injuries and Conditions, First Edition. David Bradley.
© 2014 John Wiley & Sons, Ltd. Published 2014 by John Wiley & Sons, Ltd.
Companion website: www.wiley.com/go/bradley/musculoskeletal

Section 1
Applied anatomy and physiology

Cervical vertebrae

Clearly, the seven cervical vertebrae are not the easiest of bones to start your studies with, especially if you don't have the actual bones or models of them in front of you. Still, the world is rarely a fair place, so let's do the best we can with some illustrations. But please **do your best to actually handle some bone fairly soon**: nothing can take its place.

All complex subjects are best studied by first revising what you already know. So do not take offence if I start with the basics and build from those. I have tried to include **just the amount of detail that you will need** in your new role.

However, some of the anatomical detail is not here because it is required to manage a patient's condition, but so that you can understand and keep yourself updated, reading books and journal articles.

 Activity 5.1   **Time: 10 minutes**

Can you think of seven major features that most of the cervical vertebrae have in common? List these on some paper before you go further; don't be too concerned with the exact names – they will come to you later.
Afterwards compare with my observations and illustration Figure 5.1.

Observations on Activity 5.1

The parts of a **typical cervical vertebra**:

- A basic ring of bone.
- A thickened part with surfaces, to join with inter-vertebral discs above and below (**vertebral body**).
- Hole for the spinal cord to pass through (**vertebral foramen**).

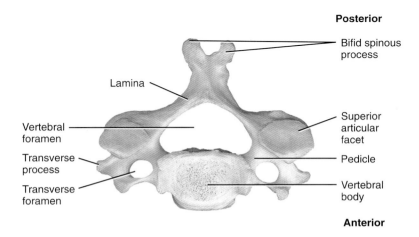

Figure 5.1 Superior view of a typical cervical vertebra (Tortora and Nielsen, 2012). This material is reproduced with permission of John Wiley & Sons, Inc.

- Small holes for arteries passing up to the brain (**transverse foramina**).
- Small joint surfaces on either side, to articulate with vertebrae either above or below (**facet joints**).
- Projections of bone sticking out backwards and to the sides for the attachment of muscles and ligaments (**spinous and transverse processes**).
- Spaces in adjacent vertebrae, which when put together form a hole (**intervertebral foramen**). These clearly show on an oblique X-ray, not lateral.

 Activity 5.2   **Time: 10 minutes**

A useful activity would be to try to draw, or trace over, the major features of Figure 5.1. Actually doing something, as well as just reading, assists retention.

Afterwards, you can then see if you can remember the names of the parts. Throughout the book, you will find that additional drawing and writing make learning so much easier than just reading.

Applications of the parts you have just learnt

Basic ring of bone

There is a progressive variation in size, from the largest seventh cervical, 'sitting' on the top of the first thoracic vertebra, through to the small atlas vertebra (C1). Just one of the implications of this concerns palpation of the vertebrae, C7 being an easily felt landmark, whereas the remainder are often difficult, especially in those with a 'thick' neck.

The separate regions that make up the ring are almost inseparable and difficult to follow; that is why it is so very important to **try to get models to study** with your book rather than just using illustrations.

The vertebral body

In a similar manner to the variation of the mass of the bone itself just discussed, the vertebral body is large in C7, trailing off to be almost non-existent in C1 (just called a '**tubercle**').

In most, the superior and inferior surfaces of the vertebral body have a circular 'lip' of bone around the edge, which the disc neatly fits into. When viewed from the side, the body is roughly rectangular in shape; this is a very important point to remember when trying to learn from an X-ray, because with injury and disease the shape can vary.

The construction of the whole of a vertebra, and especially the body, is that of cancellous (spongy) bone with a light covering of compact that we can see, very strong and very light. The body protects the spinal cord anteriorly and forms surfaces for the positioning of intervertebral discs.

Vertebral foramen

This varies in both size and shape from C1 to C7. The spinal cord is not a neat fit inside. High up in the column the space is far larger, to allow for the increased movement of the head and fatty 'padding' around the cord.

Transverse foramina

Situated on either side of each vertebra at the laminae are these small holes about 3–4 mm in diameter supporting arteries going up to the brain. The significance is that, as we age and our spinal column degenerates, the foramina can deform, sometimes compressing vessels as we make large head movements, and temporarily interrupting the blood flow.

Facet joints

These are called '**zygapophyseal joints**' in some books, but 'facet joint' is fine. These are so small, yet so important, and often cause our patients considerable pain. Mostly, each vertebra has four. All are situated laterally, two on the superior surface and two on the inferior surface. Each are completely separate hyaline joints, able to make small gliding movements. They have a small capsule and are held by small ligaments surrounded by muscle to allow tiny movements.

If looked at from the side on an X-ray, the line of the joints are almost horizontal in children, but less so in adults.

 Activity 5.3   **Time: 15 minutes**

Put the following into your web browser: 'uncovertebral joints', or 'joints of Luschka'. To avoid mix-ups, don't read about them until you have looked at several illustrations first. Few people even know of their existence!

Spinous and transverse processes

These are there for the attachment of major muscles and ligaments supporting the column and will be named a little later on. The spinous processes can usually be palpated, with the seventh far more prominent and easily seen.

Intervertebral foramen

Spaces in adjacent vertebrae, when put together, form a hole (*see* Figure 5.2). This is a view of a **lumbar vertebra** to show the foramina more clearly. They are perhaps one of the most important and significant structures that you should understand. Problems surrounding them account for a major part of cervical spine problems.

Other parts

The first two vertebrae are rather specialised and this is heightened by their being given their own names.

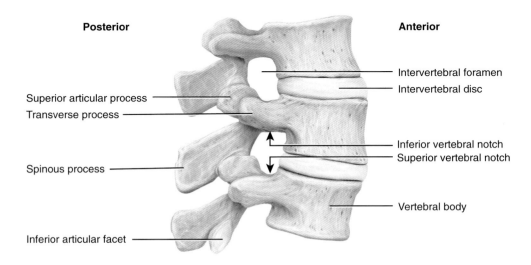

Figure 5.2 Right lateral view of articulated lumbar vertebrae, to show intervertebral foramen (Tortora and Nielsen, 2012). This material is reproduced with permission of John Wiley & Sons, Inc.

Posterior

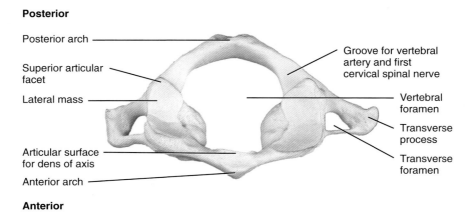

Posterior arch

Superior articular facet

Lateral mass

Articular surface for dens of axis

Anterior arch

Groove for vertebral artery and first cervical spinal nerve

Vertebral foramen

Transverse process

Transverse foramen

Anterior

Figure 5.3 Superior view of atlas (C1) (Tortora and Nielsen, 2012). This material is reproduced with permission of John Wiley & Sons, Inc.

C1 the atlas

This is literally a ring of bone, with a stumpy little bulge anteriorly (**tubercle**) instead of a body. Posterior to this tubercle is a small but vitally important articular surface for the nestling of an upward projection from the axis below called the '**Odontoid peg**' or '**Dens**'. Posteriorly is the smallest of all spinous processes (**tubercle**) (Figure 5.3).

Large, crescent-shaped articular surfaces can be seen on the upper surface articulating with similar surfaces in the base of the occiput (**atlanto-occipital joint**), allowing the head a nodding motion.

On the inferior surface are two facet joints (C1/2) for the axis vertebra below, which allow mostly the side-to-side movement of turning the head.

C2 the axis

The most prominent feature of the axis is the **odontoid peg**. There is a small 'peg' of bone projecting upwards to articulate with the atlas see Figures 5.4a and 5.4b. It is held in place mostly by the **transverse ligament** of the atlas, but there are others involved in the support of this joint.

 Activity 5.4 **Time: About an hour**

Look at some cervical spine X-rays now, either at work or at home on Google Images. Talk to your colleagues and get practice looking at the X-rays, tracing the often-confusing bone shadows and, most importantly, getting feedback.

If your chosen mentor cannot be with you at the time, why not either take copies of some X-rays, or print out copies if on a website. Doing this, you can get expert feedback at a later date.

Leave the website associated with this book until later in the chapter.

The curves of the cervical spine

These are described as being both **primary** and **secondary**. In the womb all the vertebrae, are concave anteriorly; this is called the 'primary curve' and it bends forwards in the foetal position (*see* Figure 5.5a).

Posterior   **Anterior**

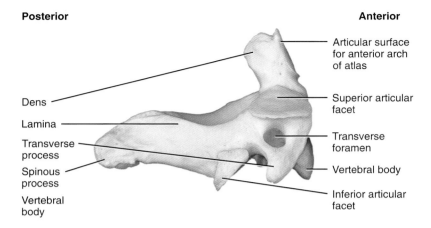

Articular surface
for anterior arch
of atlas

Dens

Superior articular
facet

Lamina

Transverse
process

Transverse
foramen

Spinous
process

Vertebral body

Vertebral
body

Inferior articular
facet

Figure 5.4a Right lateral view of axis (C2) (Tortora and Nielsen, 2012). This material is reproduced with permission of John Wiley & Sons, Inc.

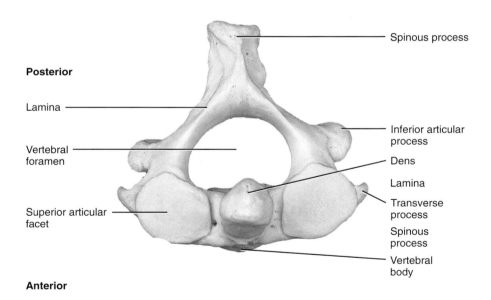

Spinous process

Posterior

Lamina

Inferior articular
process

Vertebral
foramen

Dens

Lamina

Transverse
process

Superior articular
facet

Spinous
process

Vertebral
body

Anterior

Figure 5.4b Superior view of atlas (C2) (Tortora and Nielsen, 2012). This material is reproduced with permission of John Wiley & Sons, Inc.

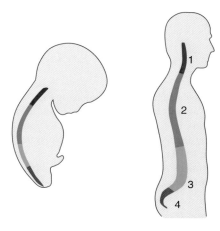

Single curve in foetus   Four curves in adult

Figure 5.5a Foetal and adult curves of the spine (Tortora and Nielsen, 2012). This material is reproduced with permission of John Wiley & Sons, Inc.

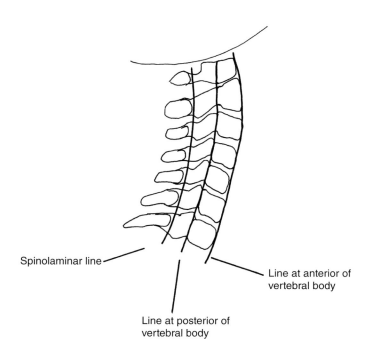

Spinolaminar line

Line at anterior of vertebral body

Line at posterior of vertebral body

Figure 5.5b Some curves of the cervical vertebrae as seen on lateral X-rays.

As the baby starts to take an interest in outside surroundings, the cervical vertebrae develop into the usual secondary curve that you are used to in normal adults, concave posteriorly (**lordosis**) see Figure 5.5 a and b. The thoracic vertebrae maintain their primary curve.

Surface anatomy

The 'soft tissues' of the neck have a great deal of 'give' in them, allowing ease of palpation to many of the structures.

As with most areas of the body, surface anatomy is made far easier if you start by looking at and palpating your own tissues. Next come friends and family, who can act as ideal specimens for your practice, so long as they are not over-weight. In these early stages of your looking and feeling for landmarks, excess fat can turn a reassuring anatomy practice into a confusing and confidence-draining session.

Sometimes palpable in the front of the neck are the major structures illustrated in Figure 5.6. These are of course overlain in part by the **sternocleidomastoid** muscles.

Paediatric differences

Especially with babies and small children, there are quite a few very important and specific anatomical differences, such as the angle of the facet joints and the shortness of the neck in general. Complexities also arise in the interpretation of epiphyses.

Intervertebral discs

Situated between the bodies of the vertebrae, these discs serve to:

- carry the weight of the body
- act as cushioning
- assist in the minute movements between each vertebrae
- help support and bind the vertebral bodies.

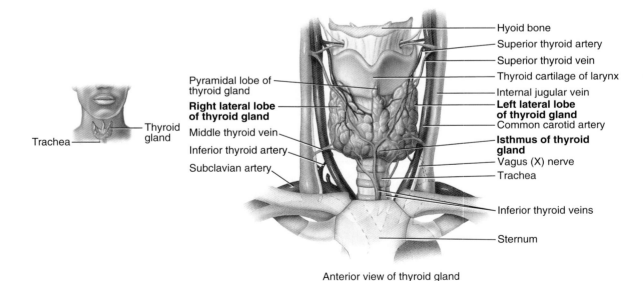

Anterior view of thyroid gland

Figure 5.6 Major structures in the front of the neck; the sternocleidomastoid muscles and some other tissues have been removed (Tortora and Nielsen, 2012). This material is reproduced with permission of John Wiley & Sons, Inc.

The discs are made of two main substances – a soft almost 'toothpaste' type of centre (**nucleus pulposus**) and an outer strong retaining tissue (**annulus fibrosus**) with a lamellar construction. In this cervical region, they are slightly bulkier anteriorly.

Spinal ligaments

- Ligamenta flava.
- Anterior longitudinal.
- Posterior longitudinal.
- Inter spinous.
- Supra spinous.
- Facet joint ligaments (*see* Figure 5.7).

You may at first think of these ligaments as a form of 'accessory' to the column, but in reality they are at its very heart because, without them and surrounding strong muscles, we are lost – the strength of the column lies within these structures.

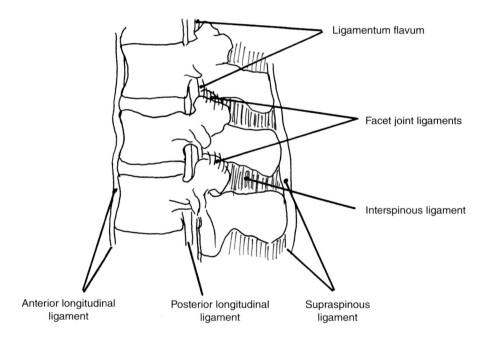

Figure 5.7 The spinal ligaments, left lateral view.

The cervical and brachial plexuses

A plexus is a complex 'interchange' of nerve fibres, situated in the neck and shoulder, looking like sections of complicated rail-track sidings.

The construction of the interconnections is not necessary for you to learn, but an understanding of some of the points is essential if you are to understand some conditions.

The spinal cord is divided into **segments**. From each of the spinal segments there is a **dorsal** (sensory) and a **ventral** (motor) **nerve root** leaving on either side. These join together and leave the spinal column through an intervertebral foramen, becoming a **spinal nerve**.

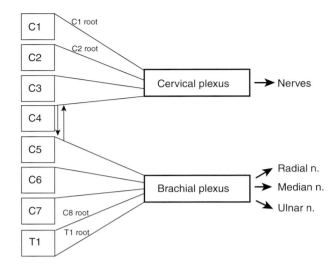

Figure 5.8 Some nerve pathways in the neck.

These cervical roots are numbered: the C1 root leaves the column by the foramen at the upper border of C1, the C2 root by the foramen at the upper border of C2, and so on as shown in Figure 5.8 until you get to C8 at the upper border of the T1 vertebra.

Roots from C5 to C8, plus T1 roots, feed into the brachial plexus and from this exit the three major motor and sensory nerves to the upper arm. These are the **radial**, **median** and **ulnar nerves**.

You do not need to learn the detail of the interconnections inside the plexus, but you should know the root levels that apply to each nerve. This is discussed further in the examination section.

Section 2
History and mechanism of injury

Now that you have revised a little about the anatomy of the neck structures, the next stage is to attempt to discover what has happened to your patient. As will be frequently reinforced throughout this book, taking a history is perhaps the major skill that you will develop. On many occasions, if done with care, it will almost hand you the diagnosis 'on a plate'. Understanding the MOI or history is a key area of study.

History

It is vital for you to remember that this book is concerned with minor injuries and conditions. **It is not intended to involve the 'clearing' of a cervical spine following severe or multiple trauma**. Here it is for you to manage the 'walking wounded' type of patient whose main problem is either a minor injury to their neck or a minor neck problem that has occurred.

The very first thing that you need to do is always eliminate any possibility of a severe spinal injury. Perhaps this is a good place for a golden rule:

GOLDEN RULE

The very first thing you must do is always to eliminate the likelihood of a severe spinal injury.

Activity 5.5   **Time: A few minutes**

How would you start to approach this elimination? Write your basic ideas down and then check with my observations for this activity.

Observations on Activity 5.5

Well, if you said something like those below the following, I would be pleased:

Ask how the problem or accident occurred and the severity of the forces involved. This is **the** major point to ascertain with any patient and is the first thing to ask following the initial 'What is the problem?' or 'How may I help you?'

Next, build on that information with a little detail. For instance, if the patient said, 'I must have twisted my neck while I was asleep, because I woke up with the pain', ask about the previous day or evening activities and a previous history of anything like the problem.

The assessment and examination of all patients should be approached in a systematic way; but that does not mean that there is only one way to go about things. Think and enquire in a logical and orderly manner, but you must know your subject well enough to be able to vary from the main pathway when necessary because all patients are individual.

Think head injury, think neck injury. A blow to the head always carries the possibility of an associated injury to the neck, so you must consider it by asking specific questions.

Sometimes the patient will not differentiate between the head and neck, thinking of them as one part. The 'headache' associated with a minor head injury will only become a 'headache and painful neck' following precise questioning by you.

Whiplash

This mechanism is foremost in the minds of most people when they think of neck injuries. A sudden forward movement of the body, allows the very heavy head to be 'left behind' and therefore **hyperextend** the cervical vertebrae (*see* Figure 5.9). Following that, the head may **hyperflex** the cervical vertebrae, causing further sets of injuries. A road traffic colli-

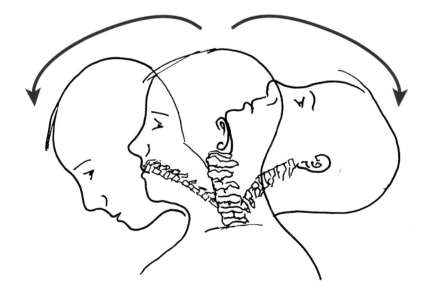

Figure 5.9 Whiplash mechanism.

sion (RTC) is the most common cause. Any resultant damage will be discussed later (in section 4); here we are just considering the mechanism, so that you will always recognise it.

Although this is the classical presentation, it must be remembered that the whiplash phenomenon can occur from any angle. It is a mechanism, not a pathology, so it can have many implications from the very minor to the very severe.

Sporting tackle

A rugby tackle can bring a player down heavily onto the shoulder and neck area, but tackles occur in other sports too.

Always be extremely wary if your patient's history involves a rugby scrum (*see* Figure 5.10). The collapse of a scrum, especially of school children or adult amateurs (both with poorly developed musculature) may easily lead to critical neck injuries.

Diving

In any situation with a history involving a diving accident or near drowning, I want you to consider that the cervical spine may have been involved as the person hit the water or base.

Skiing injury

High-speed collisions spring to mind here, both with others and objects.

Child abuse, head shaking

Thankfully not common, but as a senior nurse or paramedic you must always consider the possibility and ask the correct questions (*see* Figure 5.11).

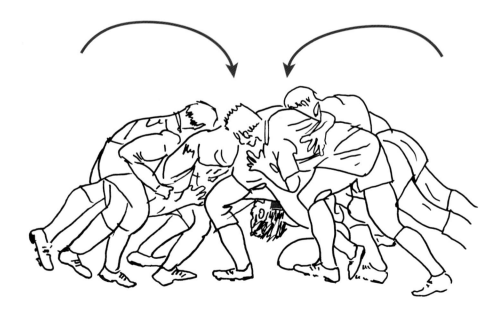

Figure 5.10 With a rugby scrum, always consider the cervical spine.

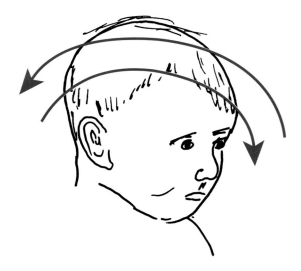

Figure 5.11 If the story sounds strange, always consider that the toddler's head may have been shaken.

Lack of support at night

Waking up in the morning with a painful stiff neck is a fairly common presentation. If the neck is not well supported with a suitably sized pillow, the soft tissues can easily be over stretched for hours and become inflamed by the following morning, see **wry neck**.

Mechanisms of major spinal injuries

Each of the common mechanisms that cause the major unstable spinal injuries can, with the use of lesser force, produce just a relatively minor injury (*see* Figure 5.12).

Acute flexion

Perhaps the movement most likely to cause damage – for example, diving into too shallow a depth of water.

Acute extension

Elderly, fall downstairs.

Vertical loading (or its exact opposite – distraction)

- Diving.
- Object falling onto head.
- Fall downstairs.

Rotation associated with acute flexion or extension

A classical example here would be falling from a horse.

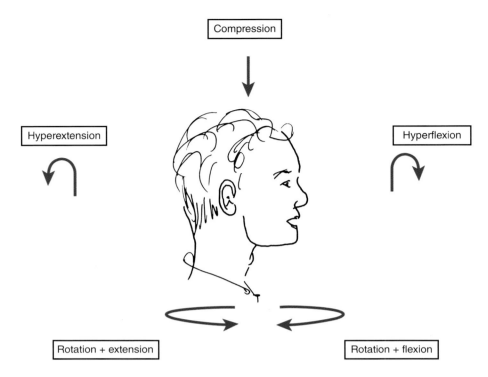

Figure 5.12 The standard mechanisms of major spinal injuries may also be the cause of minor ones.

Rheumatoid arthritis C1/C2 instability

Many parts of the body may be affected by RA, and the patient may not even realise that they have any problem in the neck. The **transverse ligament** on C1 may be weakened; this ligament was mentioned in Section 1. Be alert to signs of the disease in common joints, and question the patient with care.

Cervical spondylosis

Sometimes I think that half the population has this condition. In those over 55, up to 50% are thought to have X-ray changes that are associated with it. In all probability, most have never had more than occasional pain or stiffness in the neck, and would be surprised if you told them that they had such a condition. So, you see that this mostly has a very slow and insidious onset, 'creeping up' on the patient, unawares.

With progression, it only takes a small amount of overuse or excessive stress to the area for the features to worsen. This could be something like hyperextending the neck for a few hours while painting a ceiling, continued twisting to talk to a friend on the back seat of a car, an over-zealous twist while playing with children or a minor whiplash.

The features may vary considerably from little more than occasional stiffness and pain for a few days, easily brought under control with simple drugs, through the whole range to severe disability with severe pain, neurological deficits and severe limitation of neck movements.

Wry neck (torticollis)

There are two main presentation groups here: first, the patient who was born with the condition (**congenital torticollis**, or **wry neck**) or has had it for a long time because of some associated condition.

Second, the very common **acquired torticollis**, or **wry neck**, whose classical presentation is that the patient goes to bed fine and wakes up the next morning or in the early hours with the muscles on one side in painful spasm, dragging the neck to one side. They may be any age, but are often young children or young adults (Brukner and Khan, 2012).

Klippel-Feil syndrome

The patient is born with this condition and when undressed you will see a deformity. If you have not seen a patient with this before, it is best to have a look at pictures of several variations of the condition, so that you can look at it and instantly be aware of the diagnosis.

Activity 5.6   **Time: 15 minutes**

Try Google Images now and put in 'Klippel-Feil syndrome' to get an idea of variations in the appearance, to heighten your awareness.
    The change of activity will also aid learning.

Congenital hemi-vertebra and congenital extra rib (cervical rib)

These are usually just found on X-ray as a reason for pain, compression features or deformity.

Down's syndrome

Those with Down's syndrome may have weakened ligaments at C1/2 that could cause problems following even trivial trauma. This is not often realised by emergency staff, but close families and care workers are likely to be aware of the problem.

Sporting muscle tears

These can be caused by the shot put, for example.

Prolonged computer use

This may cause a neck problem (repetitive strain injury [RSI]) if the screen is at a poor angle to the eyes.

Referred pain (*see* Figure 5.13)

This form of pain is very common from many areas including:

- neck pain referred to shoulder
- shoulder pain referred to neck
- tension headache referred to neck
- sore throat and glands referred to neck
- temporomandibular (TM) joints.

Section 3
Patient examination

The examination of your patient's neck

You will already be comfortable with the standard protocols for the management of any neck injury and you may have supported your patient's neck with your hands while asking them the mechanism of injury or if their neck even hurts.

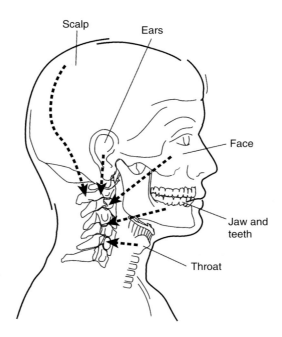

Figure 5.13 Sites of referred pain to the neck (Gross *et al.*, 2009).

These protocols are beyond the scope of this book and will not be discussed further. However, the special needs of paediatric patients with neck problems is worth your consideration (Davies, 2011).

When dealing with minor injuries, patients have usually come to a decision about themselves before they reach you, and decided the level of urgency, so to rush in supporting necks would be inappropriate, very frightening and present you in a negative light.

If you are learning about minors here for the first time, it is important to realise that, without frightening the patient, you must get an accurate MOI followed by a brief assessment to eliminate the possibility of an unstable spinal injury. If concerned, you then tactfully explain the possible problems to the patient and immobilise the spinal column.

Over the years in A&E, I can think of two patients in particular whom I have seen: one walking into minors holding onto their head and another sitting quietly for over an hour in a wheelchair in the waiting room. Both had unstable fractures.

A minor injury exists only if major ones have been eliminated.

Enough of these frightening experiences; from now on, we will presume that our patients have only stable injuries.

Observation

Although this book is about musculoskeletal problems, the neck must be considered as part of the patient as a whole. Examination starts with inspection, looking in particular for symmetry of the structures from the front, the laryngeal cartilages, musculature and swellings of the soft tissues as shown previously in Figure 5.6. The thyroid gland itself is not normally visible, but should be considered with any neck swellings. Similarly observe from the back, ensuring that into the hairline and behind the ears are included.

Palpation of structures

Initially stand behind your patient and, like with examination of the abdomen, warm your hands and be gentle. Remember that the patient cannot see what you are doing, so you must explain your moves to prevent them becoming nervous.

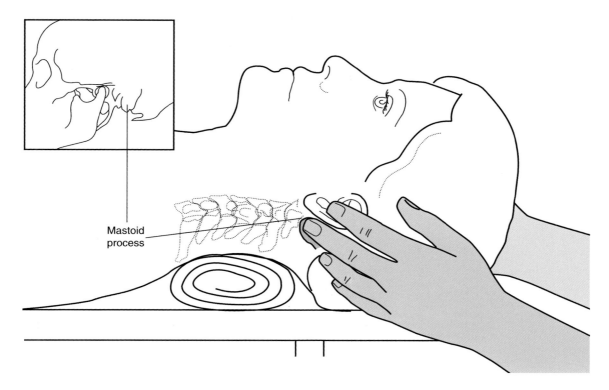

Mastoid
process

Figure 5.14 Palpation of the mastoid process (Gross *et al.*, 2009).

Although we are concerned mostly with problems of the musculoskeletal system, it would be folly to narrow our examination to only cover those structures. If you are studying to become an autonomous practitioner, **this is one of the most important points that you have to learn**. Spending a great deal of time on other systems and structures is not what I'm after; just **consider them** and make the depth of your examination match the circumstances.

Find the **spinous processes**; C7 should be the most prominent. Then, from the **mastoid processes** behind the ears (*see* Figure 5.14), travel downwards, feeling deeply towards the **transverse processes** on either side. These will be difficult and often impossible to feel, especially for the inexperienced, but do attempt it, all the time noting any tenderness.

At the base of the neck, complete your palpation of the bony landmarks by feeling the **sternoclavicular joints** on either side.

Other structures to attempt to palpate are:

• thyroid gland
• parotid glands
• cysts (the neck is a prime site for several types)
• lymph nodes; most nodes are situated both under the jaw and generally following the line of the sternocleidomastoid muscle (*see* Figure 5.15)
• larynx for form and mobility
• trachea, midline above the manubrium of the sternum.

Complete this part of your examination with palpation of the overlying musculature of the trapezius and sternocleidomastoid.

Examination of neck movements

First, see what active movements there are (*see* Figure 5.16). Because of pain, your patient may have to be encouraged to demonstrate the full extent of active movements as below:

- Flexion (put your chin to chest).
- Extension (look up to the sky).
- Rotate to the left and right (move your chin to your shoulder).
- Lateral flexion (put your ear to your shoulder) (*see* Figure 5.16).

If there is any deficit of these active movements, gentle passive movements may be tried until pain is reached.

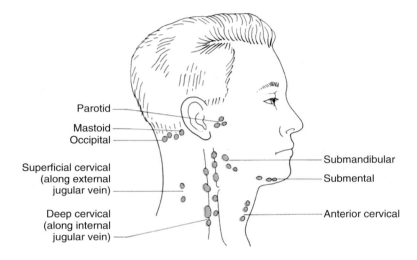

Figure 5.15 Scheme of the lymph nodes of the head and neck (Ellis and Mahadevan, 2010).

Neurological examination

The aim of a neurological examination is to find any association with nerve, nerve root or spinal cord pathology.

It is sometimes very necessary to eliminate these problems, or even, just by doing so, to indicate to the patient that you are taking their problem seriously.

Any abnormal finding should automatically be a pointer to signpost your patient's problem to a doctor.

Remember that the nerve roots to the brachial plexus are C5, C6, C7, C8 and T1. Each of these roots has sensory, motor and tendon reflex changes, which are suggestive of a problem at that particular level. Only a rough outline is given of these here and in Figure 5.17.

C5

- Sensory, outer elbow.
- Motor, flex elbow.
- Reflex, biceps.

C6

- Sensory, anterior tip of thumb.
- Motor, wrist extension.
- Reflex, brachioradialis.

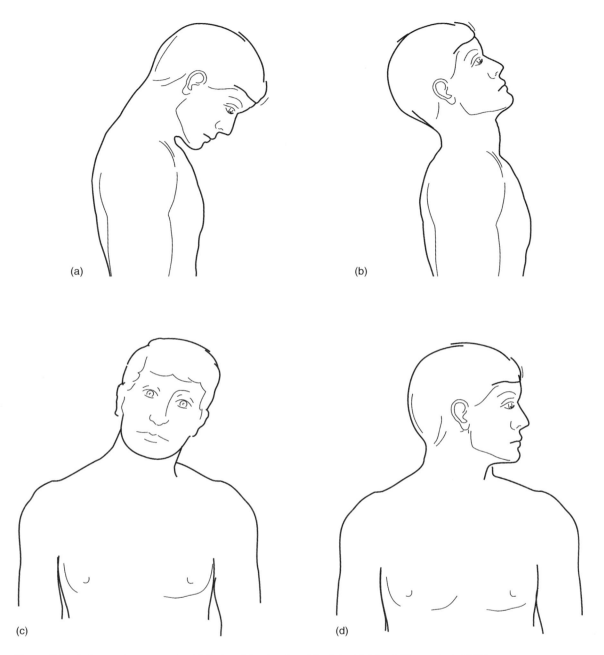

Figure 5.16 Active neck movements: (a) flexion, (b) extension, (c) rotate, (d) lateral (Gross *et al.*, 2009).

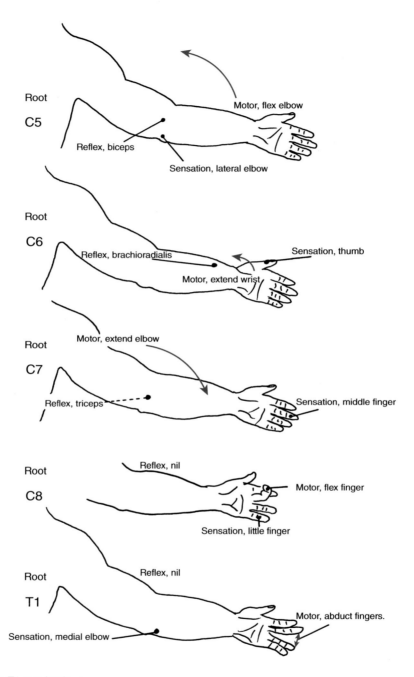

Figure 5.17 C5 to T1 root levels.

C7

- Sensory, anterior tip of middle finger.
- Motor, elbow extension.
- Reflex, triceps.

C8

- Sensory, anterior tip of little finger.
- Motor, bend fingers.
- Reflex, none specific.

T1

- Sensory, near medial condyle.
- Motor, abduction of fingers.
- Reflex, none specific.

The best (but not easiest) way of learning all this is to ask a colleague to call you to see actual patients with problems at specific levels; it will stay in your mind far more effectively.

Within each regional chapter, you will find a checklist (see Checklist 5.1) to help you keep up to date with your practical physical examination progress. For each of the major tasks, there are columns for you to sign if you have practised on yourself or friends first, to gain confidence. **This is not meant as an indicator of competency**, merely a check that you are keeping up with practice requirements.

Section 4
Minor musculoskeletal injuries

Whiplash injury

This is an MOI rather than an injury to a specific part; it is a grouping of clinical features with a similar cause, rather than a recognised injury to a single place in the neck. Several grading systems exist to classify whiplash injuries; these vary from trivial through to fractures or dislocations of the cervical vertebrae.

Forms of injury

The forces cause degrees of strain to the capsule and ligaments of the **apophyseal joints** of the cervical spine. The pain of this damage, although in many instances immediate, often isn't apparent for hours or days, simply because the features of inflammation can take that time to develop. It can be likened to a heavy day's work in the garden or home: while you are doing it, all is okay, but the next morning (after a night of microscopical bleeding) it hurts!

Depending on the severity of the force and the exact direction, other ligaments – for instance, the **anterior** and **posterior longitudinal** and **interspinous** – may also be damaged.

Surrounding muscles later come into the picture: going into spasm in an attempt to keep the painful joints still and then becoming part of the problem themselves.

Clinical features

- Neck pain is the most prominent feature, although the pain may also spread to, or present in, the shoulders, arms and hands, or between the scapulae, the upper or even the lower back.
- Tenderness throughout the cervical column.
- Limitation of movements, especially flexion and extension.

Checklist 5.1 Record of progress

Physical examination of the neck

Examination	On self	Friend practice	Friend practice	Patient practice
Patient history, a variety				
Observation:				
General				
Neck veins				
Palpation:				
SC joint				
Mastoid process				
Spinous process				
Transverse process				
Larynx				
Trachea				
Cysts				
Lymph nodes				
Thyroid				
Parotid				
Trapezius				
Sternomastoid				
Range of movement:				
Flexion				
Extension				
Side to side (ear to shoulder)				
(chin to shoulder)				
Sensations:				
(Specify root levels below)				
Circulation:				
Skin				
Carotids				
Specific tests:				
Root levels				
C5				
C6				
C7				
C8				
T1				
Others:				
Associated to throat and ears				

Many other non-specific features have been reported; the more common are:

- headaches, especially occipital
- pain in the TM joints of the jaw
- dizziness
- paraesthesia
- visual changes.

The diagnosis depends very much on the history of the incident with an accurate MOI.

Many patients will fit the criteria for cervical spine X-rays; know your own local rules for these and stick to them rigidly. Outcomes for patients can be very variable, with protracted continuation of features for 18 months or more.

Initial management, advice and referral

- Reassurance and explanation.
- Very occasionally a soft collar could be used for a few days. Alternatively, instruct the patient to sit comfortably with the neck and any hollows well supported; use a towel or cloth from around the house.
- Analgesia and/or anti-inflammatory drugs.
- The application of local warmth with something like an electric or microwavable heat pad is sometimes very soothing. Patient compliance with instructions for ice packs is unlikely to be successful!
- After a few days, active exercises should be encouraged; continuation of trying to keep the neck still will produce more severe problems (Richell-Herren, 2005).
- Some patients will require referral to physiotherapy or their GP for follow-up.
- To return SOS.

Acquired torticollis (stiff neck, wry neck)

This is a reasonably common situation, where (usually) a youngster wakes in the morning with a very painful stiff neck (Figure 5.18). There is no history of any form of injury. Here it is reasonable to presume a simple musculoskeletal cause at first. It can also sometimes occur suddenly following a sudden movement of the neck.

 Activity 5.7　　　　　　　　　　　　　　**Time: 15–30 minutes**

There are other forms of the condition with far more serious causes, and a little study of these will be beneficial to you.

Have an outline understanding of the following:

- Congenital torticollis.
- Klippel-Feil syndrome (mentioned in Activity 5.6).
- Some drug reactions showing extra-pyramidal side effects.
- Local malignancies.

Clinical features

The patient wakes up in pain, without any history of injury. Painful spasm of the sternocleidomastoid muscle occurs that often takes a week or more before resolving. It is important that your history taking is thorough. Here are just some of the simple features that may have had an influence on starting the condition off:

- Minor trauma previously, possibly holding the head in an unusual position for a long time, a stretch or twist.
- Being drunk going to bed or taking sleeping tablets; with this the possibility exists of lying for a very long time in an unnatural position.

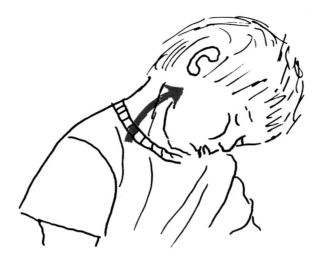

Figure 5.18 A simple cause of neck stiffness.

- Using a different pillow from usual.
- Being in a strong draught.
- A throat infection.

The sternocleidomastoid pulls the head and neck towards the affected side, with the chin twisting towards the good side.

Initial management, advice and referral

- Reassurance of the usual outcome and explanation is important.
- Analgesia.
- Support throughout the day.
- Correction of any of the causative problems listed earlier.
- Warmth.
- Occasional ice packs.
- Graded exercises.

Remember the value of SOS; although every incidence of this condition will probably have a simple cause, every patient will need referral to their GP for further investigation if steady improvement does not occur.

Postural neck pain

This is a form of RSI often seen in those doing office work (although not necessarily **at** work) with the head and neck not being held in a suitable position. Working on a computer for hours on end while studying is a frequent cause.

The head is held in an unusual position, but if coaxed the patient can usually cover a full range of neck movements.

As well as education to prevent it in the future, the management is similar to that described for wry neck mentioned earlier.

Section 5
Minor musculoskeletal conditions

Cervical spondylosis (spondylitis, OA cervical spine)

Definition

All the above names may be used, but perhaps the most accurate for you now is 'cervical spondylosis'. Not a minor condition, but exacerbations of it form a major source of patient attendances and because of this it is something that you should be familiar with.

Changes in the vertebrae occur with increasing rapidity from the age of about 30 onwards, with the majority of people from late middle age onwards showing some of the changes on X-rays. The level of **C5/6 is the most frequent site**, but the condition can spread to affect many levels.

The first changes are usually in the posterior-lateral surfaces of the **annulus fibrosus**; on X-ray the discs are seen to be narrowed when compared with those either side. This can be seen on Figure 5.19, but more detailed explanations of this X-ray and many others can also be found on the book's website.

The **anterior** and **posterior longitudinal ligaments** can become degenerate and **osteophytic spurs** form there. This and the **ligamentum flavum** damage can narrow the spinal canal.

The **facet joints** and **uncovertebral (Luschka)** joints are affected, with the joint surfaces becoming progressively deformed and destroyed (Skinner, 2006).

Osteophytes form around the margins of the vertebral bodies and may deform the intervertebral foramen, where the nerve roots exit from the spinal column.

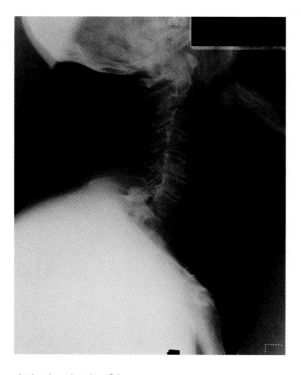

Figure 5.19 An X-ray of the cervical spine showing OA.

Clinical features

Many patients have cervical spondylosis without realising it, and are just told of the changes in the bones following a chance X-ray. Conversely, they may have severe features, but little to show for them on X-ray. This can be explained by the fact that we have what we are born with: those with slightly wider foramina will be less prone to injury.

A minor injury may act as a trigger factor causing symptoms to start or worsen.

Pain and paraesthesiae

These may be almost anywhere in the neck bridging dermatomes, even travelling up to the head giving patients an occipital headache, which could be the presenting symptom.

Pain may also travel downwards to the shoulders, or between the shoulder blades, or down the arm to the hands and fingers.

Neck stiffness

Lowered range of all movement is common.

Patients may complain that they can feel their neck grating (crepitus).

Management

- Analgesics and anti-inflammatories.
- Physiotherapy.
- Warmth.
- Support to the head and neck while sitting.
- Avoidance of large twisting movements.
- Avoidance of the use of a soft collar; if the patient is already using one, ask for it to be stopped after a few days.
- Remember your SOS at the end of the clinical notes: tumours, infections and inflammations (like RA) can all show at some stage with similar features, and your knowledge and diagnostic scope would not cover these eventualities.

Rheumatoid arthritis

The well-known saying, 'Fools rush in where wise men fear to tread' applies very well here when there is a mix of RA with a neck problem. Just as with any skin infection, one of your routine questions would be to ask if the patient has diabetes, so with a neck problem, look at their limbs for signs of RA and ask if they may have had it diagnosed.

RA starts in the soft tissues, ligaments and capsule surrounding a joint, then spreads into the joint itself. This means that the **alar and transverse ligament** holding C1 and C2 together may have become weakened, leading to the possibility of instability at the site (Fauci, 2010). Never take a risk: always refer your patient or get senior advice to ensure the patient's safety.

 Activity 5.8   **Time: About an hour**

I would finally like you to get a brief working knowledge of some conditions that, although serious in themselves and therefore beyond the scope of this book, may present to you in the early stages as a minor neck problem.

Read, highlight and possibly make the occasional note about:

- ankylosing spondylitis
- congenital extra rib
- forms of goitre
- fibromyalgia
- meningitis.

REFERENCES AND SUGGESTED READING

Brukner, P. and Khan, K. (2012) *Clinical Sports Medicine*, 4th edn, McGraw-Hill, Sydney.

Davies, F. (2011) *Emergency Care of Minor Trauma in Children*, Hodder & Stoughton, London.

Ellis, H. and Mahadevan V. (2010) *Clinical Anatomy*, 12th edn, Wiley Blackwell, Oxford.

Fauci, A.S. (ed.) (2010) *Harrison's Rheumatology*, 2nd ed., McGraw-Hill, New York.

Gross. J., Fetto, J. and Rosen, E. (2009) *Musculoskeletal Examination*, 3rd edn, Wiley Blackwell, Oxford.

Richell-Herren, K. (2005) Neck Sprains should be Mobilised Early, www.bestbets.org (accessed 24 May 2013).

Skinner, H.B. (2006) *Current Diagnosis and Treatment in Orthopedics*, 4th edn, McGraw-Hill, New York.

Tortora, J. and Nielsen M. (2012) *Principles of Human Anatomy*, 12th edn, Wiley Blackwell, Oxford.

Multiple choice questions

Before you start, take in the reasoning behind these MCQs, how to answer them and how to interpret the results, from the section at the end of Chapter 1.

1. Which (if any) of the following choices is a correct description of the normal curve of the cervical vertebrae in an adult?

   A   Concave posteriorly
   B   Cervical lordosis
   C   Convex posteriorly
   D   Convex anteriorly

2. Regarding cervical spine, which of the following is/are correct?

   A   The anterior longitudinal ligament runs along the anterior pedicles of the cervical vertebrae
   B   Apophyseal joints, facet joints and zygapophyseal joints are the same
   C   The transverse ligament holds the dens in place against the body of C2
   D   The intervertebral foramen between C3 and C4 contains the C4 spinal nerve root

3. In a classical 'whiplash' injury:

   A   Hyperextension of the cervical spine is followed by hyperflexion and both of these mechanisms may cause damage
   B   A stationary car being 'rear-ended' is a common mechanism
   C   Clinical features usually occur immediately
   D   Clinical features commonly continue for many months

4. Which of the following can significantly weaken ligaments in the cervical spine?

   A   Diabetes
   B   Down's syndrome
   C   RA
   D   Tetracycline

5. Which of the following would be the most likely cause of a patient presenting to you with a swelling in their neck?

   A   Swollen parotid gland
   B   Branchial cyst
   C   Enlarged lymph node
   D   Thyroglossal cyst

6. When a non-trauma patient presents to you with a painful, aching neck, which (if any) of the following should always be considered?

    A Stingers
    B Burners
    C Meningitis
    D Influenza

7. While examining a patient's neck, you first notice a swelling and on palpation feel a crackling sensation under the skin. Which of the following should you consider?

    A Goitre
    B Surgical emphysema
    C Lymphoma
    D History of chest trauma

8. With cervical spondylosis, which of the following apply?

    A The progress of X-ray changes accurately mirror the patient's clinical features
    B Headache is a major presenting symptom of the condition
    C A whiplash injury to a cervical spine with spondylosis may cause a 'central cord' lesion
    D A xanthine oxidase inhibitor may be used

9. The sternocleidomastoid muscle has:

    A An insertion at the mastoid process behind the ear
    B An insertion in the occiput
    C An origin in the clavicle
    D An origin in the manubrium of the sternum

10. Which of the following muscles is directly under the skin and subcutaneous tissues at the back of the neck?

    A Levator scapulae
    B Trapezius
    C Platysma
    D Scalenus

Answers are available at the end of the book. For an explanation of these answers and further resources visit the companion website at:

www.wiley.com/go/bradley/musculoskeletal

6

The shoulder

Aim

To develop an in-depth understanding of the anatomy and physiology, history, examination and early management of minor musculoskeletal injuries and conditions of and around the shoulder.

Outcomes

That, by the end of this study, and all the associated activities and clinical experiences, you will be able to:

- demonstrate an in-depth knowledge of the anatomy and physiology of musculoskeletal structures of the shoulder
- take an effective history and examine patients presenting with shoulder problems, forming a differential diagnosis
- demonstrate an in-depth knowledge of minor musculoskeletal injuries and conditions of the shoulder
- apply these skills to the early management of patients, recognising any need for referral.

Section 1
Applied anatomy and physiology

Anatomy

The shoulder has three joints to be considered:

1. The main shoulder joint itself, the **glenohumeral** joint.
2. The small **acromioclavicular** (AC) joint.
3. The **sternoclavicular** joint (SC), which, although a little distance away from the shoulder, is also best included as part of the girdle.

If you wanted to be terribly exact, you could also speak of the gliding joint between the scapula and the back of the rib cage that few think of as a joint at all, but is very important when considering shoulder movements (*see* Figure 6.1).

Managing Minor Musculoskeletal Injuries and Conditions, First Edition. David Bradley.
© 2014 John Wiley & Sons, Ltd. Published 2014 by John Wiley & Sons, Ltd.
Companion website: www.wiley.com/go/bradley/musculoskeletal

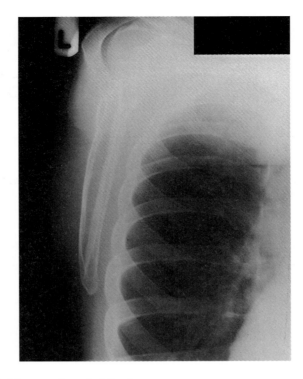

Figure 6.1 The gliding joint of the scapula against the rib cage.

First we will consider the bones and then go on to look at the individual joints in detail.

The skeleton

The bones to be detailed are the following:

- Scapula.
- Upper humerus.
- Clavicle.
- Manubrium of the sternum.

The scapula

Basically this is a triangular slab of bone with a few projections, making it easily recognisable (*see* Figure 6.2).
Both of its surfaces are for the attachment of muscles. The anterior (or costal) surface forms the **subscapular fossa**, a large flat expanse, whereas the posterior surface is divided into two fossae, the **supraspinous** and **infraspinous**, by a large and easily palpated **spine**.

The triangle of bone has three borders: one running parallel to the vertebrae (**vertebral border**), one laterally by the axilla (**axilliary border**) and finally one at the top (**superior border**).

Medially, it has two angles, superior and inferior; once again these are very easy to palpate.

The **spine of the scapula** is a large 'blade' of bone, starting on the upper third of the vertebral border; it steadily thickens to become the **acromion process** laterally, which has a small articular surface for the clavicle. The acromion is the most prominent point of the lateral shoulder.

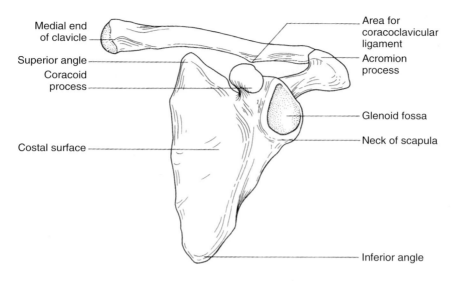

Medial end of clavicle

Superior angle
Coracoid process

Costal surface

Area for coracoclavicular ligament

Acromion process

Glenoid fossa

Neck of scapula

Inferior angle

Figure 6.2 The main parts of the scapula (Ellis and Mahadevan, 2010).

The **glenoid fossa** forms a shallow 'crater' on the lateral aspect of the neck of the scapula. Sitting on its upper rim is a small 'hill' of bone called the '**supraglenoid tubercle**'; this is for the attachment of a rather important muscle tendon (**long head of biceps**).

The **coracoid process** is like a twisted little 'finger' of bone that projects anteriorly for a few centimetres over the glenohumeral joint. It is rather difficult to palpate in all but the thinnest patients.

 Activity 6.1　　　　　　　　　　　　　　　　　　**Time: 10 minutes**

Although it is not essential from the point of view of your role that you memorise them, I've listed here some other parts of the scapula that I feel it is good that you should know:

- Suprascapular notch.
- Angle of the acromion.
- Infra glenoid tubercle.

The upper humerus

This completes the major portion of the main shoulder joint itself (glenohumeral joint) and, once you learn its parts, much of the movement will become clear to you.

Somewhat resembling an Irish shillelagh, it consists of an upper extremity of a rounded head that tilts medially and then articulates with the glenoid. There are two necks. One is '**anatomical**', situated right up close to the rim of the articular surface. The other is '**surgical**' and is where the extremity meets with the proximal shaft, a common place for fractures, especially in elderly people.

Anteriorly there are two small lumps of bone called the '**tuberosities**' (some call them '**tubercles**', but either is correct), into which muscles are inserted. The higher, larger and more lateral is called 'the greater', and the lower and more medial 'the lesser'. Between them is a sulcus called the '**bicipital groove**', because the long head of biceps tendon runs through. This groove is important for you to learn and understand.

The clavicle

This small 'strut' of bone is a little like the spokes of a bicycle wheel: they look flimsy and insignificant, but without them you are lost. So with the clavicle, the strut is a major attachment for a host of muscles and without it our upper limbs would be flail.

It is basically an elongated 'S' shape with articular surfaces at either end, one for the acromion process forming the **acromioclavicular joint**, and the other the sternum, for the **sternoclavicular joint**. It is one of the most superficial of bones; in fact, with a very thin patient you can almost get your fingers around it. This is good from the point of view that it is an easily seen and palpated landmark.

The manubrium of the sternum

On each side of the central **supra-sternal notch** on the upper border of the manubrium is an **articular facet**. These facets form small saddle joints, the **sternoclavicular joints** that are continuous with the first costal cartilages below (*see* Figure 6.3).

The joints are tightly bound by strong ligaments, especially posteriorly, yet still allowing small but important movements of the clavicle.

There is a small piece of **fibro-cartilage** inside the capsule of both joints. They are also very strong, to the extent that it is far more usual for the clavicle to fracture than for either of the joints to dislocate.

The manubrium is very superficial, often making the joint easily visible before you palpate. It is an excellent place to start your shoulder examination, before working laterally along the clavicle to the AC and then the glenohumeral joint.

Don't skimp on your study of these bones; try drawing them in outline, look at X-rays, palpate them on friends, family and then patients until you are sure of their relationships to one another.

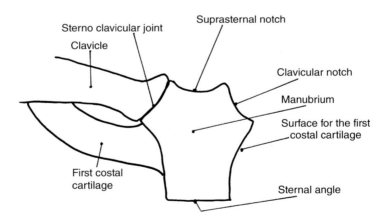

Figure 6.3 The sternoclavicular joint.

Individual joints

The glenohumeral joint

Now let us attach layers of tissue to these bones so that we can understand the joint in more depth.

The glenoid 'holds' the head of the humerus a little better, because it has a lip of cartilage firmly attached to the rim deepening it, rather like the menisci in the knee. This is called the '**glenoid labrum**'. The cartilage usually gives no trouble, but can sometimes be torn following injury.

Activity 6.2 Time: **About 10 minutes**

Instead of just showing you the labrum in an illustration, I know of an animated version that gets the message over very clearly. Go to the site of a Manchester doctor (Professor Funk): you will find this in 'References and suggested reading' at the end of this chapter.

Down the left-hand side of the screen are a series of coloured illustrations of the inside of the glenohumeral joint. The top two stills are duplicated underneath with versions that are animated, clearly showing how the labrum may be pulled away from the glenoid. This condition is called a SLAP lesion. We mention this a little later, but there is no harm in spending a few minutes on it now.

Both of the smooth articular surfaces of the bones are covered with hyaline cartilage.

The joint capsule is formed of an inner layer of synovial membrane and an outer of fibrous ligaments. However, this capsule is not very strong and the shoulder would easily dislocate were it not for the blending and strengthening of the surrounding muscles and their tendons.

Soft tissue structures

The rotator cuff

This is an ideal place to discuss a rather important shoulder structure called the '**rotator cuff**'. You will come across a great deal written about it, but not many useful illustrations. This is because it is not a single, concise object like your nose, but rather a group of muscles and tendons situated around the joint, making it difficult for someone to appreciate at first.

One easy way to visualise this is to look at your wrist; consider that it is your shoulder joint and your hand the upper humerus. Now, pull the cuff of your jacket down over your wrist to the base of your thumb and pull it tight around the hand. That is how the rotator cuff supports and protects the shoulder. Unlike your single fabric cuff, the rotator cuff is made up of four muscles and their associated tendons (*see* Figure 6.4):

1. Supraspinatus.
2. Infraspinatus.
3. Teres minor.
4. Subscapularis.

They all have tendons spreading over and therefore strengthening the joint capsule.

Each muscle runs from different points on the scapula to different points on the humerus, and it is important that you learn about them because they are often injured or diseased.

We will start the detail with the most troublesome, the **supraspinatus**. This has its origin in the **supraspinous fossa** of the posterior surface of the scapula.

 Activity 6.3 Time: **5 minutes**

It is easy to feel where the supraspinatus is on yourself. Put one of your hands over your opposite shoulder. Feel down your back with your fingertips to place them on the hard spine of the scapula. Now just draw your fingertips upwards a little into the soft flesh above the spine. That is the supraspinatus. Of course there is also the more superficial sheet of the trapezius muscle and some fat lying on top, but basically that's it.

Try it on both sides and then, if possible, on friends and relatives of different builds before you palpate patients.

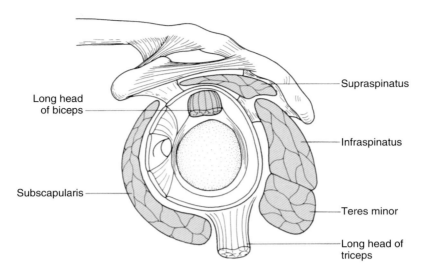

Figure 6.4 Lateral view of the left shoulder showing parts of the rotator cuff (Ellis and Mahadevan, 2010).

The supraspinatus then progresses laterally. However, the route has its difficulties. On the way it has to pass through a narrow space formed by a ligament (like a suspension bridge) spanning the gap between the acromion and the coracoid process. This is called the '**coracoacromial ligament**', getting its name from the bones on either side, as so often in anatomy.

Once under the ligament, the supraspinatus travels over the top of the humeral head and is inserted into the **greater tuberosity** of the humerus. To cushion its movement, a bursa is to be found between the tendon and the acromion above (the **sub-acromial bursa**).

The next muscle to consider is the **infraspinatus**. This has its origin in the rather large **infraspinous fossa** on the posterior of the scapula; its tendon passes laterally to also insert into the **greater tuberosity**, and in doing so strengthens the posterior of the joint capsule.

A far smaller muscle, the **teres minor**, extends from the lower part of the axilliary border of the scapula, passing upwards and posteriorly to the **greater tuberosity**.

The final muscle that is part of the rotator cuff is the **subscapularis**. This is 'sandwiched' between the posterior of the ribs and the anterior of the scapula. Its tendon passes the front of the shoulder joint and this time inserts into the **lesser tuberosity** of the humerus. This is important to know because in an anterior dislocation this muscle holds the head in adduction (*see* Figure 6.5).

Bursae

Other major soft tissue structures at the shoulder are the **bursae**. These are sacks of synovial membrane filled with a little synovial fluid, and their task is to ease friction between nearby structures. The **sub-acromial bursa** (*see* Figure 6.6) is the most problematic; as the name suggests, it is tucked under the large acromion process of the scapula and extends beyond its margins. As the supraspinatus moves, it 'gives' a little rather than rubbing directly against the bone.

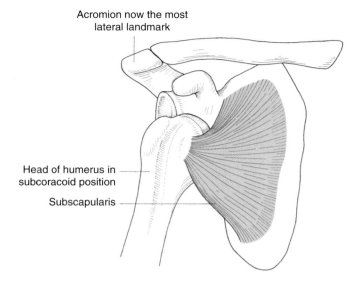

Acromion now the most
lateral landmark

Head of humerus in
subcoracoid position

Subscapularis

Figure 6.5 Subscapularis holding the dislocated head in adduction (Ellis and Mahadevan, 2010).

Activity 6.4   Time: 15 minutes

The shoulder has about eight bursae; they vary in size and may interconnect with each other or sometimes the joint capsule. For practical purposes, it is not clinically necessary for you to know about them all in detail. However, it would be advantageous to give some brief consideration to some, especially the:

- subscapular
- subcoracoid
- subdeltoid.

Use a search engine of choice to view illustrations; note how the bursae practically surround the joint and their proximity to possible areas of friction with muscular activity.

The biceps

It is important to understand the origins and track of the **long and short heads** of the biceps.

The 'short' is the larger and stronger of the two. Its origin is from the coracoid process of the scapula, where it then travels laterally over the anterior of the humeral head. The 'long' has an origin at the upper border of the glenoid rim (supraglenoid tubercle), where it forms a pencil-thin band passing over the top of the head of the humerus, through the joint capsule, and then through the **bicipital groove** between the greater and lesser tuberosities of the humerus. At the most distal part of this groove, the tendon is held in place by a ligament and then travels down to the muscle body (*see* Figure 6.6; another view is shown in Figure 6.7).

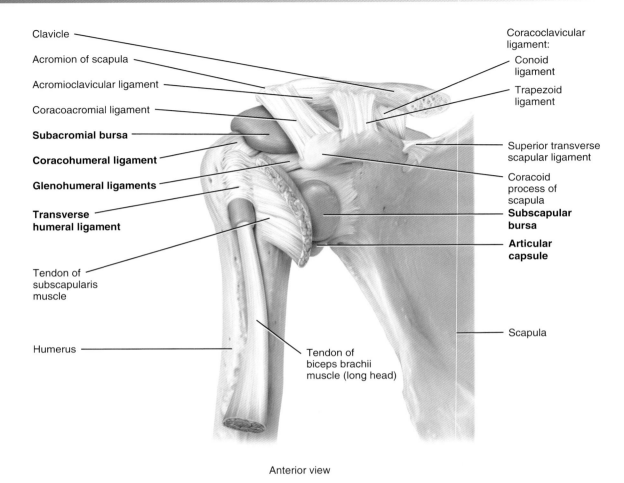

Clavicle

Acromion of scapula

Acromioclavicular ligament

Coracoacromial ligament

Subacromial bursa

Coracohumeral ligament

Glenohumeral ligaments

Transverse humeral ligament

Tendon of subscapularis muscle

Humerus

Coracoclavicular ligament:

Conoid ligament

Trapezoid ligament

Superior transverse scapular ligament

Coracoid process of scapula

Subscapular bursa

Articular capsule

Scapula

Tendon of biceps brachii muscle (long head)

Anterior view

Figure 6.6 Anterior view of right shoulder, showing bursae, AC joint and ligaments (Tortora and Nielsen (2012). This material is reproduced with permission of John Wiley & Sons, Inc.

The deltoid

This large, triangular-shaped muscle hangs like a bulky curtain over many of the deeper shoulder structures, presenting us with a smooth outer curve that is important to notice.

The muscle origin attaches to a 'curtain rail' that comprises the **spine of the scapula** posteriorly, the **acromion** laterally and the **clavicle** anteriorly (*see* (Figure 6.8).

The acromioclavicular joint

This small, mostly gliding joint is situated immediately above the glenohumeral joint and is formed by the junction of the outer end of the clavicle with the acromion process. It has a compact synovial capsule and is held very firmly by three groups of ligaments (*see* Figure 6.6):

1. Those forming part of the AC joint capsule, the **acromioclavicular ligaments**.
2. Others running between the clavicle and the coracoid process of the scapula, the **coracoclavicular ligaments**.
3. These coracoclavicular ligaments may be subdivided by some into the **conoid ligament** (laterally) and the **trapezoid ligament** (medially). All of them may become damaged.

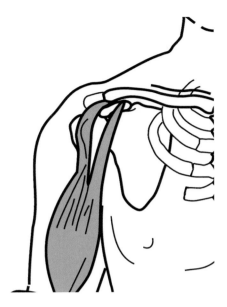

Figure 6.7 Two heads of biceps (Gross *et al.*, 2009).

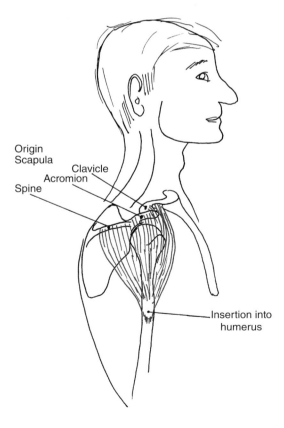

Origin
Scapula

Clavicle
Acromion

Spine

Insertion into
humerus

Figure 6.8 The right deltoid.

Section 2
History and mechanism of injury

As with all patients who attend with a minor injury or condition to their shoulder, you must not start with a set mind as to the possibilities. First, let them introduce the problem to you at their own pace and direction, so that important pointers are not missed.

 Activity 6.5   **Time: A few minutes only**

Cover up my observations on this activity before you read on.
   Can you think of two examples of instances when a more serious problem could become confused with a minor injury or condition of the shoulder?
   Write in rough note format in your notebook. Then read on.

Observations on Activity 6.5

Two examples that spring to my mind are:

1. A condition
   A gall bladder problem may give referred pain to the shoulder. This could be missed initially, because of a 'blinkered' attitude to questioning just the most obvious feature.
2. An injury
   A young patient from an RTC on a motorbike walks in with an obvious fracture of the clavicle. There is so much pain and discomfort from the fracture that questioning regarding the remainder of the body is minimal; it is an easy way to miss an abdominal bleed in its early stages.

These may have been obvious points to the more experienced of you. If so, use such instances occasionally in your teaching because those who are new to minor injuries need to learn from an early stage to sometimes expect the unexpected, and because of that always to be thorough.

Specific mechanisms of injury and backgrounds to shoulder conditions

Painful fracture

The pain of a fractured clavicle is notorious for its intensity. It is often a complete fracture with wide separation of the fragments and there is no method of effective immobilisation.
   Because of this, the discomfort of injuries elsewhere may not be noticed until later when the patient arrives home.

Increased use

Especially with elderly people, an increase in use of the shoulder – for instance, painting a ceiling the previous day – may be a significant contributory factor to damage. An example could be a degenerated rotator cuff.

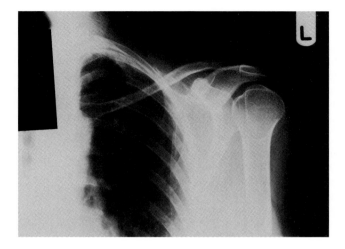

Figure 6.9 X-ray of a posterior dislocation of the shoulder.

Pre-existing problems

Finding the norm for an individual patient is essential for you to make an accurate assessment. For example, a woman in her sixties presents with a shoulder pain. If she has had ongoing symptoms in her neck from previously diagnosed cervical spondylosis, it is reasonable to question about this in detail, just in case this new pain is part of the same problem. It is common for neck problems to present in the shoulder.

The inarticulate

Superficially, you would think it difficult to miss a dislocated shoulder, especially if an X-ray has been taken. But this may happen if you do not **listen with care** to your patient. I can remember two instances when, because both patients were in their eighties and not too articulate, features were minimised and the diagnoses almost missed.

Both patients had a very heavy build, so the clinical deformity could not be appreciated. Added to that, X-rays of a posterior dislocation are notoriously difficult for the inexperienced to interpret (*see* Figure 6.9) Some think of X-rays as the 'be all and end all' of making a diagnosis. If the X-ray seems ok, there is nothing serious wrong with the patient. Whereas what I want you to think is, 'There is nothing obvious on X-ray, but they are still in a lot of pain, little movement, etc., so I must look further for a diagnosis.'

The atypical presentation

Finally, the atypical onset of a given condition is a major fear. Walk into any A&E, pale, clutching your chest with a crushing pain and everything will be done to immediately eliminate an MI and save your life. However, walk into an MIU with a vague ache in your shoulder and you would be lucky to get a sniff of an ECG within an hour. Consider another golden rule:

GOLDEN RULE

The first major step in the elimination of any major injury or condition is to get to know the whole picture surrounding your patient and the circumstances of why they have attended the unit or clinic.

Mechanisms of injury

First a word of warning! Some of the conditions mentioned here will be thought of by many as 'far from minor', so why do I even mention them in this specialist text? Remember, 'minor' is a very vague term, with patients managed in different ways throughout the country. As an advanced practitioner, you may have patients presented to you who have not been effectively triaged and you must learn the full range of conditions at every level of complexity and seriousness.

Let's now review the way that shoulder injuries are caused and the lead-up to some conditions. When taking a history, there are a few fairly standard injury mechanisms for consideration that cause the vast majority of the problems seen. These are as follows:

- Direct fall onto the shoulder (*see* Figure 6.10a).
- Fall on an outstretched hand (FOOSH) (*see* Figure 6.10b).
- Overhead, swinging, throwing or circling movement (*see* Figure 6.10c).
- Repetitive shoulder movements.
- Electric shocks.
- Fits, or severe jerks to the arm; heavy lifts.

I suppose you can remember all six of the mechanisms listed!!! With these, whether an injury occurs, and the form and severity of that injury, depends on several factors.

 Activity 6.6   **Time: 15 minutes**

Can you list what some of these factors might be? Try to think of six and write them in your notebook. When complete, check your answer with my observations.

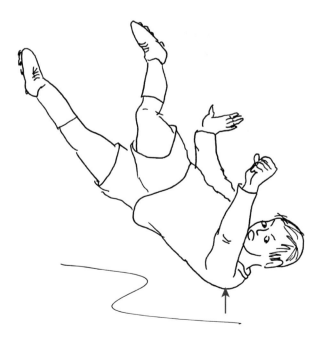

Figure 6.10a A direct fall onto the shoulder as a mechanism of shoulder injury.

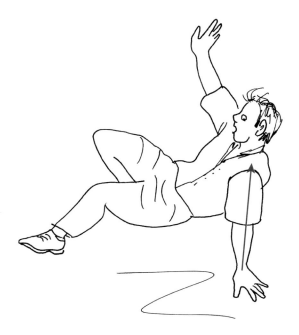

Figure 6.10b A FOOSH as a mechanism of shoulder injury.

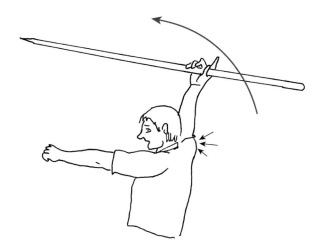

Figure 6.10c A throwing movement as a mechanism of shoulder injury.

Observations on Activity 6.6

My answer would be as follows:

- Age.
- Weight.
- Force of impact.

- Strength of bones and joint soft tissues.
- Angle of impact.
- Surface fallen onto.
- Pre-existing conditions.
- Protective clothing or sports gear worn.

That is quite a list of variables, isn't it? What you have to consider is that, with a given history, it would be logical to consider a particular set of injuries before commencing examination.

   If there is no history of an injury, it would be wise to ask about the following associations:

- Previous cervical disease.
- Inflammatory disease.
- Occupational hazards.
- Features of a tumour.
- Hepatic or diaphragmatic problem.
- Fibromyalgia.

The following listing gives you common injury and condition interconnections.

Fracture of the clavicle

This is the most common shoulder fracture and nearly always the result of a direct fall onto the shoulder.

   A FOOSH comes next, but is only an occasional cause. A FOOSH is commonly thought of just as the MOI for wrist injuries, but it is also possible for the force to carry straight up the arm and fracture the clavicle.

 Activity 6.7   **Time: 15 minutes**

What! Are you sure? Who said so? I thought a FOOSH was the most common cause of a clavicle fracture.

   Studying from textbooks such as this, you tend to trust the printed word. This activity is just a gentle reminder that one of the major things I want to encourage in you is to question everything you see – and that includes what I write!

   There will be many places throughout this book where you will be faced with facts like those just listed. I have purposely not referenced many, because this is a trend that you will see increasingly in standard texts presenting well-known and accepted information. However, even in the most prestigious publications, if you read carefully, you will find mistakes.

   Try finding a reference to confirm the main cause of a fractured clavicle. Then read the observations for this activity.

Observations on Activity 6.7

Just one reference to a piece of actual research to prove it could be Stanley, Trowbridge and Norris (1988); you will find the details at the end of this chapter. But short statements in books and journals from many prestigious practitioners can be found in minutes.

Shoulder dislocation

Following a clavicle fracture, a dislocated shoulder is the next most common serious shoulder injury. Most dislocations that you see will be anterior. Just a few will be posterior and you may perhaps see one inferior. Shoulder dislocations are uncommon in children, usual in young adults and become common again in elderly people.

   An acute injury, commonly indirect by a FOOSH, or direct by a fall onto the shoulder, are the usual causes. With the anterior dislocation, the arm will be in abduction, extension and external rotation at the time of the injury.

To get the uncommon posterior dislocation, the arm will be in internal rotation and adduction. The FOOSH, direct force, electric shock, fit or sudden severe jerk may all do this.

With the inferior dislocation, axial loading and hyper-abduction is the key position for the injury to occur.

 Activity 6.8   **Time: Ongoing in clinical practice**

It is rare in practice that a patient will be able to provide you with the detailed history of the position that their arm was in at the time of the fall, or exactly how they fell. More often than not, you have to be content with 'I slipped and fell over; it all happened so quickly I cannot remember how I landed.' Use your judgement; sometimes too detailed a questioning may upset patients.

From now on, try to fit together in your mind the jigsaw of the most likely positioning of the arm as they fell.

Can you remember what it was for the very common anterior dislocation? There were three aspects; write them down, then check with the observations.

Observations on Activity 6.8

Well, I hope that you remembered:

- abduction
- extension
- external rotation.

If you didn't get them all, it probably means that you have been just automatically reading the page without taking in all the information. The reason for that is almost always that you need a break from study. This may only be a few minutes for a drink, or possibly to do a job about the home. Frequent breaks help you to absorb information into your brain.

Other aids could be to highlight important points as you progress, underline what is new to you, or make lists:

- Abduction.
- Extension.
- External rotation.

Try not to do this when anyone is looking at you, but putting your arm into the position may also help it to remain in your memory! Anything, but don't just read.

Finally, it would be wise to mention that, if the shoulder has been dislocated previously, it can become very easy for it to re-dislocate. A simple movement of the joint, doing an everyday task like waving or catching a ball with almost no force at all, could be all that it takes.

Acromioclavicular dislocation

This injury does not occur as often as a dislocated shoulder, but is still commonly seen. The joint is usually damaged by the patient falling directly onto the point of the shoulder while their arm is adducted, commonly during sport, but a FOOSH can also be a mechanism. The injury does not occur very often in children.

Sternoclavicular dislocation

Compared with the AC joint, the sternoclavicular is not often dislocated, but may be by either indirect or direct forces acting on the joint.

It usually dislocates anteriorly, this caused by an indirect frontal force pushing the shoulder and outer clavicle backwards and moving the medial clavicle anteriorly. Examples could be a blow to the shoulder, a fall onto the shoulder or a FOOSH.

On some occasions – for instance, contact sports or RTCs – a considerable direct anterior force can cause the joint to dislocate posteriorly.

Fracture of the proximal humerus

The many categorised forms of fracture of the proximal humerus are usually caused by direct force from a fall on the side; they are often impacted with minimal displacement. An alternative mechanism is a FOOSH with the body moving on a fixed arm.

Fracture of the humeral shaft

Direct forces – for instance falls onto the side, blows with weapons and crushing – are very common and easily understood. Indirect forces from a FOOSH are also common.

Adhesive capsulitis (frozen shoulder)

The precise cause of this condition is unknown, but the following features may help you to consider it when taking a history:

- Common in women of advancing age.
- Often seen in diabetic patients, those with thyroid dysfunction and autoimmune illnesses, following an MI or cerebrovascular accident (CVA).
- Existing problems in the shoulder, such as a torn rotator cuff, bursitis or tendinitis.
- Develops after a period of inactivity.

Rupture of the long head of biceps; biceps tendinitis

Both these are separate conditions in their own right, but the background to their presentation to you is very similar and they can be associated with one another.

Your patient will more frequently be older, especially if the rupture follows slow degeneration, tendinosis or tendinitis. Other shoulder problems may increase the strain on the biceps and could be a predisposing factor in rupture.

Small repetitive movements (especially overhead) may be a factor – for example, painting a ceiling. With younger patients it's seen with forceful acute movements in sports. Degenerative calcification in the tendon may be a feature with tendinitis.

Rotator cuff problems; impingement syndrome; bursitis

Separate conditions to be discussed in later sections, but they may occur together and are often related.

They are seen mostly in late middle age, often because of repetitive movements such as painting, polishing, cleaning windows, etc., but they may also be seen in sporting youngsters with a heavy lift, swimming, bowling, etc.

A common confusion

The final listing in this section may be thought of as both injuries and conditions. I do not want to play around with words here, but:

- accumulative minor injury
- repetitive injury
- overuse injury and
- degeneration of tissues further damaged by ordinary use

must all be in your thoughts as you consider them in your mental list for possible diagnosis. For patients, however, all will be clear-cut. If you simply ask if they have injured their shoulder, they will picture in their mind something like a fall and, if that didn't occur, will say 'No', whereas injury to you can have several of the possibilities mentioned earlier. It is so easy to be misunderstood.

Section 3
Patient examination

Always remember that I subdivide the body into artificial regions to explain to you how to approach patient management. This has a danger, because you must approach your patient holistically. Pains in the shoulder may be referred, for instance, from the neck or diaphragm. So, although this chapter concentrates on the shoulder, be prepared to extend your examination depending on your history and initial examination. This is one of the differences between a qualified and an exceptional professional.

Circulation

The circulation distal to the site of the problem must be routinely checked and an excellent time to do this is by feeling the pulse and skin temperature while holding the initial history conversation with them. Do whatever is best for your individual system, so long as it is part of a routine.

Sensations

The sensations around the shoulder and the affected arm should always be examined. A good general screening for the radial, ulna and median nerves is described in Chapter 8. Also worthy of a mention is damage to the **axillary nerve** following an anterior dislocation of the shoulder. At the time of the dislocation, it can be stretched and irritated, causing paraesthesiae or numbness to the '**military badge area**' (*see* Figure 6.11) over the outer shoulder. Make it part of your routine to test this and you will never be caught out.

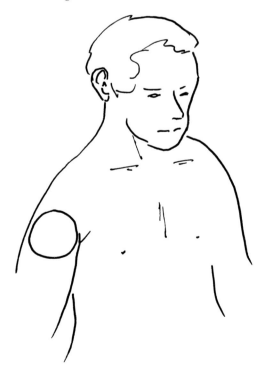

Figure 6.11 The military badge area of neuro deficiency.

Observation

While listening to your patient's answers to your enquiries, you can be getting a good overall view of **both** shoulders for comparison. Don't fall into the trap of looking at just one side. For all shoulder problems, you are looking for the following points with right and left being equal:

Anterior

- Deltoid outline.
- Trapezius outline.
- Arm positioning.
- Biceps outline (Popeye).
- AC joint.
- Line of clavicle.
- SC joint.
- Pectorals shape.
- Head and neck positioning.
- Sternocleidomastoid outline.
- Larynx.

Posterior

- Trapezius flow.
- Scapula outline (winging).
- Spine of scapula.
- Head/neck positioning.

Lateral

- The pattern of haematoma only showing below the deltoid.

 Activity 6.9   **Time: A quick question**

What would be the reason for 'The pattern of haematoma only showing below the deltoid'? Read my observations on this activity.

Observations on Activity 6.9

With a fracture of the proximal humerus, blood escapes and tracks downwards underneath the deltoid. It only shows on the surface at the lower level of the deltoid's insertion (*see* Figure 6.12).

As well as these points, the full list of items for general observation of the skin in Chapter 3 should be noted. In fact, now would be an ideal time for revision to see how many of them you could list from memory.

With a lot of practice, all these points could be covered quickly with the patient hardly realising what you have done.

 Activity 6.10   **Time: 5 minutes**

Why may it sometimes be a **disadvantage** to be very quick with your observations? Make a brief note here and then read my answer in the observations paragraph.

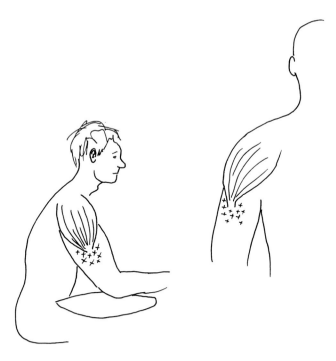

Figure 6.12 Bleeding from a fractured upper end of humerus, only showing below the deltoid.

Observations on Activity 6.10

There are several reasons, but it is important that the patient realises you are **taking an interest** in them **and listening** to what they say. You may have noticed within seconds a subtle swelling over the shoulder with 'blurring' of the underlying bony features. But, if no mention is made of this, you miss an opportunity. It's better to demonstrate that you are comparing and have noticed something that fits with what they are saying.

Palpation

Where to start? Well, nothing says you have to start anywhere in particular, but why not try the sternoclavicular joint? It's rarely injured or the source of a problem, so is unlikely to make the patient apprehensive. It is very superficial and when palpation is complete you can then 'work your way' towards the shoulder along the clavicle.

Be sure to inform the patient before you start that you have listened to what they have said and that you will 'home in' to their painful area shortly.

 Activity 6.11   Time: **A few minutes**

Palpation of the sternoclavicular joint is an easy starting point for you; perform it in isolation for a few seconds only on your practice person, or do it as part of a complete shoulder examination. Your own joint in front of a mirror is also a fine starting point for practice because it is so superficial.

As a guide, place your index fingertip in the central notch at the top of the manubrium, the suprasternal notch (*see* Figure 6.3). While there, with the other hand, trace the superficial medial clavicle to its SC joint.

Quite firm pressure should be managed with ease by the patient without any discomfort and, if the arm is moved about, small movements should be felt at the medial clavicle at the SC joint.

Once you have done this and the many other parts of the examination, mark them off on your record of progress (Checklist 6.1).

 Activity 6.12   **Time: 10 minutes**

Palpation of the clavicle and AC joint

From the SC joint, now let your fingers follow the clavicle out throughout its whole length to meet the acromion at the AC joint and feel the margin of the AC joint itself (*see* Figure 6.13). Do this on both sides and you will soon be able to go directly to the AC joint.

Once again, this is a sturdy joint and under normal circumstances the patient should have no discomfort, even if you palpate quite firmly.

To follow a clinical activity like this one from a book is not the easiest of tasks. You must choose your initial practice friends or colleagues with great care (the thinner the better) so that the bony prominences stand out clearly and can be palpated with ease. If you are unable to be sure of the AC joint at this stage, don't be disheartened; try another time with a thinner model or, if none is available, abandon these activities for a while, wait for your mentor and read to the end of the chapter.

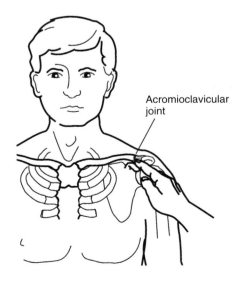

Figure 6.13 Palpation of the AC joint (Gross *et al.*, 2009).

Checklist 6.1 Record of progress

Physical examination of the shoulder

Examination	On self	Friend practice	Friend practice	Patient practice
Patient history, a variety				
Observation				
Palpation:				
SC joint				
Clavicle				
AC joint				
Acromion				
Head of Humerus				
Bicipital groove				
Coracoid proc.				
Trapezius				
Deltoid				
Supraspinatus				
Range of movement:				
Flexion				
Extension				
Abduction and adduction				
Internal and external rotation				
Scapula				
Circumduction				
Sensations:				
Upper arm				
Hand				
Fingers				
Circulation:				
To arm intact				
Specific tests:				
Painful arc				
Shape of biceps				
Other:				
Need for neck examination				
Axillary nodes				

© 2014 John Wiley & Sons, Ltd.

Activity 6.13   Time: **10 minutes**

Palpation of acromion and spine of scapula

To become familiar with 'palpating your way around', you may have to move the subject's arm while palpating, thereby feeling the movement of the humerus when your fingers are resting on it. If you are very new to this, why not make initial attempts on yourself, while looking in the mirror and having the anatomy drawings close by.

Start with your fingers on the AC joint. Now move them laterally over the rough acromion, following it posteriorly as it becomes the spine of the scapula. When over the spine, let your fingers slip off it upwards into the **supraspinous fossa**, home of the **supraspinatus**. Next, go onto the spine again and off it, downwards into the **infraspinous fossa** and the **infraspinatus**. The bodies of both these muscles can be felt underneath the overlying 'blanket' of the **trapezius**.

 Activity 6.14   Time: **10 minutes**

Palpation of the glenohumeral joint

Travel laterally along the spine of the scapula and notice how it widens and becomes the acromion. Sit a couple of your fingers firmly on the most lateral part of the acromion process. Once again, if you are unsure, just move the humerus and, if your fingers stay still, you are positioned correctly over the acromion.

Now move one of your fingers laterally until it 'falls off the end', so to speak. This is the step down onto the head of the humerus. Easy in a thin person, difficult or impossible to feel through lots of fat, so beware! Once your fingers are on the head of the humerus, feel the **greater** and **lesser tuberosities** with the hollow of the **bicipital groove** in between; this contains the **long head of biceps** tendon but don't expect to be able to feel it.

This completes a brief account of how to palpate most of the major landmarks of the shoulder joint. Your aim should be to get as much practice as possible at finding these structures on those without injuries and all body builds.

When you feel confident and have had positive support from your mentor, increase your experience, becoming familiar with all the palpations just mentioned during a full range of shoulder movement.

Examining the range of shoulder movements

So far you have gained a great deal of information on your patient by:

- taking a thorough history
- looking at the shoulder
- palpating the area,

although often this continues with the movements now to be discussed.

From the knowledge you already have, you must reach a broad conclusion and decide if there is something there like a fracture or dislocation that does not merit further disturbance, or whether to proceed to test the range of movements.

The shoulder joint epitomises the need for different forms of joint testing (*see* Figure 6.14):

- Active movements.
- Passive movements.
- Resistive movements.

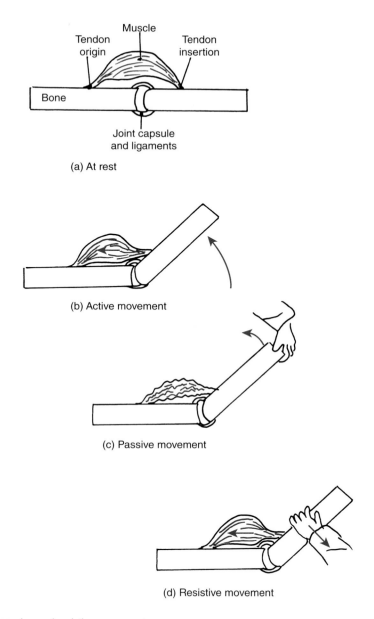

Figure 6.14 Active, passive and resistive movements.

There are additional advanced forms of movement testing, not to be discussed here, but the main three will now be individually discussed.

Testing active movements

This is where the patient does all the movement for you with their own muscles. It is the starting point in your assessment and the most common form seen, especially to 'clear' joints (see Figure 6.14b).

An addition is when the examiner sees the patient cannot perform a movement fully and encourages and assists gently with a hand to see if further movement can be obtained (**assisted active movement**).

If your patient demonstrates a full painless range of shoulder movement, you usually need to test no further. If they have pain on active movement, it does not completely answer our questions. Certainly we can say, 'Yes, there is a shoulder problem,' but it still leaves the question, 'Exactly where is the pain originating from?'

 Activity 6.15   **Time: 10 minutes**

Cover up the observations on this activity, then read on.
   Your patient actively moves their shoulder and it hurts. What are the possible structures from where the pain may be originating? Try listing at least six in your notebook and group some of them together.

Observations on Activity 6.15

My list of eight with grouping is as follows:

- Bone and cartilage.
- Joint capsule and ligaments.
- Muscles, tendons and their points of attachment to bones.
- Bursae and other surrounding soft tissues.

All the above structures should not be thought of as completely isolated and separate from one another. Consider that earlier in this chapter you discovered that the tendons of the rotator cuff are to an extent blended with the capsule of the shoulder joint to strengthen it. But testing of the joint by a different type of movement can often **cut down the possibilities** of which group of structures is the source of the pain.

Testing passive movements

This is when the patient, it is hoped, completely relaxes and you do the movement for them (although this is often impossible). If they are effectively relaxed and confident in your putting the joint through the range of movement and they feel no, or considerably less, pain, it tends to point towards the cause being from somewhere in the muscles, tendons or their attachment to the bones. The muscles will have been relaxed and 'floppy', not actively contracting and pulling on the tendons (*see* Figure 6.14c).

If, however, the pain is still severe, it tends to point more strongly to the source of the pain being in the bones, cartilage, capsule or ligaments.

Resistive testing

In this test, which may be used with the standard shoulder movements, you hold the joint still and supported with your hand and body, so that it doesn't move. At the same time you ask the patient to actively try to move the arm in a particular direction, while preventing them from doing so with your other hand. It sounds a little like all-in wrestling, doesn't it?! (*see* Figure 6.14d)

This muscle contraction, without associated joint movement, is called '**isometrics**'; you will have heard of it previously as a form of exercise.

So, if the joint is effectively held immobile and the muscles and tendons alone are trying hard to move, then pain produced by these manoeuvres point strongly to the muscles, tendons or their attachments to the bone being the cause of the pain, or structures lying next to them like a bursa.

Activity 6.16   Time: **About an hour**

Reading isn't the easiest way to learn so let's have a complete change and go to YouTube on your computer. Remember that varying what you do aids learning.

Type in 'shoulder examination' and try some of the short (3–5 minute) videos available. It is usually best to sample a couple of those from the UK first.

Notice that, although basically the same, there are slight differences in style and content; no one way is correct. Because these are teaching videos, they tend to mention many tests that would only be of use in the more specialist hospital environment. Just because they mention a particular test, it doesn't mean that you have to use it.

Videos made by a university tend to be more reliable than others, so don't take everything you see as 'gospel'.

Each of the basic active shoulder movements:

- abduction and adduction
- flexion and extension
- internal and external rotation

should be examined in turn as a routine. It is easier by far for the patient to simultaneously complete movements of both the left and right sides at the same time. This certainly aids comparison with the opposite side, especially when the differences are subtle.

However, this is not always the ideal for the patient. Consider a young man presenting with a minor pain, able to balance and move his shoulder for you with ease. Contrast that with a frail, elderly patient in quite a degree of pain who may be far more comfortable moving one side at a time to aid balance. There is no one correct way to examine: you must be the judge with your individual patient.

Additional tests

There are additional movements, usually performed by specialist professionals such as sports physiotherapists. You may find them in more specialist books.

Don't delve too deeply at this stage. It is not in the patient's best interest for you to perform these unless you can accurately interpret them.

Examining the range of active shoulder movements

Some of the basic movements are shown in Figure 6.15.

Abduction and adduction

 Activity 6.17   Time: **15 minutes**

Stand in front of your practice subject. Ask them to stand with their arms at their sides and simply raise both arms sideways above their heads as high as possible (abduction) Any deficiency on the affected side will show up clearly.

They should then bring the abducted arm back down to the body and further across to the midline (adduction), as when touching our opposite shoulder with our hand.

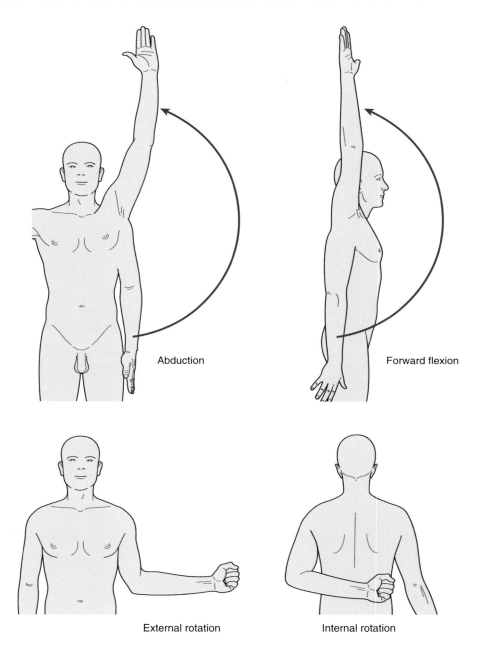

Figure 6.15 The basic range of shoulder movements (Duckworth and Blundell, 2010).

Consider that the patient may be nervous of making a particular movement because of pain, so they may have to be encouraged to see how far they can go, with you supporting some of the weight of the arm. The balance between causing them undue and unnecessary pain and finding what they are capable of is rather delicate. It is something that you need the advice of an experienced mentor to realise, because your patient's confidence in you may so easily be lost.

Sometimes pain is felt during just one particular part of the arc of abduction. This is called '**painful arc syndrome**' and can have several interpretations (discussed later). It is an important sign to elicit and you may have to gently assist the patient to abduct the arm, explaining and encouraging with progression.

Flexion and extension

 Activity 6.18   Time: **15 minutes**

For shoulder flexion, simply face your subject with their arms at their side and ask them to raise both arms towards you as high as they can.

Extension of the shoulder is more difficult to describe to people so guide their arm posteriorly or demonstrate the movement for them to copy.

Internal and external rotation

 Activity 6.19   Time: **15 minutes**

Standing in front of your subject again, ask them to place their hands behind their heads. This abducts and externally rotates the arms.

Next ask them to place both hands behind the small of their back. This will partially abduct and internally rotate the arms.

Both movements have the added beauty of needing very simple instructions.

Scapula movements

 Activity 6.20   Time: **15 minutes**

Stand behind your practice subject, remembering that this exercise will be far easier if they are on the thin side so that the outline of both scapulae can be clearly seen. How much of a part do you think the scapula plays in abduction of the arm in health? Insignificant, just a little, a great deal?

If you wish, you can just look at the scapula outline for movement, but you may find it easier to place your hand over it to feel the movement as well.

Ask your subject to actively, slowly abduct. Observe for any scapula movement.

Write a brief note in your book of what you noticed, before you read further.

Observations on Activity 6.20

Well, what should have happened is that initially the scapula remained still. The **initial abduction is at the gleno-humeral joint**. Then, when the arm was raised to about 30 degrees, the scapula would have started to rotate on the back of the chest wall, allowing the arm to abduct further. Eventually with full abduction it would have rotated about 45 degrees.

A significant point about this is that, if there is a joint problem limiting movement, that **scapula rotation can 'hide' the lack of joint movement**, so always look for this.

 Activity 6.21   **Time: A quick question**

Can you name three other shoulder movements made by the scapula? List them, then read my observations.

Observations on Activity 6.21

I can think of four:

1. Shrug, when you raise both shoulders.
2. Depression, when the shoulders hang down.
3. Arching forwards, like when wrapping your arms around your chest when cold.
4. Swinging backwards, like when you are breathing in deeply and 'throwing' your chest out.

All the above easily combine as we go about our usual tasks.

The part played by the scapulae gliding across the posterior of the chest in association with movement of the gleno-humeral joints is rather fascinating – accounting for a major part of what we think of as 'pure' shoulder joint movement.

Be sure to complete the record form (Checklist 6.1) and keep it up to date to follow your progress accurately.

Section 4
Minor musculoskeletal injuries

Shoulder dislocation

The shoulder can dislocate in three ways:

1. Anterior (almost all).
2. Posterior (a few).
3. Inferior, also called '**luxatio erecta**', I have only seen one in my lifetime.

Dislocations may occasionally spontaneously relocate, especially when the shoulder has dislocated many times in the past.

Clinical features and diagnosis

The patient always realises from the start that something is seriously wrong and may come to you saying that their shoulder 'feels out of place'.

The fact that a shoulder has dislocated once makes it far more likely to dislocate again because of previous damage to the capsule making it 'loose'. The more frequently it has dislocated, the easier it dislocates again, ending up with some joints dislocating with very minor movements like waving.

With this information you would wonder how a dislocation could be missed. There are several dangerous circumstances when you have to be careful:

• A patient whose level of consciousness is down – for instance, with a head injury, drugs or alcohol.
• A confused patient.
• An obese patient.

The features to look for with the very common **anterior dislocation** are the following:

- Patient holding their arm.
- Sharp angle deltoid.
- Anterior fullness.
- Line of the shaft of humerus displaced medially.

These are shown in Figure 6.16.

The X-ray is usually clear (*see* Figure 6.17) and easy to read; no 'Brownie points' for noticing this! Once again, the book's website has more detail for you about both of these figures.

With **posterior dislocation**, the major point is the X-ray appearance. It is one of the classical problem areas and **very easy to miss for the untrained eye** (*see* Figure 6.9). Once again the book's website has further examples for you.

The outstanding feature to look for with the **inferior dislocation** is that they present to you with their arm in the air and the hand often resting on the top of the head.

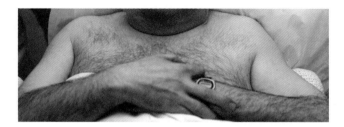

Figure 6.16 Anterior dislocation of the shoulder.

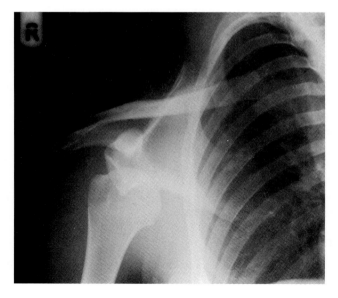

Figure 6.17 X-ray of an anterior dislocation of the shoulder.

Initial management

First-time dislocated shoulders are not something that easily 'pop' back into place as Hollywood would have you believe. An experienced operator plus adequate anaesthesia or analgesia and muscle relaxation is required if the patient is not to suffer.

They should be made comfortable and nil by mouth, until everything is ready for the reduction.

Positioning of the body and arm may be as helpful in reducing pain as the analgesia. Your patient, plus trial and error, is your best guide, with sometimes unusual positions, such as lying face down with the affected arm hanging free over the side of the trolley, being useful. Support with pillows while sitting also often wins over a sling.

Before reduction, remember to ensure that the military badge area has been tested for abnormal sensations.

 Activity 6.22   **Time: About an hour**

Reduction of a dislocated shoulder

Assisting with a reduction is preferable within a few weeks, once you have consolidated your anatomical and examination knowledge.

First, 'put yourself forward' and let others know that you want to first observe and then assist with reductions. Study the following methods of reduction:

- Kocher's technique.
- Hippocratic technique
- Gravity technique.

Use one or look at several standard orthopaedic or trauma texts. I can recommend McRae (2010) – details are in the 'References and suggested reading' at the end of this chapter.

Following reduction, a sling will hold the arm for a minimum of three weeks (Dollery, 2001).

A warning: the fact that you have studied and assisted with these reduction techniques doesn't mean that you may automatically use them. That decision is a local one, made by your employing Trust and will vary tremendously throughout the country.

Fractures of the proximal humerus

Many fracture designs are possible, with or without an associated dislocation. Figure 6.18 is an X-ray showing a design of fracture commonly seen.

In children, a greenstick of the surgical neck is the most common fracture in this region. A little less common is a fracture through the proximal humeral epiphysis with slight displacement.

Clinical features and diagnosis

Following a likely MOI, an individual's response varies, and it is impossible to form a firm diagnosis that a fracture exists unless an X-ray is taken. Impacted fractures in adults and greenstick fractures in children, where an arm can still be moved, have caught out many a professional over the years.

Initial management

Explanation, reassurance, an arm sling under clothes to avoid movement, and analgesia will be the standard form of initial comfort for the patient.

These injuries are not all supported well in a sling, so pillows on a trolley may be required while they await possible X-rays and/or reduction.

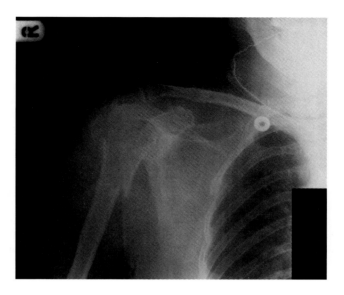

Figure 6.18 X-ray of a common form of fracture of the upper humerus.

 Activity 6.23   **Time: Just a few minutes' thought**

A quick point here, of pure nursing care, as you prepare your patient for home. As well as what I have already mentioned, what else would you consider doing?

Observations on Activity 6.23

They will thank you so much if you take the trouble to wash their armpit and apply powder and a pad to keep the skin surfaces apart. That should give them 24 hours of 'BO'-free time at home, when they do not have to disturb a painful shoulder.

Patient advice

In many instances, further advice about toileting would also be welcome; many patients are afraid to disturb anything you have applied.

 Activity 6.24   **Time: An hour**

If not available already within your Trust, why not try to write an information leaflet for patients with any form of shoulder immobilisation?

 Activity 6.25   **Time: A few minutes**

Mention would be worthwhile here of the broad arm and collar and cuff slings. Think for a moment, **why choose one rather than the other?** Write your answer first; then read on.

Although both slings hold the arm to the chest, the two work in different ways.

The broad arm sling

This is excellent for a wrist or hand that needs to be 'cradled', supported or elevated. Some of the weight of the forearm and hand is being taken around the neck. Some elbow injuries may get some comfort from it, but it would tend to press on the injured part. For problems around the shoulder, the sling would 'push' in an upwards direction through the shaft of the humerus (*see* Figure 6.19a). That would be good to keep certain surgical neck fractures in position if already firmly in place, or to ease the stresses on an injured AC joint, or for the management of most fractures of the clavicle. Note that the base (cradle) part of the sling is slightly elevated, as shown by the dotted lines.

The collar and cuff sling

This allows the weight of the arm to hang. It is useful for some fractures of the humerus, the weight of the arm tending to apply traction to the distal fragment keeping it in good alignment (*see* Figure 6.19b).

Many junior staff you may be mentoring will not have considered these points before, so explain the reasons behind all treatments that you prescribe. **Asking someone to perform a treatment gets it done at the time. Explaining the reasoning behind it helps them to understand what to do in the future in a situation that may be new to them**.

Ongoing hospital management

Comment of ongoing treatment is out of place here. Suffice it to say that the age, health, occupation and lifestyle of the patient can have a tremendous influence on the decision of the orthopaedic surgeon.

Fractures of the clavicle

These are by far the most common of all shoulder injuries and they tend to group into recognised areas on the bone. The overwhelming majority are in the middle third, with the remainder towards either extremity (a few laterally and hardly any medially).

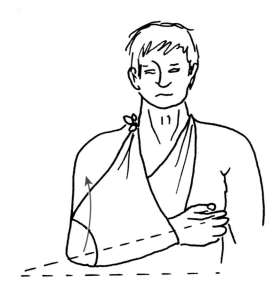

Figure 6.19a The broad arm sling.

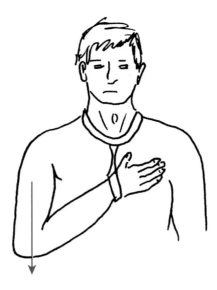

Figure 6.19b The collar and cuff sling.

Clinical features

Because the clavicle is so superficial, the clinical features hardly need mentioning; the fracture can be seen in all but the stockiest build.

Because this bone is perhaps the most difficult to immobilise, it can be exceedingly painful if displaced and result in the patient sometimes having an extremely shocked appearance, which usually settles so that they 'pink up' after a short while in the department.

The most common displacement is for the medial fragment of the fracture to be pulled upwards by the sternocleido-mastoid muscle and the lateral fragment angle downwards by gravity, taking the shoulder with it (*see* Figure 6.20).

Displacement of fractures in the outer third is discussed later in the AC joint section.

The more usual trivial outlook should not give you a false sense of security. This is especially so with displaced fractures, because of the damage that could be done to the nerves in the nearby brachial plexus and the subclavian blood vessels. Make it become second nature to check the movements, sensations and circulation to the affected limb with all clavicle fractures.

Initial management

Explanation, reassurance, sling, analgesia (Carley, 2003).

Stay ever alert for the very occasional fracture caused by a severe direct force, for instance in an RTC. This situation means that you have to go into a **major trauma** frame of mind, working through all the standard ATLS protocols.

Ongoing hospital management

The vast majority of fractures of the clavicle require no further intervention. The use of figure-of-eight bandages, appliances, etc. all have local variations and the need for operative fixation is rare.

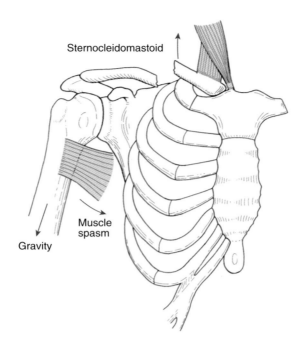

Figure 6.20 Clavicle fracture, the common movement of the fragments (Ellis and Mahadevan, 2010).

Acromioclavicular joint injury

A range of problems may occur:

- Sprains and partial tears with the joint left intact.
- Subluxations of just a few millimetres through to complete dislocations.

The resultant disruption depends on the force causing the trauma and the strength of the acromioclavicular joint ligaments and the coracoclavicular ligaments (conoid and trapezoid).

The main varieties of damage to the local ligaments are shown in Figure 6.21, but fractures of the lateral extremity of the clavicle may also occur.

Clinical features and diagnosis

All the injuries have characteristic pain and tenderness at the AC joint, along with a small swelling with a joint sprain, through to a clear step in the shoulder contour with a frank dislocation. Sometimes without an X-ray it is difficult to differentiate between lateral clavicle fractures.

Shoulder movements that adduct the arm across the body may be particularly uncomfortable, because they stress the AC joint causing local pain (*see* Figure 6.22).

Initial management

An explanation and reassurance that it is not as serious as a glenohumeral dislocation can be very comforting to the patient. They will find that the pain is not as sickening and will usually be comfortable sitting up and walking.

A broad arm sling will be all that is necessary at first, along with only moderate analgesia. Ensure that the knot is not on the injured side.

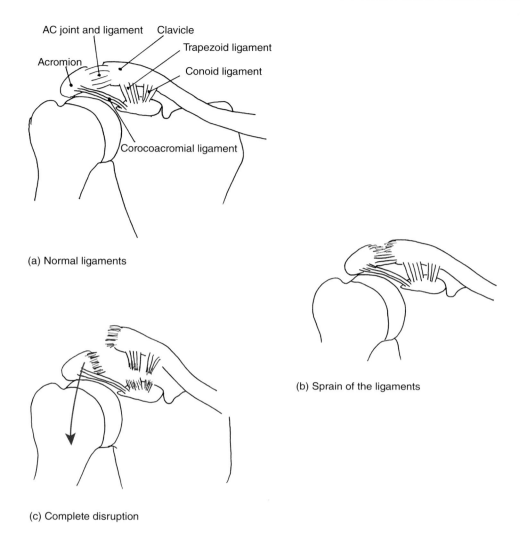

(a) Normal ligaments

(b) Sprain of the ligaments

(c) Complete disruption

Figure 6.21 Main varieties of damage to the ligaments surrounding the AC joint.

Ongoing management

Some practitioners prefer compression strapping around the shoulder and elbow for a complete dislocation of the joint, but this is far from universal.

Sternoclavicular joint damage

Both subluxations and dislocations of the joint may occur. Posterior dislocation may be a major injury, the severe forces giving the possibility of major damage to the mediastinal structures situated behind the sternum (*see* Figure 6.23). The injury can also be associated with other major trauma.

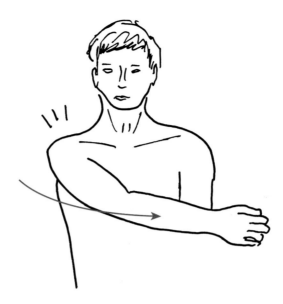

Figure 6.22 Adduction causes pain at an AC dislocation.

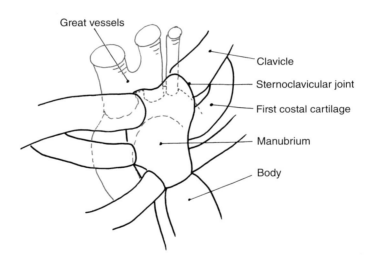

Figure 6.23 Major structures behind the sternum.

The more common anterior dislocation doesn't hold the same dangers because there is no posterior impingement.

Clinical features and diagnosis

With the joint being superficial, with either form of injury the one-sided swelling is usually obvious, although deciding on whether there's a sprain, subluxation or dislocation is difficult without an X-ray.

Immediate management

Decide first if this is major trauma requiring ATLS protocols? Next, even if not major trauma, the patient's breathing should be assessed because this is damage to the thoracic cage. Only then manage the local circumstances.

Movement of the affected arm will increase pain, so a broad arm sling will be required for your patient's comfort. That may be accompanied by analgesia and possibly ice packs over the area to reduce swelling.

Ongoing hospital management

All but obvious anterior sprains will require immediate orthopaedic discussion to decide on the severity of the damage and need for reduction and follow-up.

Rotator cuff injuries

These are very common. Although here under the main heading of musculoskeletal 'injuries', in many ways they could equally be called musculoskeletal 'conditions'. This is because the rotator cuff can easily tear under the stress of a sudden large force; but it is far more likely that there has been some predisposing problem in the cuff building up over months or years to weaken it.

The problems that may be seen here and in other regions are in Figure 6.24:

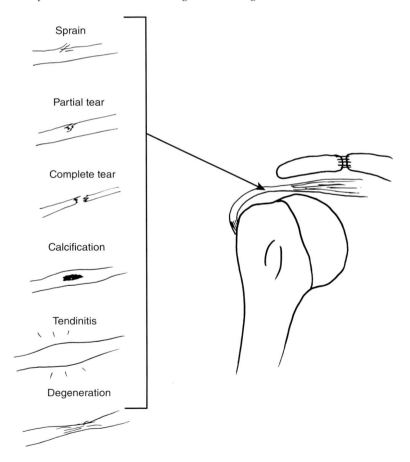

Figure 6.24 Forms of damage that may occur in the rotator cuff.

- Sprain.
- Partial tear.
- Complete tear.
- Tendinitis/osis (possibly caused by a repetitive injury).
- Degeneration of tendon.
- Calcification inside the tendon.

These are well worth learning by heart, for application elsewhere.

Clinical features and diagnosis

The part of the cuff by far the most commonly injured is the **supraspinatus tendon**, since it glides over the head of the humerus. Because of this, the features and management will apply to this injury and you will have to access far more specialised volumes to get to grips with the more uncommon injuries.

Difficulty with abduction is the major problem. The supraspinatus initiates the first degrees of abduction, so, if it is completely torn through, the patient will either not abduct their arm or will have found a 'trick' of letting it swing outwards; then the movement will be taken up by other structures such as the scapula and deltoid.

Immediate management and information

An explanation of the problem is perhaps the best that you can do for your patient in the short term. Simple drawings or showing them on a model is a must; remember the cuff is a difficult concept.

Offering a sling is not a good idea because other shoulder movements need to be encouraged. Analgesia, anti-inflammatory drugs and occasional use of ice or heat are worthy of a try.

Ongoing hospital management

The mainstay of management will be an initial orthopaedic referral for a definitive diagnosis, usually followed by physiotherapy sessions. Further on, there could be steroid injections into the damaged tendon, but repair is not a simple decision.

Section 5
Minor musculoskeletal conditions

Thrombosis of the axillary and/or subclavian vein

This is a rare major condition in everyday circumstances, the vein becoming thrombosed. Sometimes it just happens and at other times it may occur following some form of stressing trauma where the arms are doing some repetitive heavy overhead work.

Clinical features and diagnosis

There will be congestion and swelling of the arm distal to the thrombosis, sometimes with a red/blue hue and obvious distended superficial veins. The patient will also have a severe ache in the shoulder with tenderness in the axilla and upper arm. The temperature may be raised, but a lot of the severity of features depends on how long the condition has been developing.

The strength of the pulse on the affected side may be affected by swelling.

Activity 6.26   Time: **A few minutes' thought**

Cover up the observations on this activity and then proceed.
Can you think of anything else to routinely cover in your clinical examination of this problem?
Write a few notes in your book; then look at my observations.

Observations on Activity 6.26

Well, I would have wanted you to remember to consider the chest, in particular for features of a pulmonary embolus. Always consider your patient as a whole; they may not have connected any chest pain or cough with their shoulder problem. If you missed it this time, it was perhaps because you have never seen one. Make a note about this or maybe highlight the section for revision and you will probably remember it. Also think of the problems associated with it as similar to the more common deep vein thrombosis (DVT) in the calf.

Immediate management

Immediate referral upon suspicion of this condition is important.
Analgesia plus a sling or elevation of the arm on pillows may make the patient comfortable.

Impingement syndrome

This is a group of clinical features with several causes, rather than a single condition. The gap between the underside of the acromion process and the top of the humerus is narrowed (*see* Figure 6.25c). The supraspinatus tendon of the rotator cuff is a major cause of the problem as it becomes thickened with disease, but other causes are shown in Figure 6.25d:

- Forms of arthritis, all with osteophytic lipping of the acromion.
- Previous bony injury.
- The acromion just having grown in an unusual way (just as some of us may have a large nose)!
- Bursitis, the tissues becoming inflamed and thickened.
- Bicipital tendinitis.

Although, looking at this list, it is obvious that this condition is far more common in elderly people, it can also be seen in younger adults, especially those training hard for overhead sporting activities (Hyde and Gengenbach, 2007). As I write this, it is the first week of Wimbledon, so tennis springs to mind as a prime example.

Clinical features and diagnosis

Some of the glenohumeral movements, especially abduction, are minimised and cause the patient significant pain (painful arc syndrome).

Immediate management

Advice, rest, analgesia and anti-inflammatory drugs are the first line of attack.
Although your elderly patients will mostly do as you say, in many instances (especially youth deeply into a sport) patients will not give the injury the rest needed to give it a chance to settle.
You will have to summon all your skills to help them **get a balance that is right for them**, between short-term sporting activity and long-term damage to their joints. With some of the extremes, the standard NHS care will not suit and the best advice, **for them**, may be through private care.

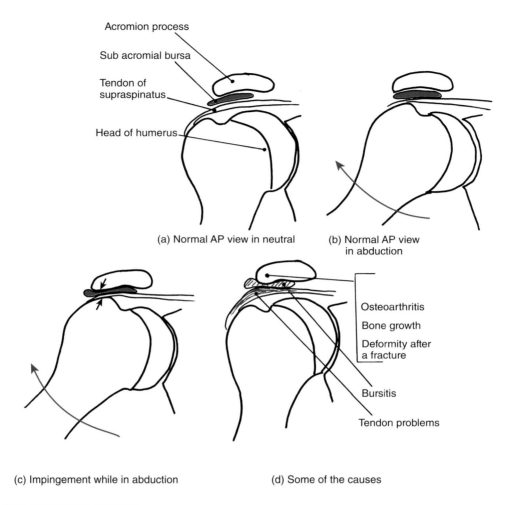

(a) Normal AP view in neutral

(b) Normal AP view in abduction

(c) Impingement while in abduction

(d) Some of the causes

Figure 6.25 Impingement syndrome.

Activity 6.27   Time: **A few minutes' thought now**

As the opportunity arises in the next few weeks, discuss the following with colleagues:
  Do they consider that NHS money should be used for athlete patients, if they continue hard with their particular sport, clashing with your advice to ease their condition?

Ongoing hospital management

- An ultrasound scan usually shows the problem clearly.
- Physiotherapy
- Steroid injections into the supraspinatus tendon or other nearby inflamed tissues.
- Tidying up operations on the bone or soft tissues.

Torn long head of biceps and biceps tendinitis

This injury occurs in two circumstances. First and most commonly, there is the older person whose muscles have weakened over the years. Also in young adults, a good example of this would be a sporting injury; they have simply applied too large a force and the muscle has given way.

Although the muscle can give way anywhere along its course, it is most common to see the long head damaged. This final tearing of the tendon sometimes follows an ongoing chronic problem like biceps tendinitis.

The long head of biceps tendon in its intracapsular position over the head of the humerus takes up a lot of local movement and is therefore prone to irritation, inflammation or even slipping out of its bicipital groove.

Clinical features and diagnosis

The belly of the muscle sags downwards towards the elbow, reminiscent of the old cartoons with **Popeye the sailor** flexing his muscles after eating spinach. Pain and tenderness on movement is a feature, usually in the **bicipital groove**, but there is still the short belly attached to give some movement.

Immediate management

Rest in a broad arm sling for a few days until the main pain has eased should suffice, along with analgesics if necessary and possibly some ice. Information will vary with the patient's age and required future use of the arm. In your initial explanations, be sure not to make an elderly patient feel as though nothing will be done for them, purely because of their age.

Ongoing management

Operation is a complex decision requiring much experience, and many factors have to be considered.

Frozen shoulder

Also called '**adhesive capsulitis**', this is a very common incapacitating and unpleasant condition. The capsule of the glenohumeral joint becomes inflamed and as it progresses parts of it adhere to one another.

Clinical features and diagnosis

More commonly seen in the fifties plus age group, this presents usually without any previous injury as an initially very stiff shoulder (active and passive) in all directions, with an increasing amount of pain, often described as a severe ache.

The pain is often worse at night, although this is a common situation with many shoulder conditions.

Some authors say that it passes through three phases:

1. Initial stage of inflammation (lasts months).
   Pain worsening.
   Shoulder movements decreasing.
2. Second stage (may last up to a year).
   Stiffness progresses.
   Pain starts to ease.
3. Third stage (lasts months to a couple of years).
   Slow recovery.

Immediate management

- Explanation of what is wrong, to reassure and comfort.
- Analgesia and anti-inflammatory drugs.

Activity 6.28   Time: **10 minutes' thought**

Cover up the observations on this activity.

At this early stage in the management of a patient, how far do you feel that you should go with an explanation of the likely progression of the condition?

Write just a few rough lines in your notebook and possibly discuss with others either in class or in clinical practice.

Observations on Activity 6.28

It is certainly a temptation to describe the typical lengthy outcome so that they 'know where they stand' and that it will eventually get at least significantly better.

But think for a moment: might it not be better to give them some **hope** that their problems may be comparatively short-lived, and 'go very easy' on the prognosis drifting into **years**? Their GP may be a far better person to talk to them about this.

Ongoing hospital management

Physiotherapy, steroid injections into the joint and occasionally operation can be offered to some patients. But, if on a desert island, most would eventually heal themselves and regain a reasonable function.

Arthritis

Forms of the condition

RA springs to mind here as a reasonably common cause, but other forms of polyarthritis – for instance, sarcoidosis – occasionally present.

Although the shoulder joints are non-weight bearing, the common osteoarthritis is sometimes seen in the gleno-humeral, AC and SC joints. This may be associated with a previous injury such as a fracture or damage to the rotator cuff.

 Activity 6.29   Time: **Future study**

The three joints in the shoulder are related, with problems in one sometimes affecting others: for instance, the main glenohumeral inducing stresses on the AC. Complex orthopaedics here, but nevertheless something to bear in mind.

Such mechanics are far more noticeable with large weight-bearing joints like the hips and knees, with arthritis in one increasing the weight taken by another, increasing problems there.

Clinical features and diagnosis

Pain in the shoulder and down the arm, which increases with movement and eases with rest. This interferes increasingly with daily activities. As with many conditions we have mentioned, it is often worse at night, interfering with sleep.

Immediate management

Explanation of the possibilities along with suggestions of rest, hot or cold packs, relief of pain and inflammation with drugs, is about the maximum for a minor injury facility.

Ongoing hospital management

Refer to the GP for X-ray, maybe bloods and then follow up depending on the outcome.

Bursitis

Forms of the condition

There are many bursae around the shoulder as you discovered in a previous activity. Inflammations are common and usually associated with a nearby mechanical cause – for instance, a supraspinatus tendon or long head of biceps that is degenerated, swollen and inflamed will irritate surrounding tissues like the subacromial bursa making the whole situation far worse. It would be unusual for the bursa to become inflamed as the primary condition.

With developing inflammation, the bursa swells and thickens. Both acute and chronic forms may occur.

Clinical features and diagnosis

Features will initially be of the causative condition in the middle aged, but with progression the features of the added bursitis will compound the problem. The patient will have a deep-seated aching pain, holding the arm in slight abduction and resisting any further adduction or abduction. Tenderness will be present just off the edge of the acromion process over the greater tuberosity of the humerus.

Management

Initial management will consist of:

- explanation of the condition and advice to minimise specific activities
- analgesic and anti-inflammatory drugs to ease the discomfort
- referral for definitive diagnosis of background condition.

Ongoing management will be via physiotherapy or the orthopaedic department.

Tumours

A text on minor injuries and conditions, yet here we are considering tumours, why?

Well, my answer is, it happens.

In the days when I thought that I knew it all, I came across a middle-aged woman presenting with a classical painful arc syndrome. To cut a long story short, I thought of all the usual things and did all the usual things. Much later, by chance, I found out that it was a secondary deposit; I thank the Lord for 'SOS' in my documentation.

Clinical features and diagnosis

Further discussion is not relevant at our level; we just have to be aware that very unusual conditions are just occasionally seen. Also that very serious conditions commonly start in a small way with an obscure ache or pain, and that this could be the case with the next patient in your waiting room. But this is part of the fascination of your role, isn't it, and why you have to study so hard?

Activity 6.30   **Time: 15 minutes**

In this final activity, I would like you to read briefly around some conditions that are useful for you to just know of, rather than to study in any detail. They are:

- winged scapula
- Sprengel's shoulder
- Klippel-Feil syndrome

About five minutes' study on each would be adequate.

REFERENCES AND SUGGESTED READING

Carley S. (2003) No Evidence for either Collar and Cuff or Sling after Fracture of the Clavicle, www.bestbets.org (accessed 24 May 2013).

Dollery, W. (2001) First Anterior Shoulder Dislocations Should be Immobilised for at least Three Weeks, www.bestbets.org (accessed 24 May 2013).

Duckworth, T. and Blundell, C.M. (2010) *Lecture Notes on Orthopaedics and Fractures*, 4th edn, Wiley Blackwell, Oxford.

Ellis, H. and Mahadevan, V. (2010) *Clinical Anatomy*, 12th edn, Wiley Blackwell, Oxford.

Funk, L. (2002) SLAP Lesions, http://www.shoulderdoc.co.uk/patient_info/shoulder-slap.asp (accessed 24 May 2013).

Gross J. Fetto, J. and Rosen, E. (2009) *Musculoskeletal Examination*, 3rd edn, Wiley Blackwell, Oxford.

Hyde, T.E. and Gengenbach, M.S. (2007) *Conservative Management of Sports Injuries*, 2nd edn, Jones and Bartlett, Sudbury.

McRae, R. (2010) *Practical Fracture Treatment*, 5th edn, Churchill Livingstone, Oxford.

Stanley, D., Trowbridge, E.A. and Norris, S.H. (1988) The mechanism of clavicular fracture. *Journal of Bone and Joint Surgery*, 70B (3), 461–464.

Tortora, G.J. and Nielsen, M.T. (2012) *Principles of Human Anatomy*, 12th edn, Wiley Blackwell, Oxford.

Multiple choice questions

Before you start, take in the reasoning behind these MCQs, how to answer them and how to interpret the results, from the section at the end of Chapter 1.

1. **With an anterior dislocation of the shoulder, which of the following may occur:**

    A   An angle at the deltoid outline, rather than a gentle curve
    B   Line of humeral shaft points medial to the glenoid
    C   Anterior fullness
    D   A 'lightbulb' sign on an anteroposterior X-ray

2. **Which group of four muscles are involved in the formation of the rotator cuff?**

    A   Supraspinatus, deltoid, biceps, teres major
    B   Teres major, infraspinatus, subscapularis, deltoid
    C   Biceps, brachioradialis, teres minor, subscapularis
    D   Supraspinatus, infraspinatus, teres minor, subscapularis

3. **Which of the following bursae are most commonly inflamed?**

    A   Subcoracoid
    B   Subacromial

C Subdeltoid
D Subscapular

4. **Which of the following may indicate a problem with the supraspinatus tendon?**

A Tenderness over the supraspinous fossa of the scapula
B Shoulder flexion
C A 'painful arc'
D X-ray shows calcification superior to the acromion

5. **Which of the following may indicate a problem with the biceps?**

A Have a short head attached to the coronoid process of the scapula
B Have a long head attached to the upper rim of the glenoid
C Insert into the radius
D Have a short head running through the bicipital groove of the humerus

6. **Which of the following may indicate a problem with the adhesive capsulitis?**

A Mainly affects adduction of the arm
B Is usually an acute condition settling down within a few days
C Has acute flare-ups, but is more of a chronic condition lasting weeks to months
D Is another term for frozen shoulder

7. **Which of the following may indicate a problem with a fractured clavicle?**

A Always occurs as a result of a fall onto the shoulder
B If caused by a direct blow to the region, should alert you to the possibility of a major chest trauma
C Is commonly compound because it is so superficial
D Could damage the brachial plexus, so the nerve supply to the arm should always be examined

8. **Which of the following may indicate a problem with fractures of the neck of the humerus?**

A Are associated with paraesthesiae in the military badge area over the deltoid
B Are associated with a dropped wrist
C Commonly occur in elderly people, because of osteoporosis at the site
D Often show bruising further down the arm because of the deltoid

9. **Which of the following should be considered as a cause of shoulder pain?**

A Acute MI
B Acute pancreatitis
C Some causes of acute abdomen
D Arthritis in the neck

10. **Which of the following may cause difficulties with abduction of the arm?**

A Impingement syndrome
B Calcification inside the supraspinatus tendon
C Partial tear of the supraspinatus tendon
D Tendinitis

Answers are available at the end of the book. For an explanation of these answers and further resources visit the companion website at:

www.wiley.com/go/bradley/musculoskeletal

7

The elbow

Aim

To develop an in-depth understanding of the anatomy and physiology, history, examination and early management of minor musculoskeletal injuries and conditions of and around the elbow.

Outcomes

That, by the end of this study, and all the associated activities and clinical experiences, you will be able to:

- demonstrate an in-depth knowledge of the anatomy and physiology of musculoskeletal structures of the elbow
- take an effective history and examine patients presenting with elbow problems, forming a differential diagnosis
- demonstrate an in-depth knowledge of minor musculoskeletal injuries and conditions of the elbow
- apply these skills to the early management of patients, recognising any need for referral.

Section 1
Applied anatomy and physiology

Another fairly complex set of joints for you to learn, but, if you take it step by step with me, you should end up with a thorough understanding.

Bones

The elbow comprises three bones (*see* Figure 7.1):

- Humerus.
- Ulna.
- Radius.

Managing Minor Musculoskeletal Injuries and Conditions, First Edition. David Bradley.
© 2014 John Wiley & Sons, Ltd. Published 2014 by John Wiley & Sons, Ltd.
Companion website: www.wiley.com/go/bradley/musculoskeletal

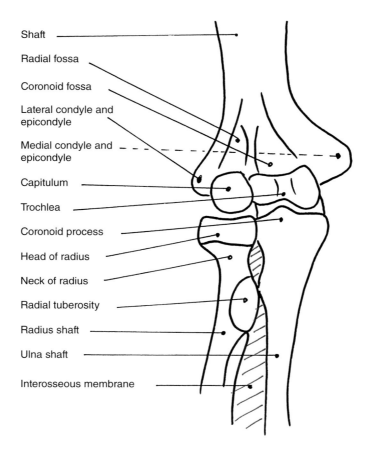

Shaft

Radial fossa

Coronoid fossa

Lateral condyle and epicondyle

Medial condyle and epicondyle

Capitulum

Trochlea

Coronoid process

Head of radius

Neck of radius

Radial tuberosity

Radius shaft

Ulna shaft

Interosseous membrane

Figure 7.1 The bones of the elbow, anteroposterior view.

Humerus

Anteriorly, the distal shaft forms the **medial and lateral supracondylar ridges** flowing downwards to form large masses of bone, the **medial and lateral condyles**. Each of these condyles is mounted by an **epicondyle**, both of which are very important origins for some of the forearm muscles.

Between the condyles are two complex-shaped articular surfaces. The more centrally situated trochlea looks like a bobbin and receives the **trochlea notch** of the ulna. The more lateral surface, the **capitulum** (some call it the 'capitellum') is almost spherical and receives the **head of the radius**.

Immediately superior to the trochlea is a hollow, shaped to receive the coronoid process of the ulna, the **coronoid fossa**, seen best on the lateral view (*see* Figure 7.2). Likewise, superior to the capitulum is a smaller one for the radius, the **radial fossa**.

 Activity 7.1   Time: **30 minutes (for those with some artistic skills)**

Help the information just given to stay clearly in your mind by trying to draw the main features of the anterior view of the bones of the elbow. Even if your drawing skills are minimal, follow the faint outlines using the simple shapes that I show you in Figure 7.3, followed by the final outline. Not only will doing simple sketches like this help your memory, it will also help illustrate points to some of your patients and enthuse anyone you are mentoring.

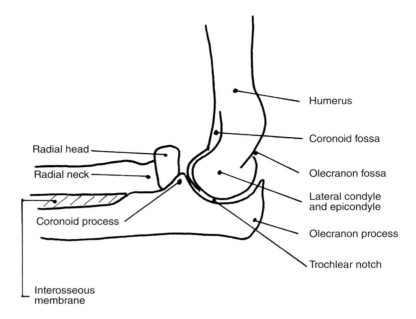

Humerus

Coronoid fossa

Radial head

Olecranon fossa

Radial neck

Lateral condyle
and epicondyle

Olecranon process

Coronoid process

Trochlear notch

Interosseous
membrane

Figure 7.2 The bones of the elbow, lateral view.

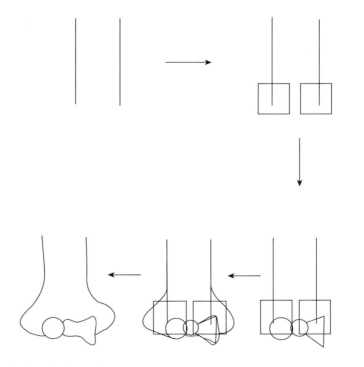

Figure 7.3 A simple way to draw the lower humerus.

Posteriorly, the lower humerus is simpler, with the same condyles, epicondyles and trochlea showing. Above the trochlea is a large hollow for the expanded end of the ulna, the **olecranon**, called the 'olecranon fossa'.

Ulna

Laterally, the proximal extremity of the ulna is formed into a large hook-shaped articular surface, the **trochlea notch**. The distal end of the hook comes to a point, the **coronoid process**. The lateral border of the trochlear notch has a small articular surface for the head of the radius to rotate against when the forearm is supinated or pronated, the **radial notch**.

Posteriorly, the proximal ulna is just a large mass of bone, the olecranon, or the **olecranon process**. This is one of the easiest of all bony landmarks to find and feel. If you sit with your elbows on the table, it is the olecranon that you lean on.

Radius

Anterior and posterior views of the proximal radius are similar, with the slightly concave **head of the radius** that articulates with the **capitulum**. Below is **the neck** and medial and distal to that is the projection of the **radial tuberosity** where the biceps muscle inserts.

The lateral view of all three bones is also important for you to become orientated with. Note how the capitulum is very much anterior and articulates with the radial head.

The bones in children

The multiple centres of ossification of these three bones have significant and complex changes throughout childhood, making interpretation of elbow X-rays in children an absolute 'minefield' unless you are very experienced. This is not an area for the occasional traveller; it is very possible to have a grossly displaced fracture with little to show for it on X-ray.

Figure 7.4 shows just one example of how a fracture (in this case of the medial condyle of the humerus) may appear small and insignificant on X-ray because only a small part of the centre of ossification (shaded) can be seen on X-ray.

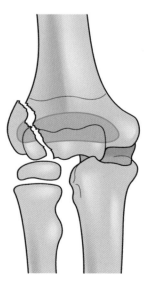

Figure 7.4 Fractured medial condyle of the humerus, through the centre of ossification (shaded) (Duckworth and Blundell, 2010).

Understanding of this general concept is important here, rather than the detail of the ages and shapes of the centres being firmly in your memory.

Joints

Although we tend to talk of the elbow as one joint, the reality is that it comprises three:

1. Humeral ulna joint.
2. Humeral radial joint.
3. Superior radio-ulnar joint.

All are interconnected and in general conversation we speak of them collectively as the elbow joint. Their articular surfaces are covered with hyaline cartilage.

Humeral ulna joint

This is the main 'hinge' part of the elbow joint between the trochlea of the humerus and the trochlear notch of the ulna, allowing us to move the joint from its 0° at full extension to approximately 150° flexion (*see* Figure 7.5).

The carrying angle

The angle of the forearm to the midline of the humerus when the elbow joint is in extension (carrying angle), is different between the sexes (*see* Figure 7.6). In females with their wider hips, there is a need for a few more degrees of valgus so that the arms may swing easily at the side. A variation from the normal for either a male or female is called either '**cubitus varus**' or '**cubitus valgus**'.

 Activity 7.2   **Time: A few minutes**

Cover up the observations on this activity.
   This is a quick question for you, not essential, but of general interest. In the preceding paragraph is the word 'cubitus'; what does it mean and what is its origin?

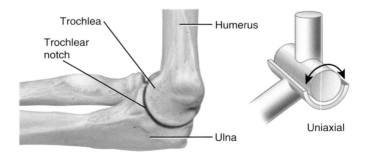

Hinge joint between trochlea of humerus
and trochlear notch of ulna at the elbow

Figure 7.5 The humeral ulnar joint, with the hinge motion highlighted (Tortora and Nielsen, 2012). This material is reproduced with permission of John Wiley & Sons, Inc.

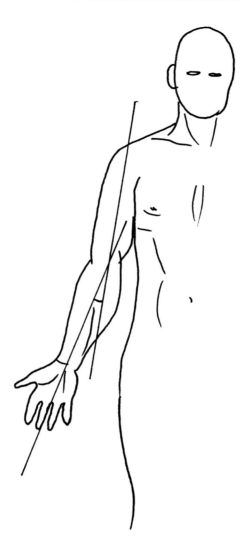

Figure 7.6 The carrying angle.

Observations on Activity 7.2

'Cubitus' means pertaining to the forearm; it comes from the word 'cubit', an ancient measurement approximately the length of a forearm. Some also use it as referring to the elbow.
If ever you come across something like this, but are not familiar with the use of the word, always look it up or ask. It is a tremendous aid to the retention of facts.

Humeral radial joint

This, on the lateral aspect of the arm, is a far less important part of the hinge mechanism. In fact, following serious damage, the proximal radius can be removed and the elbow still function. The concave, circular head of the radius slides against the almost spherical capitulum.

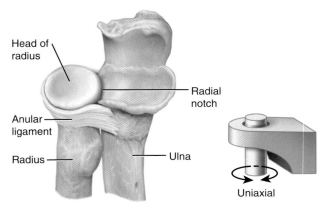

Pivot joint between head of
radius and radial notch of ulna

Figure 7.7 Superior radio ulnar joint, with rotation highlighted (Tortora and Nielsen, 2012). This material is reproduced with permission of John Wiley & Sons, Inc.

Another movement at this joint is the rotation of the radial head against the capitulum, as seen with the pronation and supination of the forearm. This movement is also aided by the superior radio-ulnar joint discussed next.

Superior radio-ulnar joint

This tiny pivot joint, sometimes also called the 'proximal' radio-ulnar joint, allows us to pronate and supinate our forearm with ease. It occurs with the head of the radius rotating against the radial notch of the ulna (*see* Figure 7.7). The joint capsule communicates with the other two aspects of the elbow joint, and can be considered as one.

Soft tissues

Capsule

The elbow joint has a fibrous capsule that lines the edges of the hyaline cartilage and is itself lined by an extensive **synovial membrane** (*see* Figure 7.8a). This loose-fitting synovium is reflected onto the radial, coronoid and olecranon fossae of the humerus and the neck of the radius with annular ligament (*see* Figure 7.9).

 Activity 7.3   **Time: 10 minutes only**

Take Figure 7.8a and colour in the synovium of the elbow. This activity may at first seem simplistic, but it is an excellent method for understanding and retaining the concept of the folds.

Just as the loose skin on the surface of the elbow allows for extensive swelling following trauma or inflammation, so the extensive synovium of the joint allows significant effusions inside the joint capsule (*see* Figure 7.8b).

The capsule is strong at either side, strengthened by the medial and lateral ligaments, but comparatively weak anteriorly and posteriorly.

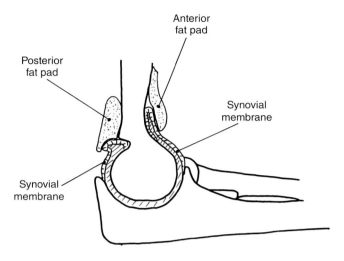

Figure 7.8a Sagittal section of the elbow, showing the normal position of fat pads and synovium.

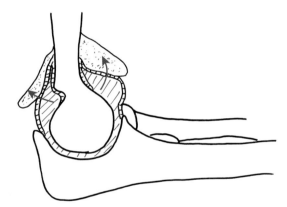

Figure 7.8b Sagittal section of the elbow, showing the movement of the fat pads with a haemarthrosis.

Ligaments

The elbow is quite a stable joint, made so by the strength of its ligaments:

- Medial (or ulnar) collateral ligament.
- Lateral (or radial) collateral ligament.
- Annular ligament.

These surround and blend with the joint capsule to strengthen it.

The **medial collateral** is the strongest, taking most of the stresses of the joint when in heavy use (*see* Figure 7.10a). It is delta shaped, arising from a point at the medial epicondyle and fanning out in three bands:

1. Anterior.
2. Intermediate.
3. Posterior.

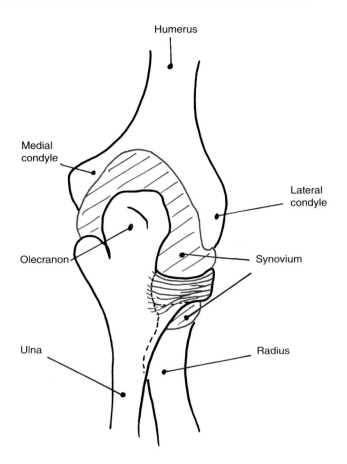

Figure 7.9 Posterior view of the right elbow synovium.

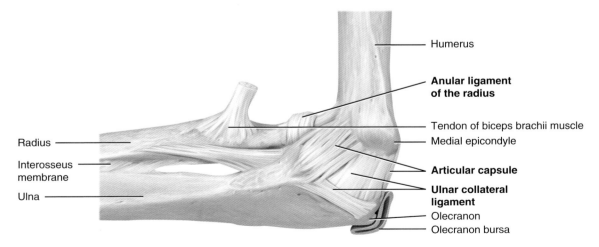

Figure 7.10a Medial aspect (Tortora and Nielsen, 2012). This material is reproduced with permission of John Wiley & Sons, Inc.

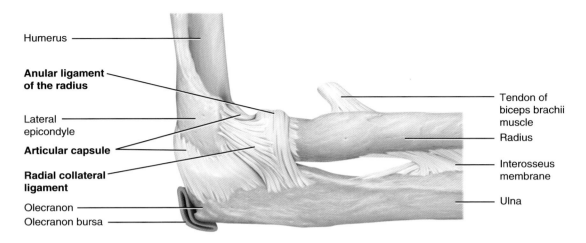

Figure 7.10b Lateral aspect (Tortora and Nielsen, 2012). This material is reproduced with permission of John Wiley & Sons, Inc.

These run to the coronoid process and through to the olecranon of the ulna.

The **lateral collateral ligament** is smaller and runs from the lateral epicondyle of the humerus to the annular ligament; it is not as strong as the medial (*see* Figure 7.10b).

As a general rule in children, all the above **ligaments tend to be stronger than the surrounding bone**. So following a fall, the supracondylar region of the humerus is more likely to fracture than the ligaments to tear. In adults, this situation is reversed and one tends to see fewer supracondylar fractures.

Strangely, the **annular ligament** is lined by some joint cartilage and synovium allowing easy rotation of the radial head. Part of the ligament is sometimes called the '**quadrate**' ligament.

Fat pads

Some 'island' pads of fat surround the elbow, most commonly in the bony fossae:

- Olecranon fossa.
- Radial fossa.
- Coronoid fossa.

These are inside the thin fibrous capsule of the joint, sandwiched between the fibrous tissue and the synovium, but obviously outside the joint's synovial cavity (*see* Figure 7.8b). When viewing X-rays of the elbow, a clear understanding of their position can be important for your interpretation of the films.

The major muscles of the elbow are now listed, although there are others not mentioned that have a less significant effect.

Muscles – flexors

Biceps (biceps brachii)

This is the main flexor of the elbow. The biceps tendon inserts into the radial tuberosity. Try to place your thumb on the tendon, which is in the fold of the elbow when displaying the biceps deep tendon reflex. It can sometimes be torn (like the long head of biceps) but this is unusual.

Brachialis

An associate flexor of the forearm, this originates in the lower humerus and inserts into the proximal ulna at the coronoid process and tuberosity.

Brachioradialis

From its origin in the lower shaft of the humerus, this is one of the lesser flexors of the elbow. Its tendon inserts into the distal shaft of the radius at the styloid process.

 Activity 7.4   **Time: A few minutes**

What is the practical significance of knowing about the brachioradialis?

Observation on Activity 7.4

Hitting over this tendon with a hammer displays the brachioradialis deep tendon reflex.

Because of their varying attachments, each of these three muscles assumes a different flexion performance, depending on the positioning of the forearm, arm and shoulder at the time.

Muscles – extensors

Triceps (triceps brachii)

This has three closely sited origins: one on the scapula just below the glenoid, a second on the upper posterior shaft of the humerus and finally one on the postero-medial aspect of the humeral shaft. The single strong insertion is into the olecranon process and once again is near the site of the deep tendon reflex.

Lateral extensors and medial flexors

Some of the details of these two groups of muscles are to be studied further with the wrist and hand in Chapter 8. However, for the time being, I want you to understand that both epicondyles are major sites for the origins of many muscles:

Medial epicondyle: the **F**lexors and **P**ronators originate here. Remember just '**MFP**' or possibly by using a phrase of your own, like 'My favourite pal'.

Lateral epicondyle: the **E**xtensors and **S**upinators originate here. Remember just '**LES**' like the name.

Just listed are the major muscles of the elbow; there are others not mentioned that have a less significant effect.

Bursae

The elbow has several bursae, used to minimise friction. However, only one (the **subcutaneous olecranon bursa**) is likely to become a problem for you. This is situated in the subcutaneous tissue overlying the olecranon process (*see* Figure 7.11).

Another (the **subtendinous olecranon bursa**) is situated immediately proximal to the triceps insertion, between the triceps tendon and the bone of the olecranon, but this is far less likely to be troublesome. Perhaps you could draw it into the small space in Figure 7.11 before you read on.

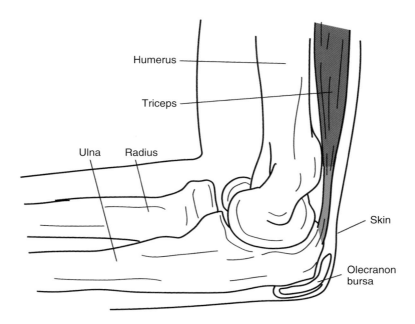

Figure 7.11 The subcutaneous olecranon bursa. Space has been left for you to draw in the subtendinous bursa, between the olecranon fossa of the humerus and the triceps tendon (Gross *et al.*, 2009).

Nerves

Ulnar nerve

This passes through a groove behind the medial epicondyle of the humerus, then through the **cubital tunnel** (*see* Figures 7.12a and 7.12b). The tunnel is formed from the medial collateral ligament, olecranon and fibrous tissue. The nerve then emerges from the tunnel between the two heads of the flexor carpi ulnaris (FCU) muscle on its way down the arm. Anywhere there is an enclosed space, such as in this cubital tunnel, there is the opportunity for swellings and entrapment of a nerve.

Radial nerve

Unlike the ulnar, both the radial and median nerves near the elbow are anteriorly placed and seldom suffer any problems unless by direct penetrating trauma.

However, the **radial nerve** is most vulnerable above the elbow as it traverses the **spiral radial groove** halfway down the shaft of the humerus (*see* Figure 7.13). Here it may be damaged by fractures, but is more likely to be seen as a minor injury following prolonged pressure on the arm.

The **radial tunnel** is about 5 cm long, situated antero-laterally in the forearm between the supinator muscles, more or less over the radial head and neck (*see* Figure 7.14). Once again, where there is a tunnel you can get compression, and this is the most common site of damage to the radial nerve. There are several places in this area where damage may be caused to the nerve by pressure from muscle or fibrous tissue.

Blood vessels

A rich network of branching blood vessels surrounds the elbow joint. The precise positioning is not of much clinical importance to you except that with supracondylar fractures of the humerus you must realise that arteries may occasionally become:

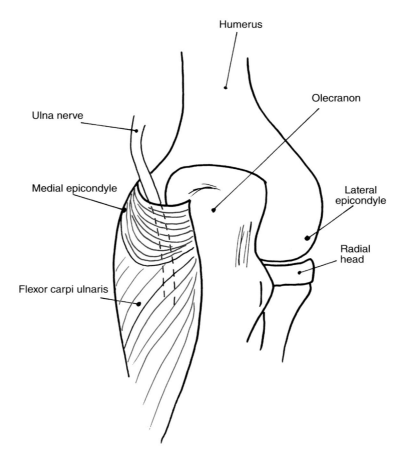

Figure 7.12a The cubital tunnel traversed by the ulnar nerve – right posterior view.

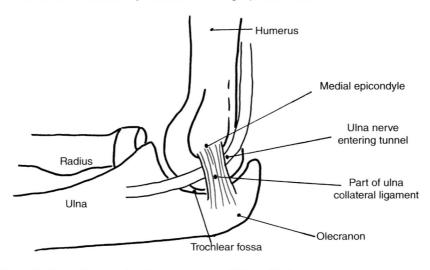

Figure 7.12b The cubital tunnel traversed by the ulnar nerve – right medial view.

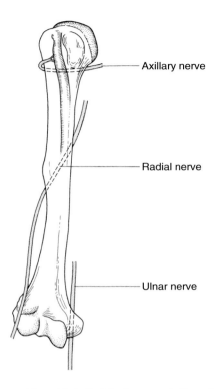

Axillary nerve

Radial nerve

Ulnar nerve

Figure 7.13 The radial nerve winds around the mid shaft of the humerus in the spiral radial groove (Ellis and Mahadevan, 2010).

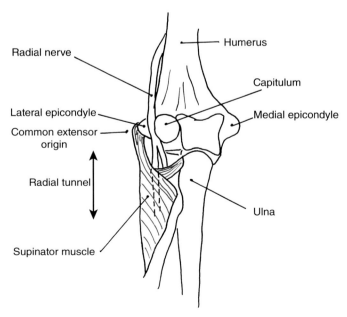

Radial nerve

Humerus

Capitulum

Lateral epicondyle

Medial epicondyle

Common extensor origin

Radial tunnel

Ulna

Supinator muscle

Figure 7.14 The radial tunnel.

- torn
- compressed
- stretched
- irritated,

all of which may cause degrees of compromise to the circulation of the arm distal to the injury.

Section 2
History and mechanism of injury

Listening carefully to your patient is absolutely essential if you are to arrive at a correct diagnosis, or even a reasonable differential diagnosis.

   Patient problems associated with repetitive injury also mean that you will have to study linking a given joint movement with a specific activity. As an example of this, the movement **supination of the forearm** occurs with the use of a screwdriver tightening up a screw or a hand screwing a bottle top down. Similarly the reverse of unscrewing is mostly pronation.

Activity 7.5   Time: **10 minutes**

Cover up the observations on this activity.
   Can you think of any other example of an activity that can cause repetitive injury?

Observations on Activity 7.5

Some examples (although there are many):

- Throwing, as with a ball game, which demonstrates the use of the triceps to extend the elbow.
- Tennis, the overuse of wrist extensors.

Common mechanisms

Here are some common mechanisms that can lead up to various injuries. By becoming familiar with these, you could have a differential diagnosis in your head before you even touch your patient:

Microtrauma caused by overuse

- Repetitive wrist flexion or extension.
- Forearm rotation.
- Vibrating machinery.
- Prolonged posture.

Fall onto an outstretched hand

Perhaps the most common MOI for many elbow injuries is the FOOSH, with the associated forces carrying up the shafts of both the radius and ulna. Exactly how much of a force and up which of the two bones is very variable, as are any associated torsional forces and possible heavy landings on the elbow.

Common injuries and conditions

Posterior dislocation

This is often caused by a FOOSH.

Coronoid process fracture

It can easily be seen how the coronoid can sometimes be pushed off distally by the trochlear as the elbow dislocates posteriorly.

Without an associated dislocation, it can occur as a hyperextension avulsion by the joint capsule type of mechanism

Radial head and neck fractures

These are often caused by a FOOSH. The force travels up the radius, smashing the head against the capitullum.

Supracondylar fracture of humerus

Most of these are caused by a FOOSH of one kind or another, with the elbow in some flexion (*see* Figure 7.15), but a direct fall onto the elbow in flexion may also be a mechanism.

Intercondylar fractures

Here it is easiest to think of the ulna driving hard between the condyles, following trauma like a fall or heavy blow. They are more common in patients of late middle age.

Monteggia fracture

This may be caused by a direct blow to the ulna, or a FOOSH accompanied by a twist, pronating the forearm.

Ulnar nerve lesions

Compression over the medial epicondyle can cause these.

Radial nerve lesion

This may be the result of an arm pressing over a chair (while sleeping, often after alcohol).

Pulled elbow

The mechanism here is always either the swinging of a small child by their arm or arms, or sharply dragging them while holding their hand (*see* Figure 7.16).

Fractured olecranon

- Direct fall onto the elbow or, less frequently, a direct blow.
- FOOSH on a flexed elbow.

Olecranon bursitis

Frequent compression by leaning on the elbow, or friction, is the commonest mechanism. However, it is not unusual to see a bacterial bursitis caused by an overlying (often minute puncture) wound.

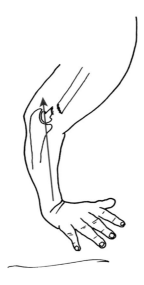

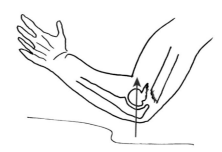

Figure 7.15 MOI of supracondylar fractures: (a) direct fall onto hand (b) direct fall onto elbow.

Biceps tendinitis

- Lifting.
- Repetitive hyperextension plus pronation as in throwing.

Triceps tendinitis

- Sports, including tennis.
- Effect of steroids or some antibiotics.
- Forceful elbow extension plus supination.

Lateral epicondylitis (epicondylosis , or tennis elbow)

The lateral epicondyle is perhaps **the most common place to find elbow pain**. Overuse, repetitive strain of the wrist extensors, is the most likely cause.

Patients are mostly in their forties or fifties, with a slow onset of increasing pain and tenderness at, or just distal to, the epicondyle.

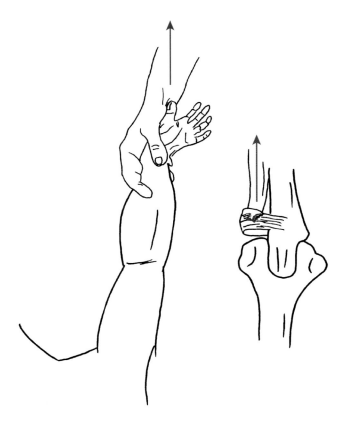

Figure 7.16 A pulled elbow.

Many who play tennis will show the features, but it is far from the only cause. Extending the wrist and supinating the forearm against resistance increase the features, with the extensor carpi radialis longus (ECRL) being the most frequently affected muscle.

Medial epicondylitis (some call it an epicondylosis, or golfer's elbow)

- Overuse.
- Pain on resisted flexion of the wrist.

Osteochondritis dissecans

Here we are considering mostly teenagers. The features of this uncommon condition may include sudden locking of the joint.

It is most frequently seen in athletes, for instance gymnasts pushing their elbows to the extremes.

Ulnar collateral ligament damage

- Overhead throwers.
- Repetition.

Radial tunnel syndrome

- Features distal to lateral epicondylitis and often mistaken for lateral epicondylitis.
- Pain over the head and neck of radius.
- A severe ache rather than the sharp pain of epicondylitis.
- Pain-resisted supination.

Cubital tunnel syndrome

- Throwing.
- Medial elbow or forearm pain.

Pronator syndrome

- Pain-resisted pronation.
- Local tenderness.

Section 3
Patient examination

The elbow is quite straightforward to examine. It is easy to access on your patient, has relatively few movements and is very accessible and superficial for you to palpate.

Examination follows the same routines as in earlier chapters. Take a detailed history and MOI as in the previous section, then assess sensations and circulation. Finally, complete your examination with observation, palpation and assessment of joint movements.

Circulation

The distal circulation must be routinely checked and an excellent way to do this is by feeling the radial pulse and skin temperature while holding the initial history conversation with the patient. Do whatever is best for your individual system, so long as it is part of your routine.

Sensations

The state of the sensations distal to the site of the problem should always be examined. A good general screening of the dermatomes for the radial, ulna and median nerves is described in Chapter 8 and should never be omitted.

What to look for?

Consider the extensive observations listed in the Chapter 3 examination. Specific pointers at the elbow include the wealth of skin available to encourage swelling. Anywhere in the body where you get an excess of loose tissue, there is the possibility of extensive swelling. Compare both sides so that you miss nothing and beware of the danger of just rolling a tight sleeve up, thereby hiding signs 'just out of sight'. Finally, as with all regions, the posterior surfaces often get the briefest of glimpses, but danger may lurk around every corner.

Activity 7.6   Time: **Just a few minutes**

Cover up the observations on this activity before you progress.
  Can you think of a condition that is commonly seen on the posterior surfaces of the elbows and could have connections with the joint itself and even the eyes?

Observations on Activity 7.6

Although the elbow joints themselves are not a common site for psoriatic arthritis (the fingers and toes are the most commonly affected), the patient sometimes gets an associated conjunctivitis. Patients can have the arthritis without any associated rash.

  Now we are to consider the remainder of the examination. After you have completed each of the examination activities at different levels, go to the record of progress (Checklist 7.1) and make a note of them – it is so easy to miss out aspects when there are so many to consider.

Palpation of the elbow

Elbow palpation is often comparatively easy, because with most patients the bones are superficial and the soft tissues lax. Examine your own elbows first, then progress to colleagues and finally patients.

The bones

I would suggest starting palpation with the tips of your index and middle fingers behind the elbow on the tip of the **olecranon**. Only in obese patients or the most swollen of elbows will there be any difficulty. If necessary, confirm this by simply leaning on your elbow, the contact point is the olecranon.

  Once you have this starting point, the remaining structures can be added. The **medial and lateral epicondyles** are the next most logical points. They are difficult to confuse because they are respectively the most lateral and medial points on the elbow. Try holding them both at the same time between your middle finger and thumb of one hand. If you flex and extend your elbow while doing this, you will notice that there is no bone movement at the fingertips confirming the position.

 Activity 7.7   Time: **A few minutes**

Cover up the observation on this activity before you read further.
  Consider the three strategic points of the elbow, the point of the olecranon and the two epicondyles. What differences would you be able to see in them if your patient had:

- a supracondylar fracture
- a posterior dislocation?

Observations on Activity 7.7

There is an important feature to notice with the elbow at a right angle. While you hold onto the two epicondyles, touch the tip of the olecranon, at the same time noticing that the isosceles (two equal sides) triangle made by you is in the same upright plane. With a supracondylar fracture, this triangle remains, but, if your patient has a posterior dislocation, it is disrupted by the posterior movement of the olecranon, a very useful diagnostic point. These three same points are in a straight line with the elbow extended (*see* Figure 7.17).

Checklist 7.1 Record of progress
Physical examination of the elbow

Examination	On self	Friend practice	Friend practice	Patient practice
Patient history, a variety				
Observation				
Palpation:				
Olecranon				
Medial epicondyle				
Lateral epicondyle				
Head of radius				
Capitullum				
Biceps tendon				
Range of movement				
Flexion				
Extension				
Supination				
Pronation				
Sensations				
Radial				
Ulnar				
Median				
Circulation				
To arm intact				
Other:				
Anterior cubital nodes				
Axillary nodes				

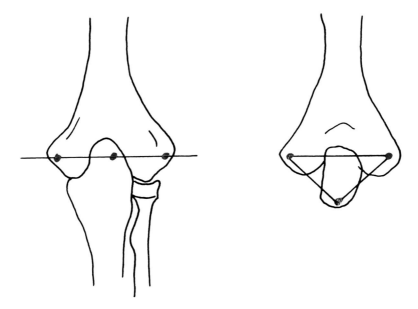

Figure 7.17 Posterior views, with elbow flexed and extended, of the diagnostic triangle at the elbow.

Although the olecranon process fills the olecranon fossa of the humerus in many positions, if the arm is held in about 45 degrees of flexion and you simply slide your finger off the proximal point of the olecranon process, most of the fossa can be palpated.

With your left elbow extended and supinated, trace the whole **shaft of the radius** from the styloid at the wrist towards the head at the elbow. Place the pulp of your right index or middle finger over what you think is the **head of the radius** (*see* Figure 7.18). Then pronate and supinate the arm; if your finger moves with the forearm rotation, you know you are in place. Once sure, move your finger a couple of centimetres proximally onto the **capitulum** of the humerus. Finally, repeat the pronation and supination; your finger being still will once again confirm the position.

Find a small groove (**sulcus**) in the **medial humerus**. It is home to the **ulnar nerve** as it winds its way behind the medial epicondyle through to the forearm, and it can be palpated between the olecranon and the medial epicondyle. With a thin patient, the nerve itself can be palpated, but do this gently or it will give the unpleasant pins and needles sensation down to the little finger.

The whole of the **shaft of the ulna** is best palpated from the easy to find olecranon downwards to the head at the wrist.

The soft tissues

The anterior surface at the bend of the elbow is called the 'antecubital fossa'. Prominent among these soft tissues is the **tendon of the biceps**.

 Activity 7.8   Time: **A quick question for you; a few minutes**

Depending on your individual roles, why should this structure be very familiar to many of you, and what is the connection with C5.

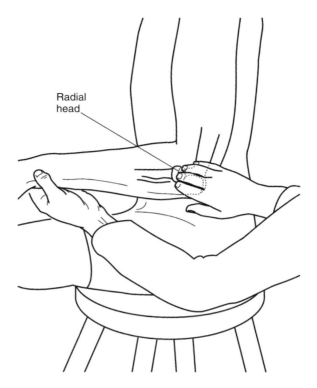

Radial head

Figure 7.18 Palpating the head of the radius (Gross *et al*., 2009).

Observations on Activity 7.8

The tendon journeys to its insertion into the radial tuberosity. Many of you will already have palpated this landmark, pressing on it while testing the biceps deep tendon reflex. C5 refers to the root level associated with that particular reflex.

These reflexes are not part of a normal elbow joint examination, but may be needed in your future examination – for instance, of minor head injuries.

The antecubital fossa is also the site to find some tender and enlarged lymph glands, following a distal infected focus; slight flexion of the joint will aid palpation by relaxing the tissues.

Three major ligaments of the elbow – the lateral and medial collateral ligaments and the annular ligament – are not directly palpable. However, from Figures 7.10a and 7.10b, shown earlier, you can see their extent and be able to elicit tenderness over their position. Finally, stress testing of the joint will demonstrate localised pain when an injured ligament is stressed.

Assessment of elbow movements

This is very straightforward. The movements to be examined are first the degree of flexion and extension, followed by supination and pronation of the hand. If suitable, ask your patient to show the extent of their active movements first and, if necessary, follow their attempts with you putting the joint gently through a passive range. Finally, resisted movements may be used to assist in the differentiation and localisation of some conditions.

Comparison with the opposite side will make a deficiency more obvious. This is especially true regarding forearm movements when the arms will often have to be viewed simultaneously for subtle differences to be obvious. Side comparisons, especially with an older age group, may demonstrate bilateral limitations possibly due to widespread arthritis. Finally, be sure to make use of the examination list (Checklist 7.1).

Section 4
Minor musculoskeletal injuries

Supracondylar fractures of the humerus

Forms of fracture

These are very common especially in children, because their ligaments at this site are stronger than the underlying bone (Simon, 2011). In their simplest undisplaced form, they may be considered a minor injury. However, they may also present with severe displacement of the fragments and the rare, but always present, possibility of damaging the blood supply to the distal limb forming an orthopaedic emergency. Because of this, they should all be treated with the greatest of respect and not trivialised.

These fractures occur here particularly because the bone is weakened by the three fossae. The distal fragment is usually displaced posteriorly as in Figure 7.19, but may also present with anterior displacement, all depending on the exact angles of the MOI.

Clinical features

Satisfaction comes with the recognition of the possibility when there is very little to show. Any child with a painful and/or swollen elbow following a fall should be **presumed to have a supracondylar fracture until it is eliminated**. With minimal greensick buckle (torus) fractures, the child may still be able to move the elbow a little and it could be easy to miss on X-ray unless you are quite experienced. Fine fissure fractures can be invisible on standard X-rays, thereby introducing you to the 'fat pad' phenomenon.

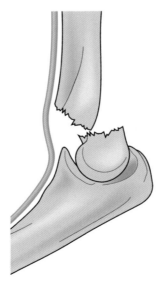

Figure 7.19 Common displacement of a supracondylar fracture (Duckworth and Blundell, 2010).

Activity 7.9   Time: **About half an hour**

Cover up the observations on this activity before going further.
Fat pad: why is this significant with a fracture? Write a brief answer in your notebook.

Observations on Activity 7.9

These elbow fractures are frequently difficult, if not impossible, to see on an X-ray. The bleeding following a fracture builds up inside the joint synovial cavity (haemarthrosis). If severe enough, pads of fat, which usually lie tucked away inside the olecranon, capitellar and trochlear fossae, but outside the joint cavity, get pushed outwards. Fat being of a different consistency from other soft tissues will sometimes show as darker areas on lateral X-rays (*see* Figure 7.8b).

Initial management

Strong effective pain management is important at first, to settle your patient down sufficiently.

The standard supracondylar fracture with posterior displacement of the distal fragment is usually stable in flexion with a collar and cuff sling, which must be under clothes, but, as with all elbow injuries, **always feel the radial pulse while flexing the joint to be certain that the strength (or existence) of the radial pulse has not been affected**.

Advice to the patient and/or their relatives for going home must include significant emphasis on observation of the circulation. The advice you tell them must be backed up in writing to reinforce matters.

I would want **you** to have considered the following:

- Weak or non-existent pulse.
- Colour changes to the limb.
- Temperature change.
- Capillary refill change.

 Activity 7.10   Time: **Half an hour's study**

What will happen if the circulation, instead of being immediately stopped, is slowly decreased over a period of hours – for instance, by increased local swelling pressing on the arteries? Write your thoughts in your notebook.

Observations on Activity 7.10

It is easier to compare such a patient with one with angina pectoris. The myocardium doesn't get an adequate blood supply (ischaemia) so the patient gets severe chest pain from the ischaemic muscle. With the flexor muscles in the forearm, if the blood supply is impeded, it may lead to severe ischaemia with pain in the forearm and the flexor muscles starting to contract. This usually (but not always) forces the fingers into a characteristic clawed position called '**Volkmann's ischaemic contracture**'. This shows with extension of the metacarpophalangeal (MP) joints and flexion of the proximal interphalangeal (PIP) and distal interphalangeal (DIP) joints due to muscle imbalances. Trying to straighten these fingers out, actively or passively, will cause the patient excruciating pain in the forearm and is a most effective pointer to ischaemia of these muscles.

These problems may start within a few hours, so you have to be vigilant with your observations. Always look for the following features that point to forearm ischaemia:

- Pulselessness, or a weakened pulse.
- Pallor of the hand or venous engorgement, depending on the stage.
- Pain in the forearm, especially on extension of the fingers.
- Paralysis of the fingers.
- Pins and needles, especially ulnar and median.

Note that they all start with the letter 'P', so to help your memory call them '**The five "P"s**'.

Ongoing hospital management

Many patients will require closed reduction and immobilisation in plaster under general anaesthetic. Further complicated fractures will require open reduction and internal fixation.

Intracondylar fractures and chips of the epicondyles

These are a vast area of interest, and much is written about them. I want to mention just a few specific points.

In children, a large proportion of the distal humerus is uncalcified cartilage making fractures invisible to X-ray. The great danger here is that a fracture is completely missed, or the severity of a fracture cannot be easily appreciated. Figure 7.4 shows how a major fracture with considerable displacement may appear to be trivial.

It is bad enough to miss fractures like this in an adult with the resultant problems, but with a fracture through a child's epiphysis there is the added risk that growth of the bone will continue in an abnormal position producing a disabling deformity.

Fractures of the radial head and neck

Some of these are very minor with little movement at the fracture site and no involvement of the articular surfaces. These varieties have to be actively sought, whereas many others with comminution and gross displacement are very obvious injuries from the outset (*see* Figure 7.20). More images may be seen on the website associated with this book.

Clinical features and diagnosis

Usually caused by a FOOSH, there is sometimes a more serious injury accompanying these fractures – for instance, a Colles – distracting the patient from possible radial head and neck injuries. I can remember several patients with radial head fractures only discovered later at a fracture clinic, when a more senior doctor has examined the patient thoroughly rather than looking at just the presenting injury.

Because the radius rotates along its length during pronation and supination, these are the two movements that produce significant pain in the elbow with these fractures. With gentle and accurate palpation, pain will also be elicited over the fracture site to confirm.

 Activity 7.11   **Time: A few minutes only**

Apart from the clinical examination of your patient's elbow, can you think of another diagnostic situation in which you should routinely look further after finding one injury?

Observations on Activity 7.11

Well, the most obvious is the patient's X-rays. After finding the obvious injury, never congratulate yourself and relax. Always systematically continue looking through the whole X-ray making sure that nothing else is wrong or suspicious. See lots more on the book's own website.

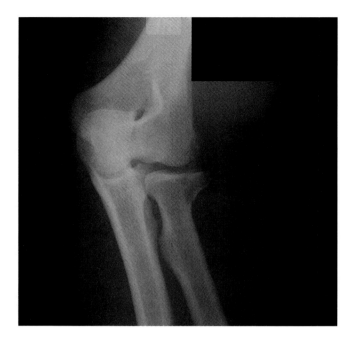

Figure 7.20 Fracture of radial head.

Pulled elbow

This is a very common injury with toddlers, especially in the summer months while at play.

Roughly in the 2–5 years' age group, the annular ligament holding the radius into the side of the ulna is not fully developed. As previously shown in Figure 7.16, the usual mechanism for this injury is a sharp tug to the extended arm, or indeed the child being swung around as in play. This can sometimes allow the radial head to partially slip distally. This subluxation is incredibly painful for the child who stops using the joint, usually leaving the arm hanging motionless at their side.

Clinical features and diagnosis

Let us start here with an activity.

 Activity 7.12　　　　　　　　　　　　　　　　**Time: Just a few minutes**

You are a 3-year-old with this injury, sitting on your mother's knee, arm dangling at your side and quite unhappy at this disruption to your life.

You know that the arm will hurt if it is moved, you are in a very strange environment and a huge uniformed figure is approaching.

What are the things that will upset you the most? Try listing some in your notebook and then read the observations.

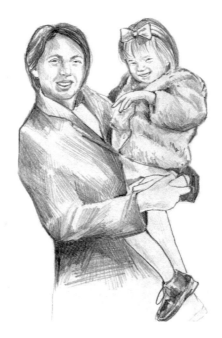

Figure 7.21 Try not to remove a child from the parent (Dustagheer *et al.*, 2005).

Observations on Activity 7.12

I would be disappointed if you did not think of all of these:

- Being removed from your mother would be number one on your list of hates.
- Moving your painful elbow.
- A huge stranger getting too close wouldn't be too good either, especially if they are not too nice!
- Clinical surroundings would make you feel uneasy.

What can we learn from this little exercise? That to manage children effectively you have to be able to empathise with them and adjust your actions accordingly:

- Treat them in pleasing surroundings for their age group.
- Don't remove them from the adult accompanying them (*see* Figure 7.21).
- Don't get too close or touch them first; wait for them to get accustomed to you.
- Talk to the adult first, explaining your approach and how they may be able to ease matters.
- If possible, don't immediately touch the site of injury.
- Use the child's own level of language; see if they want to communicate with you or if you are still 'the enemy'.
- Toy 'props' will assist matters, drawing, balloons, etc.
- Staff of a different sex or age group may be successful achieving rapport if you fail.

You must have all these points in mind when dealing with any children's injuries, but let's leave this now and detail the examination for this specific injury.

  The diagnosis will usually be evident from the MOI but you must still not presume until you have examined the patient thoroughly. Let them become used to you by examination of the uninjured side first. Explain this to the adult so that they do not think that you have made a mistake in the side of injury. Often you may have to break off and 'distraction play' with the child until they are ready to continue with your examination; this can take minutes.

Next, gently palpate the whole of the injured limb, starting either at the shoulder or hand. There should be only a little tenderness at the site of injury; pain is usually mostly on movement, and movements which you expect to be free of pain can then be made.

All this should have effectively 'cleared' the remainder of the arm and the likelihood of a dislocation, leaving just the final flexion of the elbow associated with pronation and supination, which are likely to cause the child severe pain.

These final examination movements, especially pronation with or without elbow flexion (Lewis, 2003), will usually relocate the head if it is still subluxed, with the patient almost instantly having a tremendous reduction in their pain levels. However, with a considerable number of patients, no subluxation is present and the patient just has the residual pain from initial slight tearing of the ligament, easing over the coming days. A collar and cuff sling under clothes is all that is required.

Ongoing hospital treatment and investigation

If there are any unusual presentations or remaining pain levels, gain orthopaedic advice there and then.

Olecranon fracture

Another common injury, only relatively minor.

Clinical features

Immediate and intense pain following the usual fall directly onto the point of the elbow should alert you to the likelihood of a fracture.

Because of the lax skin and soft tissue coverage of the joint, swelling will usually be early and considerable, but beware: don't jump to conclusions – a large swelling does not necessarily indicate fracture. Full examination under such circumstances is rarely an option and even attempting to place the arm in a sling is seldom advisable; the patient is usually far happier with the arm slightly flexed resting on their lap before X-ray. Occasionally, if just an undisplaced fissure fracture occurs, a reasonable elbow examination can be made.

Immediate care

For trivial forms, the usual explanation, reassurance and pain relief will be necessary, followed by immobilisation in a collar and cuff sling under clothes. With any elbow injury like this, when you flex the arm, feel for the radial pulse during movement and afterwards to ensure that your intervention hasn't compromised the circulation.

Although seldom a problem, get into the routine of also testing the limb for movements and sensations to the hand to be sure that all the nerves are intact.

Ongoing hospital management

Displaced fractures will usually be operated on immediately with a screw or wires to hold the fragments. Undisplaced or comminuted varieties can usually be totally managed in a sling. The patient's age, activity, health, interests and occupation will always be a consideration before such a decision is made, so be flexible in what you say.

Dislocated elbow

Forms of injury

Most dislocations of the elbow are when the olecranon is forced posteriorly in relation to the trochlear of the humerus (*see* Figure 7.22), and this is the only form to be covered in this book. The joint between the radial head and the capitulum usually dislocates with it. Most have some degree of associated medial or possibly lateral displacement as well.

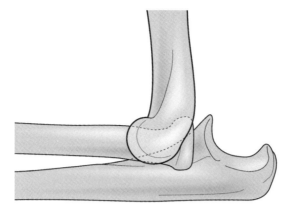

Figure 7.22 Posterior dislocation of the elbow (Duckworth and Blundell, 2010).

The features are fairly obvious and pointers have previously been discussed. In children the injury is relatively uncommon (Patel, Greydanus and Baker, 2009).

Importantly, **none of these dislocations is what you could label a 'minor injury'**; they are in this book because (as with so many other injuries and conditions) they are only **comparatively** minor.

 Activity 7.13   Time: **A quick question for you**

How may regularly looking at dislocations on X-rays lead you to think less about the total actual damage caused to the joint? Write a few words in your notebook and then continue.

Observations on Activity 7.13

Well, all you see on X-ray is the bone disruption, but for this (often severe disruption) to occur the associated ligaments and joint capsule also have to be torn. This soft tissue damage can be considerable and lead to long-term problems for the patient.

Clinical features and examination

Confusion sometimes occurs with a swollen elbow when you try to decide if the injury is a supracondylar fracture or a dislocation. Have you remembered Figure 7.17? It demonstrated one easy way to differentiate the two by palpation of three points.

Immediate care and advice

Do not try to force the arm into a position to fit it into a collar and cuff sling; if it does not adjust naturally, simply support it against the patient's body. As with all elbow injuries, confirm that an adequate radial pulse is present. Immediate orthopaedic referral is the next stage.

Monteggia fracture with a dislocation of the head of the radius

This is not a terribly common injury. The upper shaft of the ulna fractures and the force also dislocates the head of the radius anteriorly; it is not a minor injury for you to learn about in detail.

Clinical features and examination

The standard features present with pain, swelling, tenderness, loss of movement, etc. Much further examination other than light palpation would be inappropriate. An X-ray will show the extent of the injury, but a warning here: it is very easy to see the obvious fracture of the ulna and initially miss the dislocation of the head of the radius. After finding one injury, still systematically scrutinise the whole X-ray.

Associated radial nerve injuries are occasionally seen, so this is a prime reason for never letting up on your routine examination of the limb movements and sensations.

Immediate care and advice

Recognition and referral to orthopaedics should be routine, with supportive management and observations.

Isolated collateral ligament sprains and ruptures

Lesser forces acting on the elbow joint can commonly sprain, partially rupture or completely rupture the medial or lateral collateral ligaments. Of the two, the medial is by far the most robust, but complete tears of either are extremely uncommon.

Clinical features and examination

Direct palpation over the ligament and stressing will highlight the site of injury, but X-ray will be required in some instances to eliminate small fractures.

Immediate care and advice

Immobilisation with a collar and cuff sling, under clothes at first, is all that is required, plus the standard explanation, reassurance and possibly some analgesia.

Ongoing hospital management

Operative repair would be very uncommon in a non-weight-bearing joint like this (I have never known it). Prolonged discomfort would more likely require active physiotherapy and anti-inflammatory drugs

Section 5
Minor musculoskeletal conditions

Nerve problems

Few nerve conditions can be managed completely within an MIU; in most instances, your task will be to diagnose the likelihood of the condition and then signpost the patient to specialists.

Activity 7.14   Time: **About half an hour**

Study the differences between the three conditions listed here in any basic textbook or website. In descending order of seriousness, they are:

- neurapraxia
- axonotmesis
- neurotmesis.

A basic understanding of these will make you more comfortable with the conditions now discussed.

Ulnar nerve problems

Perhaps the most simple, straightforward and manageable problem to consider is pressure on the ulnar nerve where it passes behind the medial epicondyle of the humerus. In everyday life, we have all had a brief experience of this, banging our 'funny bone', causing paraesthesiae in the little finger, of the ring finger and the ulnar border of the hand.

More severe or prolonged trauma to this site will mean that the disturbance is prolonged and will draw the patient to you for advice. Diagnosis will depend on a careful history and neurological examination. When I say 'careful history', I really mean 'careful'. Rarely, even fractures near the elbow from **YEARS** previously can cause this problem (look up 'Tardy' ulnar nerve problems on the internet).

Cubital tunnel syndrome is also a reasonably common condition concerning the ulnar nerve; but here the pressure occurs in the 'cubital tunnel', which is a soft tissue structure just distal to the ulnar groove.

Radial nerve palsy

Mid-humerus the radial nerve winds around the bone, partially in a spiral-shaped groove. Because of this extra support, if there is any pressure against the nerve, it cannot move out of the way as it can in other parts of its tract, and damage may occur more easily. This is the most common cause of radial neuropathy.

Now, this pressure is a prolonged force rather than momentary, so the condition builds up with time (hours).

Activity 7.15   Time: **A few minutes only**

Why does the force become prolonged? Write your brief answer in your notebook and then read my observations.

Observations on Activity 7.15

The hint is in the everyday title on the condition ('Saturday night palsy'). We are creatures primarily designed for movement; even as you sit reading this book, your body is sensing small irritations and making you move a little to avoid pain and damage.

Set this against a patient who sleeps awkwardly with pressure over the radial nerve. This could be caused, for instance, by their arm hanging over the back of a chair. If they have had alcohol and/or taken sleeping tablets, the stimulus to make them move position may be blocked, resulting in varying degrees of nerve damage from neurapraxia to axonotmesis.

Clinical features and examination

The result is a sensory loss over the thumb web space of the back of the hand. There is usually also a motor loss, with an inability to extend the wrist and fingers (drop wrist).

Immediate care and advice

Reassurance, explanation and referral are routine because, although we understand that it is not too serious a condition, it will be very alarming for the patient. If the referral appointment is not immediate, splinting the affected wrist in slight extension and a sling will be helpful.

Radial tunnel syndrome

This is the result of the radial nerve becoming entrapped and compressed in a soft tissue 'tunnel' on the lateral side of the forearm, just below the lateral epicondyle. Examine carefully so as not to confuse the features with a lateral epicondylitis.

Your patient will not display the radial sensory loss, but rather have lateral upper forearm aching pain worsened especially by the 'screwdriver' motion of forced supination.

Non-operative management at first is the norm, with education, physiotherapy exercises and anti-inflammatory drugs.

Olecranon bursitis (subcutaneous and subtendinous)

This may be caused by both bacterial infection, usually from a minor overlying wound, or, most commonly, inflammatory reaction caused by friction (leaning on the elbow – the so-called 'student's disease'!).

Clinical features and diagnosis

The cause is usually fairly obvious from the appearance of the elbow, with the swelling of the inflammatory response being pronounced and well circumscribed, whereas it may be more diffuse and 'angry' with infection.

In both cases the elbow may be hot to touch, with extreme overlying tenderness. Flexion of the elbow will obviously tighten the inflamed tissues increasing the pain; but extension will relax the tissues easing the condition. If the problem were in the joint itself, all movement would cause pain. With infection, routinely look for a rise in body temperature, the patient feeling toxic and the possibility of enlarged lymph glands in the armpit.

Finally, consider the less common reasons for the bursitis: ask about past flare-ups, pains and swelling in other joints pointing to the possibilities of rheumatoid, or gouty, arthritis.

Initial management

Explain what bursae are and of the generally good outcome; the patient will probably not have heard of them before and will be relieved.

Stick to your department's standard protocols, which should include:

- rest and a collar and cuff sling
- analgesia and/or anti-inflammatory drugs
- a follow-up appointment, with the GP or at a fracture clinic.

Ongoing hospital management

- Both the subcutaneous and subtendinous forms of the condition may require aspiration and culture if the diagnosis is not clear (Choudaray, 2004).
- Oral antibiotics if required.
- Sometimes steroid injections into the sac of the bursa.

Epicondylitis

Two forms of the condition occur: **lateral epicondylitis** (tennis elbow) and **medial epicondylitis** (golfer's elbow). Both have the same pathology, are common and do not necessarily occur with the specific sports as the names suggest.

Remember that the epicondyles act as insertion points for forearm muscles, the extensors and supinators laterally (LES) and the flexors and pronators medially (MFP). Wherever such attachments occur, overuse, excessive repetition or a severe force can cause irritation and inflammation. Actual inflammation at the site tends to be a small part of the condition, so many now call it 'an epicondyl**osis**'.

Clinical features and diagnosis

The typical patient is middle aged. The condition starts with an ache; both forms will usually have sharp and often severe pain and tenderness directly over the epicondyle concerned or just distal to it. Specific movements will further cause pains from there down the forearm. There may be slight swelling, but this is not a major feature.

Initial management

- Rest of the part is rather obvious, minimising the specific movements that irritate the problem.
- Anti-inflammatory drugs.
- Referral.
- Some find some relief with an epicondylar clasp (Callaghan, 2007).

Ongoing hospital management

Physiotherapy will be the cornerstone of the patient's management and the condition does not cure overnight; often many months are required for it to resolve. Other treatments may be a steroid injection directly into the tender spot. Rarely, operative intervention is required.

Tendinitis

Tendinitis may occur near to the insertion of either the **biceps** or **triceps** tendons. This condition can be seen in either the older patient, because, as the tissues degenerate, even moderate overuse can instigate the problem, or in the younger patient with acute overuse associated with sports or heavy work conditions.

A sequel to this can be a **torn biceps tendon** near the site of its insertion, but this is not as common as the long head rupture.

Clinical features and examination

With tendinitis, pain, especially against resisted action of the muscle, plus tenderness on palpation, will be associated with swelling or a slight fullness of the area.

Immediate care and advice

Explanation, reassurance, rest, anti-inflammatory drugs.

 Activity 7.16   **Time: A few minutes**

Many middle-aged patients do not realise that, as they are becoming older, some muscles and tendons will not have the same ability to recover and repair. Which other areas of the body besides the elbow are common to such tendon problems?

List a couple of your ideas, then read through my observations.

Observations on Activity 7.16

Well, the Achilles is the most obvious and hot on its tail is the shoulder with supraspinatus problems.

When we manage patients with these conditions, it is important to educate them to the pathology, so that they do not expect a miraculous cure but get an opportunity to regulate their lives to minimise recurrence.

Ongoing management

Physiotherapy would be a further stage for persistent cases of tendinitis.

Conservative management would also be the choice for biceps insertion rupture, unless the patient is requiring a more substantial long-term result because of their occupation or interests.

Other conditions seen in the elbow

The following briefly discusses conditions occasionally seen in the elbow. They should always be considered in a differential diagnosis, especially if the clinical features do not completely fit the more common conditions detailed previously. Even rarities such as soft tissue sarcomas occasionally fool the unwary.

Osteochondritis dissecans of the capitulum

The most common age group for this condition is the teens. Those involved in athletics are especially susceptible. Forces causing degrees of excessive compression of the capitulum may be a cause, resulting in an eventual local necrosis and disintegration of the bone (Patel, Greydanus and Baker, 2009).

Pain on the lateral aspect of the elbow over the capitulum usually starts insignificantly and then grows with the bone destruction. Differentiation will need to be made, especially with lateral epicondylitis.

Chondromalacia of the head of radius

This may occur in young teens and lead to loose body formation with locking of the joint.

Myositis ossificans

This is most common in the thigh following a fracture of the femur. Osteoblasts get laid down inside the haematoma of a torn muscle. Bone is then formed producing a firm swelling that progressively limits the elbow movements. I have not seen this in the elbow, so because of its rarity just bear it in mind.

Osteoarthritis

Non-weight-bearing joints of the upper limbs are not as prone to OA as with lower joints such as the knees and hips. OA will not be foremost in your mind as a differential diagnosis, but always have it in the background and ask the relevant questions. A previous fracture (possibly years ago) that has not healed in a particularly good position is a major cause, because of the weight bearing of the joint being thrown out of alignment and therefore too much stress being placed onto one segment of cartilage.

 Activity 7.17   **Time: A few minutes**

What else can you think of that could damage the articular cartilage leading to OA? Write your ideas briefly in note format, then read my observations.

Observations on Activity 7.17

My answer would be considerable overuse of the part on a long-term basis as seen with a keen sports person pushing the elbow to the limits. A tissue can only take so much stress.

Other causes could be previous diseases that lead to destruction of the bone and cartilage; osteochondritis dissecans would be an example here. However, often the condition is idiopathic, with no particular circumstances being obvious.

Rheumatoid arthritis

The elbow may be affected as part of the generalised disease process, but this should be obvious from your history taking.

Gout

Occasionally gout may present in the elbow, but at this stage it has usually been elsewhere in the body first; this is yet another example of why it is so important to always take a thorough history and listen to your patient. Severe pain and sometimes gouty tophi occur, often at the olecranon bursa.

REFERENCES AND SUGGESTED READING

Callaghan, M. (2007) Tennis Elbow and Epicondyle Clasp, www.bestbets.org (accessed 24 May 2013).

Choudaray, V. (2004) Diagnostic Needle Aspiration in Olecranon Bursitis may be Indicated to Define the Underlying Cause, www.bestbets.org (accessed 24 May 2013).

Duckworth, T. and Blundell, C.M. (2010) *Lecture Notes on Orthopaedics and Fractures*, 4th edn, Wiley Blackwell, Oxford.

Dustagheer, A., Harding, J. and McMahon, C. (eds) (2005) *Knowledge to Care: A Handbook for Care Assistants*, 2nd edn, Blackwell, Oxford.

Ellis, H. and Mahadevan, V. (2010) *Clinical Anatomy*, 12th edn, Wiley Blackwell, Oxford.

Gross, J., Fetto, J. and Rosen, E. (2009) *Musculoskeletal Examination*, 3rd edn, Wiley Blackwell, Oxford.

Lewis, D. (2003) Reduction of Pulled Elbows, www.bestbets.org (accessed 24 May 2013).

McRae, R. (2010) *Clinical Orthopaedic Examination*, 6th edn, Churchill Livingstone, Edinburgh.

Patel, D.R., Greydanus, D.E. and Baker, R.J. (2009) *Pediatric Practice Sports Medicine*, McGraw Hill, New York.

Simon, R.R. (2011) *Emergency Orthopaedics*, 6th edn, McGraw-Hill, New York.

Tortora, G.J. and Nielsen, M.T. (2012) *Principles of Human Anatomy*, 12th edn, Wiley Blackwell, Oxford.

Multiple choice questions

Before you start, take in the reasoning behind these MCQs, how to answer them and how to interpret the results, from the section at the end of Chapter 1.

1. **Which, if any, of the following statements regarding the olecranon process are correct?**

    A   It is at the point of the elbow and articulates with the radius.
    B   It has a centre of ossification in the patient's teens
    C   It is in the same plane as the medial and lateral epicondyles of the humerus
    D   It serves as an attachment for the origin of the triceps tendon

2. **The radial head in the elbow:**

    A   Forms part of the distal radio-ulnar joint
    B   Articulates with the trochlear of the lower humerus and the proximal ulna
    C   Is most commonly fractured by a FOOSH mechanism
    D   In a normal lateral X-ray, remains anterior to a line drawn down the anterior border of the shaft of the humerus

3. **In the condition called 'tennis elbow':**

    A   The site of the attachment of pronators of the hand is affected
    B   Tenderness occurs at the origin of the supinators
    C   Infection of the lateral epicondyle occurs
    D   Confusion with diagnosis may occur with the condition called 'radial tunnel syndrome'

4. **A supracondylar fracture of the humerus:**

   A Is common in children
   B Is recognised as a cause of increased danger to the circulation of the limb
   C If not directly visible on X-ray, may be suspected by the movement of fat pads
   D Is often associated with considerable swelling around the elbow because of the abundance of loose soft tissue

5. **If the ulnar nerve is trapped/compressed at the elbow, you would initially expect:**

   A Paraesthesiae to the little finger and half of the ring finger
   B Paraesthesiae of the radial palmar surface of the hand
   C It to have occurred in a groove behind the medial epicondyle of the humerus
   D It to be from a penetrating injury on the medial aspect of the elbow

6. **The condition called 'pulled elbow':**

   A Is fairly common in children in the 7–10 years age group
   B Has a mechanism of injury of a sudden applied force acting along the axis of the radius
   C Occurs when the radial head tears the lateral collateral ligament, becoming completely dislocated
   D Is associated with a general laxity of ligaments throughout the patient's body

7. **A Monteggia fracture:**

   A Is a fracture of the proximal ulna with an associated dislocation of the head of the radius
   B Mostly has a mechanism of injury of a direct fall onto the elbow
   C Occurs in both adults and children
   D Produces paraesthesiae to the skin of the hand, in a medial nerve distribution

8. **Which of the following should be considered in a patient who has lateral elbow pain?**

   A Osteochondritis dissecans
   B Lateral epicondylitis
   C Fractured radial styloid process
   D Ulnar collateral ligament sprain

9. **Which of the following are correct?**

   A The coracoid process may be implicated in anterior elbow pain
   B The radial notch articulates with the humerus
   C Myositis ossificans only occurs in the thigh
   D Displacement of pads of fat in the elbow, as sometimes seen on X-ray, can indicate bleeding inside the joint cavity

10. **The ulnar collateral ligament:**

    A Reinforces the capsule of the elbow joint medially
    B Supports the joint against a varus stress
    C Is delta shaped and roughly formed of three 'bands'
    D Blends with the annular ligament

Answers are available at the end of the book. For an explanation of these answers and further resources visit the companion website at:

www.wiley.com/go/bradley/musculoskeletal

8

The wrist and hand

Aim

To develop an in-depth understanding of the anatomy and physiology, history, examination and early management of minor musculoskeletal injuries and conditions of and around the wrist and hand.

Outcomes

That by the end of this study, and all the associated activities and clinical experiences, you will be able to:

- demonstrate an in-depth knowledge of the anatomy and physiology of musculoskeletal structures around the wrist and hand

- take an effective history and examine patients presenting with wrist and hand problems, forming a differential diagnosis

- demonstrate an in-depth knowledge of minor musculoskeletal injuries and conditions of the wrist and hand

- apply these skills to the early management of patients, recognising any need for referral.

Section 1
Applied anatomy and physiology

This area is perhaps the most frequently injured part of our bodies, so this chapter should have 'well-thumbed' pages and be thoroughly studied. Although the parts concerned are intricate and there is much detail that you have to digest, the overwhelming advantage is that the wrist and hand are so accessible.

On with the work now, but remember: if you are able to acquire some bones, your study will be so much easier. If you are only able to borrow some for a few hours, read through some of the basic bony anatomy, trying to commit it to memory first.

Bones

- Lower radius and ulna.
- Carpals.
- Metacarpals.
- Phalanges.

Managing Minor Musculoskeletal Injuries and Conditions, First Edition. David Bradley.
© 2014 John Wiley & Sons, Ltd. Published 2014 by John Wiley & Sons, Ltd.
Companion website: www.wiley.com/go/bradley/musculoskeletal

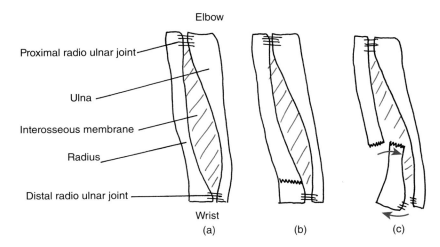

Figure 8.1 The concept of the two forearm bones, attached to each other proximally and distally: (a) the normal arrangement (b) with an un- or minimally displaced fracture, the remaining structures are unharmed (c) with a displaced fracture, either another bone or a joint must give way.

The lower radius and ulna

In the elbow the radius is small and the ulna large, but the exact opposite occurs at the wrist.

Before learning the parts of the lower radius and ulna with all their peculiarities, it is important that you understand some major principles of the arrangement of the two in general. This is most effectively put over in a very simplified way, as follows, to be built on later.

The lower radius and ulna are joined firmly at the top and bottom (the **proximal** and **distal radio-ulnar joints**) (*see* Figure 8.1) Further, stability is increased with a strong fibrous membrane (**interosseous membrane**) stretching between the two. If one of the bones is fractured and displaced, or if either the proximal or distal radio-ulnar joint is disrupted, then for that movement to have taken place there must be movement elsewhere in the system. A similar situation occurs with the 'ring' of the pelvis: if it is fractured and displaced, there must be movement somewhere else in the pelvic ring.

The lower radius is expanded to form the **radial styloid** process. Posteriorly is a small promontory called the '**dorsal (Lister's) tubercle**', which forms a clear and palpable landmark (*see* Figure 8.2).

The articular surface of the radius accommodates both the scaphoid and lunate, usually showing a distinct division.

Particular note should be made that the distal surface of the ulna is not level with the radius and does not articulate directly with the lunate and triquetrum. Instead, there is a small triangular **pad of fibro-cartilage** (*see* Figure 8.3) situated on top of the ulna, bringing the articular surface to the same level as the articular surface of the radius. This pad is firmly attached, making it 'as one' with the radial articular surface and continuing to the **ulna styloid** process. It also covers over the space between the two bones leading to the distal radio-ulnar joint. Surrounding and attaching to this pad are numerous ligaments including the:

- ulnar collateral
- radioulnar
- ulnolunate
- ulnotriquetral.

As a grouping with the cartilage, these may be termed the '**Triangular fibrocartilage complex**' or 'TFCC'. The individual names of the ligaments are not of importance to you, but all parts of the complex act in unison to keep the wrist stable. **Just understand the concept**.

At the medial base of the ulnar styloid process is a small depression, called the '**ulnar fovea**'. It has clinical significance (sometimes) when you come to examine a wrist (*see* section 3 of this chapter).

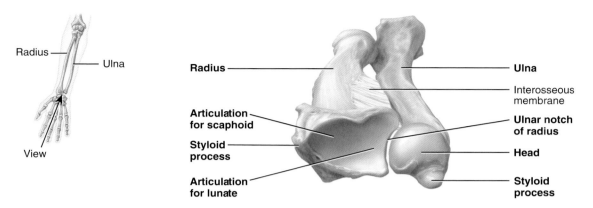

Figure 8.2 Inferior view of the distal ends of the radius and ulna (Tortora and Nielsen, 2012). This material is reproduced with permission of John Wiley & Sons, Inc.

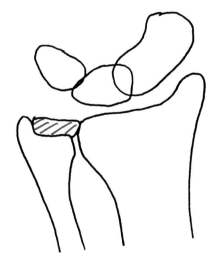

Figure 8.3 Small triangular pad of fibro-cartilage (shaded) on top of ulna.

The carpal bones

- Scaphoid.
- Lunate.
- Triquetrum (some call it 'triquetral').
- Pisiform.
- Trapezium.
- Trapezoid.
- Capitate.
- Hamate.

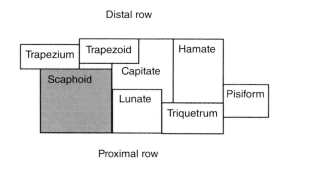

Figure 8.4 Basic layout of the two rows of carpal bones.

This is quite a number for you to remember both the names and some details of each. You must know of them all, but in reality only three will have any great practical significance for you, so it is these that you must concentrate your efforts on.

The bones are arranged into two rows of four. Because of their irregular sizes and articulations, even two rows are a little difficult for a newcomer to appreciate (*see* Figure 8.4). It is important to note how the scaphoid partly projects into the distal row, strengthening the grouping, but also while doing that places itself in a more vulnerable position when the carpus is stressed.

Both 'rows' are also formed into an arch like in a wall, concave anteriorly. This is further converted by fibrous tissue into a partial tunnel, the **carpal tunnel** (*see* Figure 8.5).

As well as the general arching of the carpal bones, they all interlock quite tightly because of their individual shapes, holding well together like a Rubik's cube.

Scaphoid

This is quite the most important for you to study in depth and gain a thorough understanding of. It gets its name from the ancient Greek meaning 'boat-shaped', possibly from a drunken Greek who saw some resemblance! My nearest approximation to this would be Figure 8.6.

Easily seen and of importance is a clearly defined narrowing called the '**waist**' with many holes for blood vessels to enter and leave called '**nutrient foramina**'. It can also be thought of as having a proximal and distal pole (*see* Figure 8.7). Recently, opinions have varied regarding the detail of the blood supply. In essence, the distal pole (supplied by volar vessels) gets a very good supply, whereas the more proximal areas (supplied by dorsal vessels that enter distally) get a precarious supply.

In Chapter 7, I mentioned that the elbow had fat pads that could sometimes be seen on X-ray. There is an associated tiny fat pad on the radial border of the wrist alongside the scaphoid; it can sometimes be seen on X-ray and therefore gives a clue to an occult fracture; ask an 'orthopod' to show it to you.

 Activity 8.1   **Time: A few minutes**

Considering the Rubik's cube analogy mentioned earlier, can you think of two practical considerations of this containment effect?

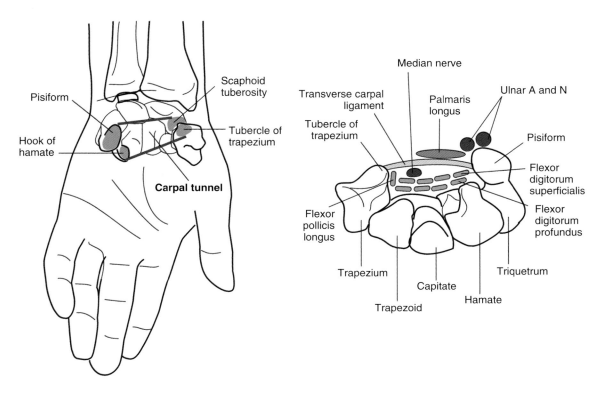

Figure 8.5 The formation of the carpal tunnel (Gross *et al.*, 2009).

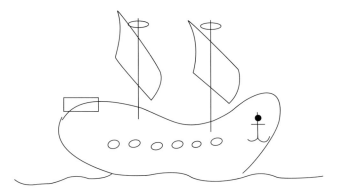

Figure 8.6 The scaphoid gets its name from the Greek meaning boat-shaped. This is the only way I can see a boat!

The scaphoid of all the bones in the body is notorious for hiding a fracture. There can be a fracture and, no matter how many X-rays are taken from different angles, it just will not show up. This is because sometimes the bone ends are simply just so tightly held together by the surrounding structures that there is no gap between the fracture surfaces.

Second, the scaphoid is 'boxed in' by the other bones, especially if the wrist is slightly dorsiflexed and radially deviated. This means that it is in an excellent position to immobilise the fractured bone while healing; hence this is the standard position of the wrist for application of a scaphoid plaster.

The **tubercle** projects distally on the palmar surface.

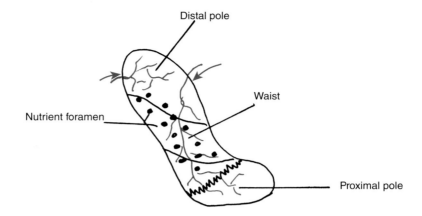

Distal pole

Waist

Nutrient foramen

Proximal pole

Figure 8.7 The blood supply to the scaphoid and the nutrient foramen. The more proximal the fracture is, the more likely it is to damage the blood supply to the proximal fragment.

Lunate

Next to the scaphoid is the lunate. The naming of this bone couldn't be more appropriate: it simply looks like the crescent moon when you view it laterally on X-ray (*see* Figure 8.8) and in the jumble of overlapping shadows it can be a clear landmark. Another landmark, nestling into the lunate's crescent is the largest of the carpal bones – the relatively massive capitate.

Triquetrum

The Latin name means three cornered and is a fine description of the bone's basic shape. It is tucked away next to the lunate and the ulna and its only claim to fame is that it occasionally gets a flake type of fracture.

Pisiform

Generally pea shaped and about the size of a little finger nail, the pisiform sits against the triquetrum, anteriorly on the ulna side of the wrist. Its function is to form attachment for some of the wrist tendons (and on X-ray to panic junior doctors and nurses into thinking that there is a dislocation!) (*see* Figure 8.8). The **flexor carpi ulnaris** inserts into the pisiform, as well as other structures nearby, and because of this the pisiform is classified by some as a **sesamoid**.

 Activity 8.2   **Time: About 15 minutes**

Can you think of any tiny sesamoid bones on the palmar surface of the hand that you will certainly have seen on X-rays, but probably missed? Go to a hand X-ray now, either on Google or this book's website. Enlarge the view and look carefully for small rounded bony ossicles, about 1 or 2 mm in diameter. Which tendons will they be in? Write your answer in your notebook before continuing.

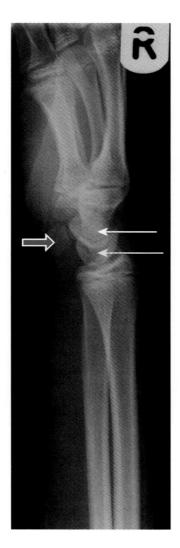

Figure 8.8 Lateral X-ray of the wrist showing the crescent-shaped lunate (thin yellow arrow), with the capitate (thin white arrow) nestling in the crescent. The block arrow points to the pisiform.

Observations on Activity 8.2

Ossicles are commonly seen in the tendons of flexor pollicis brevis (FPB) and adductor pollicis, both near the MP joint.

Trapezium

This is the first of the carpal bones on the radial side in the distal row. The origins of the word and its 'next door' partner, the trapezoid, is contentious, so let's go no further with it except to say that it is a broadly irregular box. It is firmly wedged between the base of the thumb metacarpal, the scaphoid and the trapezoid. Because of this, it is rarely injured.

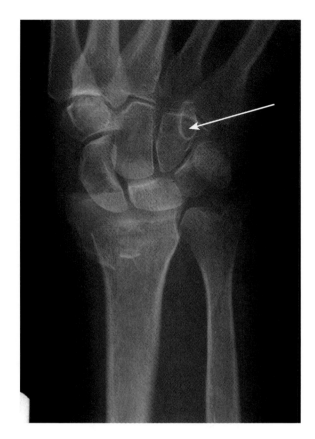

Figure 8.9 X-ray showing the hook of the hamate.

Trapezoid

This is another irregular-shaped bone, firmly held on all sides by the other carpals and the metacarpals.

Capitate

This, the largest of the carpal bones, is in part shaped like a head (hence the name) and this head articulates with the distally pointing concave surface of the lunate. This articulation is important for you to be able to recognise on a lateral X-ray, so that you can recognise forms of wrist dislocation.

Hamate

Another fairly large bone, wedge shaped with an easily seen projecting hook attached to the anterior (palmar) surface (*see* Figure 8.9).

Branches of the ulnar nerve pass nearby and may occasionally be pressed on and irritated by the hook following repetitive movements.

Metacarpals and phalanges

The individual bones are grouped as examples of the strange term 'short long bones' displaying a shaft and two extremities. The distal extremity is called the 'head', with a neck immediately below and the proximal the base; see the stylised

AP view   Lateral view

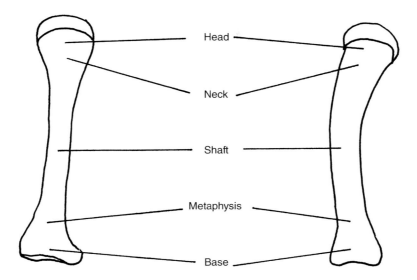

Head

Neck

Shaft

Metaphysis

Base

Figure 8.10 A typical 'short long bone' such as a metacarpal or phalanx.

view in Figure 8.10. The end of the shaft nearest to the base is called the 'metaphysis' (a **metaphyseal** fracture is common). The distal phalanges are the exception, with an almost non-existent shaft surmounted by a terminal tuft.

The wrist joint

The joints that form what we talk of as 'the wrist' are many and complex. But they basically consist of three.

Radiocarpal joint

Activity 8.3   **Time: A few minutes**

Cover up my observations on this activity before you continue.
   Why is it called the radiocarpal joint, with no specific mention here of the ulna? Write a brief comment; then continue.

Observations on Activity 8.3

The lower end of the ulna only comes in contact with the carpal bones indirectly through a small triangular piece of cartilage shown previously in Figure 8.3. This is why the ulna is not mentioned here in the joint name.

Lower (distal) radio-ulnar joint

This small synovial pivot joint is between the concave ulnar notch of the radius and the convex head of the ulna. It is essential for the supination and pronation movements, and is clearly demonstrated if you look back at the earlier Figure 8.2.

Intercarpal joints (including the midcarpal joint)

There are small synovial joints between all the carpal bones, each with interconnections. They act in unison and for our practical purposes can be thought of as a single joint between the proximal and distal rows of bones – the midcarpal joint.

Between them all are the following movements:

- Flexion.
- Extension.
- Supination.
- Pronation.
- Ulnar deviation.
- Radial deviation.
- Rotation.

The joints of the hand

It is essential that you can name every bone and joint in the hand and wrist (*see* Figure 8.11). This is so that you can accurately identify them when discussing and documenting injuries.

You must keep to the recognised naming of the digits as follows:

First, state the side: left or right. Next, use the everyday names of the digits: thumb, index finger, middle finger, ring finger, little finger.

When naming the metacarpals, use the name of the digit that it is attached to – for instance: thumb metacarpal, index finger metacarpal, little finger metacarpal, etc.

Because of long historical use, the metacarpals are sometimes also numbered, from the thumb metacarpal (first), through to the little finger metacarpal (fifth). Although possibly leading to some confusion, this is still a useful system in some circumstances and should not be dismissed out of hand. For example, popular use shows that almost everyone says that a patient has 'a fractured fifth metacarpal'. Also, with multiple fractures of the metacarpals, numbering helps discussions.

Another allowed difference is the naming of the phalanx at the tip of the finger as either distal or terminal; the detail of an individual digit is shown in Figure 8.12.

Metacarpophalangeal joints

There's one of these joints for each digit. All are synovial hinge joints and have movements of flexion and extension through 0° to approximately 90°, plus a minimum degree of adduction and abduction.

However, through two to four digits, they are held firmly by the intermetacarpal ligaments.

Interphalangeal joints

Each finger has two IP joints (proximal and distal) whereas the thumb has one. Although tiny, their free movement is important for the everyday minute movements required.

In each of the PIP joints, the distal extremity of the proximal bone has two tiny condyles articulating with the concave bases of the distal bone of the joint.

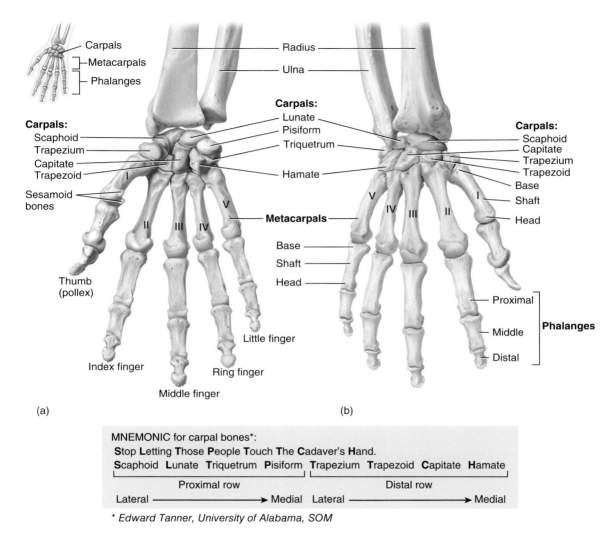

Carpals
Metacarpals
Phalanges

Carpals:
Scaphoid
Trapezium
Capitate
Trapezoid

Sesamoid
bones

Radius

Ulna

Carpals:
Lunate
Pisiform
Triquetrum

Hamate

Carpals:
Scaphoid
Capitate
Trapezium
Trapezoid

Base

Shaft

Head

Metacarpals

Base

Shaft

Head

Thumb
(pollex)

Little finger

Index finger

Ring finger

Middle finger

Proximal

Middle

Distal

Phalanges

(a)

(b)

MNEMONIC for carpal bones*:
Stop **L**etting **T**hose **P**eople **T**ouch **T**he **C**adaver's **H**and.
Scaphoid **L**unate **T**riquetrum **P**isiform **T**rapezium **T**rapezoid **C**apitate **H**amate

Proximal row   Distal row

Lateral ⟶ Medial   Lateral ⟶ Medial

Edward Tanner, University of Alabama, SOM

Figure 8.11 Bones of the right wrist and hand (a) anterior view (b) posterior view (Tortora and Nielsen, 2012). This material is reproduced with permission of John Wiley & Sons, Inc.

All the joints are synovial hinge joints, showing flexion and extension: PIP joints to approximately 115 degrees and DIP joints to about 45 degrees.

All have loose-fitting synovial capsules so, if there is an increase in the synovial fluid with injury or disease, a spindle-shaped swelling will occur. These capsules are strengthened and stabilised by:

- flexor and extensor tendons, sometimes with associated sheaths
- collateral ligaments
- accessory collateral ligaments
- (in some cases) tendon 'pulleys'.

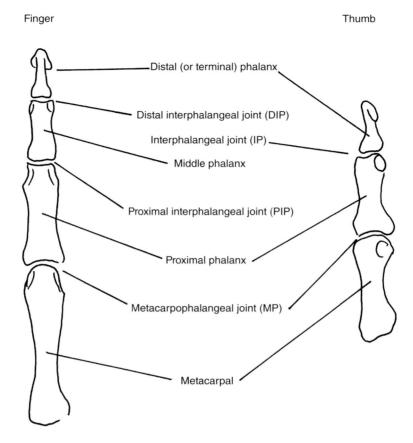

Finger   Thumb

Distal (or terminal) phalanx

Distal interphalangeal joint (DIP)

Interphalangeal joint (IP)

Middle phalanx

Proximal interphalangeal joint (PIP)

Proximal phalanx

Metacarpophalangeal joint (MP)

Metacarpal

Figure 8.12 Names of the bones and joints of the digits.

 Activity 8.4   **Time: 15 minutes**

Now label the 15 points in the following list onto Figure 8.13.
  You may photocopy the drawing if you don't like writing in books. Then check over your answers carefully.

1. MP joint, little finger.
2. Distal phalanx, middle finger.
3. MP joint, thumb.
4. Little finger metacarpal.
5. Proximal phalanx, thumb.
6. Middle phalanx, index finger.
7. IP joint, thumb.
8. DIP joint, index finger.

9. Thumb metacarpal.
10. Proximal phalanx, ring finger.
11. Carpometacarpal joint, thumb.
12. Radiocarpal joint.
13. Distal phalanx, thumb.
14. Base of ring finger metacarpal.
15. PIP joint, middle finger.

Note: Further detail can be added to identify areas by using the term 'radial border' (thumb side) or 'ulnar border' (little finger side) to state which side of a hand or digit is affected.

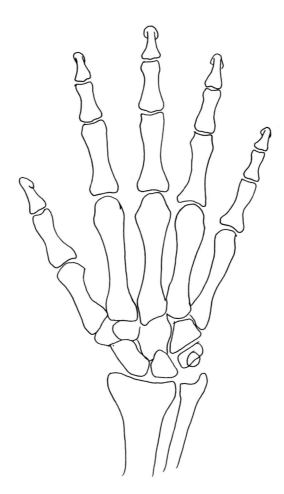

Figure 8.13 Diagram of the hand and wrist for labelling.

The structure of all the IP and MP joints is further detailed by a small piece of fibro-cartilagenous tissue called the '**volar plate**' (*see* Figure 8.14), which is built into the anterior (palmar) surface of the capsule; this strengthens the anterior surface of the joint capsule aiding joint stability, especially to avoid hyperextension.

Carpometacarpal joints

These CM joints, between the distal row of the carpal bones and the bases of the metacarpals, are mostly fairly rigid unyielding structures. They have only the smallest of movements occurring in their interconnected, irregular synovial surfaces, assisting the palm to be able to 'cup'.

That is except for the CM joint of the thumb. This joint has considerable movement because of its saddle shape, and is an essential part of the mechanism giving our hand its opposing movement.

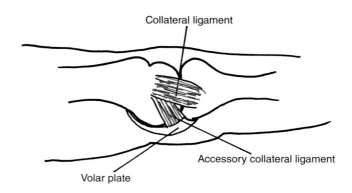

Figure 8.14 Lateral view of the volar plate in a MP or PIP joint.

Muscles of the wrist, hand and fingers

Muscle names

The naming of the individual muscles and their abbreviations at first glimpse seems horrific, but is in fact very logical and easily learnt. In most circumstances, the following rules apply.

First, they are named by their action – for example, Flexor (F), Extensor (E), Adductor (Add), Abductor (Abd); next, by the name of the part that they concern – for example:

- Digitorum (D): digit.
- Pollicis (P): thumb.
- Palmaris (also P): palm.
- Carpi (C): carpal bones.
- Indicis (I): index finger.
- Radialis (R): radius.
- Ulnaris (U): ulna.

Finally, a description of their form. Some examples are as follows:

- Longus (L): long muscle.
- Brevis (B): shorter muscle.
- Minimus (M): small.
- Sublimis (S): superficial.
- Profundus (P): deep.

I am now listing the forearm and hand muscle groups, marking with an asterisk (*) those that I feel are the most important for your initial study.

There are comparatively few muscles actually in the hand (**intrinsics**) and the names are all easily understood. Most of the movements of the hand and fingers are made by muscles in the forearm (**extrinsics**).

Intrinsic muscles

- Interossei (palmar and dorsal)*.
- Lumbricals*.

Those near the thenar eminence:

- Opponens pollicis.
- Abductor pollicis brevis*.
- Adductor pollicis*.

Those near the hypothenar eminence:

- Adductor digiti minimi.
- Abductor digiti minimi.
- Palmaris brevis.
- Flexor digiti minimi brevis.
- Opponens digiti minimi.

Extrinsic muscles

 Activity 8.5   **Time: 10 minutes**

I have listed the extrinsic muscles in an abbreviated format and once again marked (*) those I feel you should study first. To help retention, try to write the full name alongside before you continue.

If these names are new to you, you may need to refer to the earlier listing. From now on, you must take every opportunity to associate the name of a muscle with a particular movement. It is only with this clinical involvement that the names will 'stick'.

The extensor muscles

- ED*.
- EPL*.
- EPB*.
- ECRL.
- ECRB.
- EDM.
- ECU.
- EI.
- Abd. PL.

The flexor muscles

- FDS*
- FDP*.
- FPL*.
- FPB*.
- FCU.
- FCR.
- PL.

Your way forward with muscles

Eventually, as you progress, an in-depth knowledge of the muscles will have to be assimilated. At the present developmental stage of your career, the origins, insertions and nerve supply to the major intrinsic and extrinsic muscles are all that are necessary. This is because any patient demonstrating a lack of, or weakness in, movements of the hand or wrist will need senior referral for an in-depth assessment. Your role is to find a deficiency or problem and, if necessary, refer on for a definitive diagnosis.

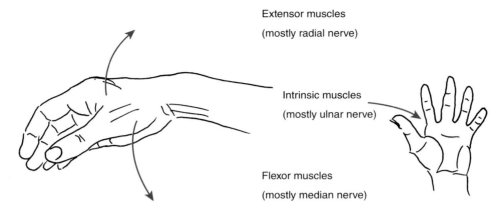

Figure 8.15 The general scheme of nerve supply to the forearm and hand muscles.

The nerve supply to the muscles is the first and easiest aspect to remember (*see* Figure 8.15); it is simply that (almost) exclusively:

- **extensor muscles,** which are situated on the posterior of the forearm, are controlled by the **radial nerve**
- **flexors**, situated on the anterior surface of the forearm, are controlled by the **median nerve**
- **intrinsics** are controlled by the **ulnar.**

Major extensor of the fingers

Extensor digitorum

Although primarily a finger extensor, because it passes the wrist, this will also have a secondary action there. Some call it the 'extensor digitorum **communis**', highlighting the fact that it is a muscle that is **common** to all fingers.

Don't be put off by variations in the names of muscles; preferences vary between both continents and authors.

This muscle belly is situated on the posterior surface of the forearm and, as you already know, is controlled by the radial nerve. The exact origin you have hopefully already learnt.

 Activity 8.6   Time: **A quick revision question**

Where is the origin of ED? Write your answer in your notebook or possibly try a brief sketch.

Observations on Activity 8.6

Do you remember the condition '**tennis elbow**' from the previous chapter? It centred around the **lateral epicondyle** of the humerus and it is here that the ED muscle originates, at **the common extensor/supinator origin** (LES).

The muscle tendons, easily seen on the dorsum, insert in a complicated fashion into the proximal, middle and distal phalanges of all the four fingers (*see* Figure 8.16).

There is no synovial sheath for these tendons in the fingers, because the majority of the 'heavy' work is in finger flexion. This changes, as you will see later, in the wrist.

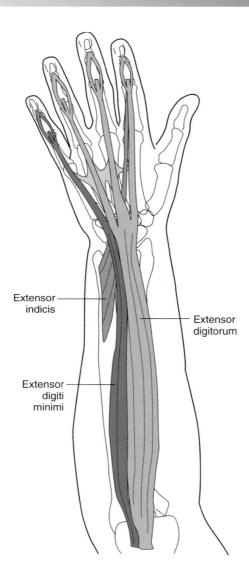

Extensor
indicis

Extensor
digitorum

Extensor
digiti
minimi

Figure 8.16 The extensor digitorum (Gross *et al.*, 2009).

Major flexors of the fingers

Flexor digitorum superficialis

Primarily a finger flexor and, because it passes the wrist, it will also have a lesser flexing action there. As the name suggests, this is the most superficial (near to the skin) of the two flexors and, if you also remember **golfer's elbow** from the previous chapter, you will recall that the medial epicondyle of the humerus is the common origin for the flexors and pronators (MFP), but the FDS also has origins in the coronoid of the ulna and parts of the radius. Not that this detail is strictly necessary for your diagnosis and patient management: just remembering the medial epicondyle will be sufficient (*see* Figure 8.17).

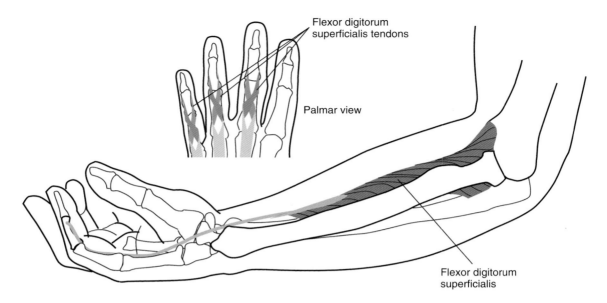

Figure 8.17 Flexor digitorum superficialis (Gross *et al.*, 2009).

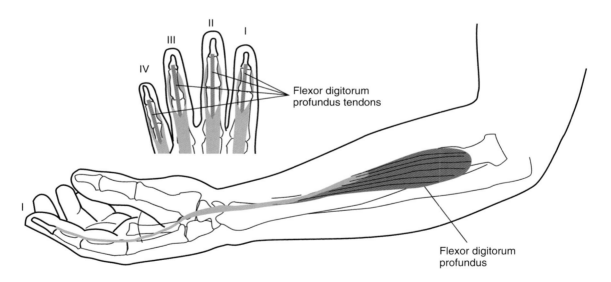

Figure 8.18 Flexor digitorum profundus (Gross *et al.*, 2009).

The tendons divide and insert anteriorly into both sides of the shafts of all the four middle phalanges enabling the PIP joints to flex while the DIP joints remain extended. Try it on yourself now. Clever, eh?

Flexor digitorum profundus

Primarily a finger flexor, this muscle will also have a flexing action as it passes the wrist. It originates from the ulna and interosseous membrane in the anterior forearm. The nerve supply is from the median (index and middle fingers) and ulnar (ring and little fingers) nerves (*see* Figure 8.18).

To remember the position of these tendons, consider someone deep in profound thoughts. Profound/profundus; the tendon lies deep to the superficialis and also continues further, to be inserted into the base of the distal phalanges of all four fingers. This arrangement gives the ability to flex the DIP joints while the PIP joints remain extended.

Muscles that extend the thumb

Extensor pollicis longus and extensor pollicis brevis

Both these muscles, on the posterior surface of the forearm, extend the thumb and are extrinsics, with EPL originating on the ulna and EPB on the radius. Both have small attachments to the interosseous membrane. The longus, being a slightly longer muscle, originates further up the arm than the brevis (brief).

The tendons are both prominent on the dorsum of the thumb, the brevis being placed centrally and the longus taking a more ulnar route. As they separate, they form a hollow, **the anatomical snuff box** (*see* Figure 8.19), which lies over the scaphoid bone. The brevis is inserted into the base of the proximal phalanx, whereas the longus takes a longer route to the base of the distal phalanx.

 Activity 8.7   **Time: A few minutes**

Examine the back of your own hand now so that you are sure of the positioning of the snuff box; in the future this will be of great practical significance.

Muscles that flex the thumb

Flexor pollicis longus

This is an extrinsic muscle, originating at the common flexor origin, plus the shaft of the radius and the interosseous membrane on the anterior surface. It travels the whole length of the thumb, inserting into the base of the distal phalanx, therefore having the effect of flexing both IP and MP joints of the thumb. It is controlled by the medial nerve.

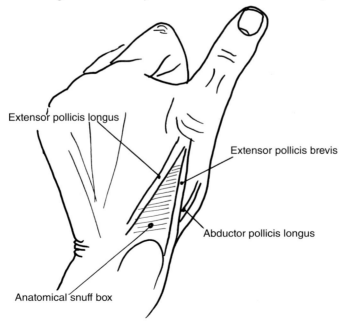

Extensor pollicis longus

Extensor pollicis brevis

Abductor pollicis longus

Anatomical snuff box

Figure 8.19 The formation of the anatomical snuff box.

Flexor pollicis brevis

Unlike FPL, this is a tiny intrinsic muscle originating from the **transverse carpal ligament** (the one forming the carpal tunnel) and the **trapezium**. Some think that other bones in the carpus are involved; minor anatomical variations often occur to many of the bones and muscles that we are considering. FPB inserts into the base of the proximal phalanx and has a mixed nerve supply (median and ulnar). Its primary function is to flex the MP joint; it also assists with several other movements of the thumb.

 Activity 8.8   **Time: 10 minutes**

What are the three remaining thumb movements not detailed so far? Write them down and alongside name the main muscle concerned with each. If you have never studied the muscles, still have a try; using the rules mentioned earlier in this section about muscle names you could still do quite well. Afterwards, read my observations.

Observations on Activity 8.8

Similar to flexion, there is **opposition**: the movement of the thumb towards the little finger. This is mainly made by a small intrinsic muscle called '**opponens pollicis (OP)**' (*see* Figure 8.20), although others are included. It is controlled by the medial nerve.

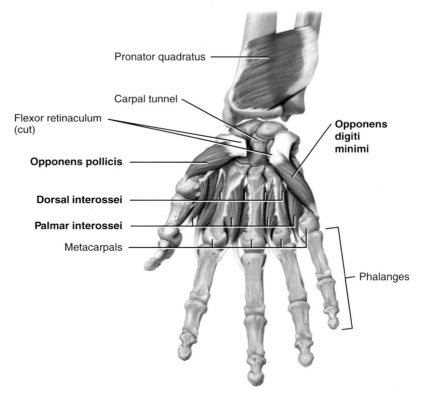

Figure 8.20 Some muscles in the palmar surface of the hand, including opponens pollicis, plus the dorsal and palmar interossei (Tortora and Nielsen, 2012). This material is reproduced with permission of John Wiley & Sons, Inc.

Next comes **adduction**; this is performed mostly by the **adductor pollicis (Add.P)** under the control of the ulnar nerve.

Finally, you should have **abduction** and there are mostly two muscles that achieve this – **adbuctor pollicis longus (Abd.P.L)** and **adbuctor pollicis brevis (Abd.P.B)**

All except Abd.P.L, which arises from the posterior forearm and is controlled by the radial nerve, are small muscles helping to make up the bulk of the thenar eminence.

Muscles affecting the wrist

As with several areas in the hand and wrist, many muscles can have an influence on a particular movement, but here I am just mentioning some primary muscles whose main function is a particular movement.

Flexors (on the anterior of the forearm)

- Palmaris longus and the flexor carpi radialis (both controlled by the median nerve).
- Flexor carpi ulnaris, controlled by the ulnar nerve.

 Activity 8.9　　　　　　　　　　　　　**Time: A few minutes during a break**

If you do not know already, talk to a surgeon colleague during the next few weeks and ask, 'What use is sometimes made of palmaris longus?'

Extensors (on the posterior of the forearm)

- Extensor carpi radialis (longus and brevis).
- Extensor carpi ulnaris.

These are controlled by the radial nerve.

The muscles of the central palm

Lumbricals

These are controlled by the ulnar and median nerves.

They are unusual muscles in that they originate from the tendons of FDP in the palm rather than on bone. They have a complex action assisting the extension of the IP joints through their insertions into the ED, plus some flexion at the MP joints (*see* Figure 8.21).

Dorsal and palmar interossei.

These are controlled by the ulnar nerve.

The two groups of muscles (*see* Figure 8.20) serve to separate the extended fingers (abduction) and close them (adduction). This will have clinical significance for you later in this chapter.

 Activity 8.10　　　　　　　　　　　　　　　　**Time: Half an hour**

Make a note now from my earlier large list of muscles not detailed so far in this book. Then stage yourself into the future, noting when you are going to learn details of these. The ideal is to cover them as and when you come across a patient who has an appropriate injury.

An accurate and easily available source of relevant information is www.eatonhand.com.

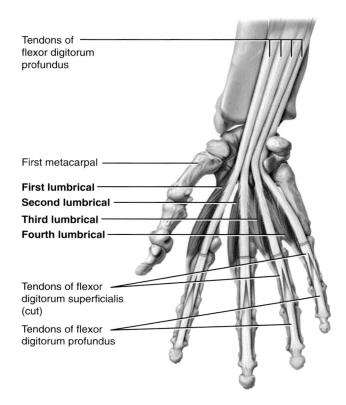

Tendons of
flexor digitorum
profundus

First metacarpal

First lumbrical
Second lumbrical
Third lumbrical
Fourth lumbrical

Tendons of flexor
digitorum superficialis
(cut)

Tendons of flexor
digitorum profundus

Figure 8.21 Anterior intermediate view of lumbricals (Tortora and Nielsen, 2012). This material is reproduced with permission of John Wiley & Sons, Inc.

Tendon sheaths

Following on from the muscles, here would be an ideal place to make a brief mention of the associated tendon sheaths. This network of synovial sheaths essentially lubricates the passage of many tendons throughout the hand and fingers, considerably minimising friction.

 Activity 8.11   **Time: A few minutes**

The advantages of such a system of tendon sheaths are obvious. Can you think of a major disadvantage that can occur with finger infections?
  Write a brief answer in your notebook before you continue with my observations.

Observations on Activity 8.11

First note the way that each finger is segmented into three (thumb into two) at the level of the IP joints as shown by the skin creases (*see* Figure 8.22).

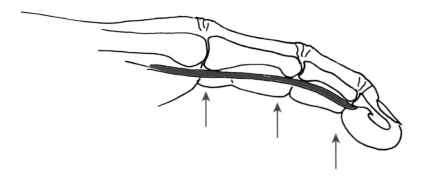

Figure 8.22 The fibrous divisions of a finger, showing the flexor tendon sheath passing through them all.

For the spread of infection from a distal focus in the finger, the 'route' is rather difficult; the bacteria have to try to pass the fibrous compartmental divisions of the finger. However, if the bacteria enter the tendon sheath (**tenosynovitis**), the infection can spread rapidly through the whole length of the finger and beyond. The analogy of a slow country road, to get from 'A' to 'B', compared with a motorway, is useful here.

Fibrous tissues

Carpal tunnel

As mentioned previously (*see* Figure 8.5), the carpal bones fit together like the stones in the arch of a wall. A sheet of unyielding fibrous tissue, the **transverse carpal ligament** (flexor retinaculum) stretches across this arch, converting it into a tunnel. Through this tunnel pass all of the flexor tendons working the fingers along with the median nerve, all very close fitting.

Guyon's canal

On the palmar surface of the hand towards the ulnar border is another far smaller canal. It is formed from fibrous tissue attached to the hook of the hamate bone. It is important because the ulnar nerve is directed through it (*see* Figure 8.23).

The deep palmar space

This is a contained area deep in the palm underneath the extensive and strong **palmar fascia** (palmar aponeurosis) (see Figure 8.24). Both the space and the fascia have great clinical significance, which will be discussed under **Dupuytren's contracture** and **collar stud** in section 5.

Pads of fat

These pads of fat or **pulp spaces** are situated over the palmar surfaces of all the distal phalanges, giving essential cushioning to our grip of fine objects. Although seemingly of little practical interest, **their exact anatomical design is critical to your understanding of some common soft tissue infections** of the fingers (*see* section 5, 'Pulp space infection (Felon)'.

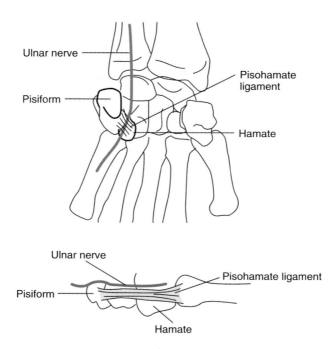

Figure 8.23 Guyon's canal (Gross *et al.*, 2009).

Figure 8.25 is a lateral view of a finger terminal (distal) pulp. The fat in the pulp space is sectioned off like the holds of a ship into compartments by sheets of fibrous tissue acting like bulkheads (dotted lines). This gives the pad a degree of firmness. Also note that the tiny digital arteries supplying the distal phalanx have to travel through these 'bulkheads' to supply the bone.

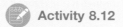 **Activity 8.12**   **Time: A few minutes**

With the information that I have just provided, what are the negative implications for such a design?

Observations on Activity 8.12

Imagine that you prick your finger and bacteria take hold in one of these tiny sealed compartments, increasing the pressure inside. As the tissues swell, the pressure inside will very rapidly become more than that of the blood pressure in the tiny branches of the digital artery. This will significantly diminish the blood flow to areas of the distal phalanx.

The mixture of bacterial infection, plus areas of tissue with no blood supply, do not go well together and the result is often **osteomyelitis** of the distal phalanx, the most common place in the body for osteomyelitis.

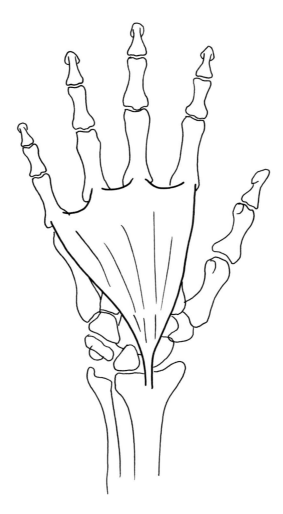

Figure 8.24 Palmar surface of the right hand, showing the palmar fascia.

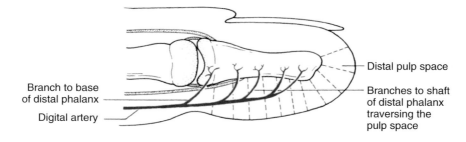

Distal pulp space

Branch to base
of distal phalanx

Digital artery

Branches to shaft
of distal phalanx
traversing the
pulp space

Figure 8.25 Distal pulp space of the finger, lateral view (Ellis and Mahadevan, 2010).

Section 2
History and mechanism of injury

Taking an accurate history or detailing the mechanism of injury are just as important here as with other areas of the body, and possibly more so. This is because of the frequent way in which general conditions often show up with features in a patient's hands. Ensure you don't cut your patient out of such thoughts; if appropriate, include them in your reasoning. This will both gain their support and explain, what is to them, an unusual line of questioning.

Beware of a 'light' occupation found at questioning. It is very common for someone with an office type of job to have very different interests in their leisure time, such as heavy gardening or sport, which may stress the hand and wrist.

Common mechanisms of injury

Of all the MOIs concerning the hand, the FOOSH is certainly the most common, so we will start there.

Fall onto an outstretched hand

The definition is that the **palmar surface** of usually one hand is put out by a patient, to save themselves or lessen the effect of a fall. This hand and arm may be put forwards, sideways or backwards (*see* Figure 8.26). The exact angle that the hand hits the floor or ground will vary considerably, as will the amount of force applied and the amount of flexion of the elbow. Another factor will be the positioning of the weight of the body above the arm.

All the above factors blended with others, such as the exact shape and strength of bone and the surface the patient falls onto, have the effect of producing a large variety of possible fractures, dislocations and degrees of displacement, etc.

You must also never simply accept that a patient has fallen. If they do not volunteer the information, always ask what made them fall.

There is a basic selection of injuries that commonly occur with a FOOSH and you must become completely familiar with them, looking for them in every instance.

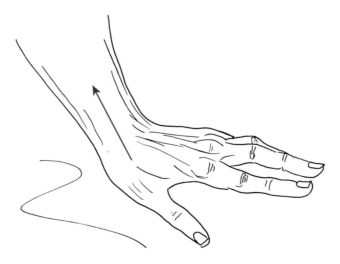

Figure 8.26 The fall on an outstretched hand (FOOSH).

Activity 8.13   **Time: 30 minutes**

Cover up my observations on this activity.

Thinking back to previous chapters, can you name fractures and other injuries caused by a FOOSH? Revising like this really will help your memory. Try to list them in your notebook and then read through my list.

Observations on Activity 8.13

I would have expected you to remember this list:

- Clavicle fracture.
- Fractured head or neck of radius.
- Posterior dislocation of the elbow.
- Supracondylar fractures of humerus.
- Monteggia fracture.
- Olecranon fracture.
- Dislocated shoulder.
- AC joint dislocation.
- Sternoclavicular dislocation.
- Shaft and proximal humerus fractures.

We will now leave this list and consider the **hand and wrist injuries** caused, exclusively or in part, by a FOOSH:

- Colles fracture.
- Scaphoid fracture.
- Radial styloid fracture.
- Ulna styloid fracture.
- Fractured shafts of the lower radius and/or ulna.
- Bennett's fracture.
- Dislocations of the lunate and the wrist.
- Some fractures of the phalanges and metacarpals.

Quite a list, isn't it? You could almost receive any serious wrist and hand injury with this mechanism.

Add to the equation that a patient may not know exactly how they fell and you are left with the situation in which **you could be thought negligent unless you actively looked for all these injuries** following any fall onto a hand. An experienced operator, with a cooperative and prepared patient, can easily roughly palpate all the areas inside a minute.

Another variety of FOOSH occurs when a patient jumps down heavily, landing mostly upright on their heels and then falling forward. This is part of what is fancifully known as the **Don Juan syndrome**, the lover jumping out of the bedroom window to escape the returning husband! Here we have the possibility of bilateral fractures as discussed earlier, but also the possibility of widespread major fractures to the remainder of the body, *see* Chapter 11.

Fall onto a hand not outstretched

The classical circumstance here is the less common Smith's and Barton fractures, the fall tending to the dorsum of the wrist (*see* Figure 8.27) rather than the palm.

The punch

This mechanism is not necessarily caused by fighting as the name suggests, but could be punching a surface in anger. Even some awkward falls can end up with the forces concentrated on a flexed finger. However, most are caused by lads having drunken 'swings' on an evening out. The neck of the little finger metacarpal is the most common site, but others are common.

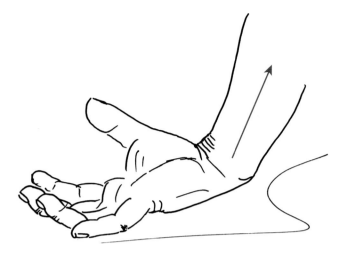

Figure 8.27 A fall, mostly on the dorsum of the wrist.

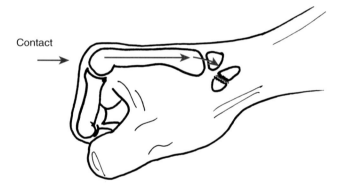

Figure 8.28 Occasional punch mechanism for a scaphoid fracture.

Although not well known, this is also an occasional mechanism for a scaphoid fracture (*see* Figure 8.28). The force travels down the second metacarpal, through the trapezoid and onto the distal pole of the scaphoid.

Common injuries and conditions

Vibration injury

Think of a workman operating a drill or hammer for hours on end as part of their daily life. This can lead to problems with the circulation to the hand and neurological changes (Heaver *et al.*, 2011).

Overuse injury and repetitive strain injury

With an overuse injury, a movement is made very frequently, causing irritation and damage to the tissues.

Activity 8.14 Time: **10 minutes**

Cover up my observations on this activity before you proceed.
  Give me an example of an overuse injury to the wrist and/or hand.

Observations on Activity 8.14

You should be familiar with events as the body ages; the tissues often cannot cope and repair themself to the same extent as in youth. So, an activity that would be nothing to you would be beyond the capability of someone older. Just one example could be an elderly patient having to do heavy DIY. The next day there is synovial inflammation with thickening and pain on the back of the wrist because of this overuse. It will settle in a few days following rest, but is initially an unexplained event to the patient.

Another example could be a youngster pushing themselves very hard while competing in sports, with the tissues just being pushed too far.

Repetitive strain injury (RSI) is a little different: there is an often-repeated minor set of movements by a person of any age. The classical example here would be a wrist problem associated with using a computer, commonly a synovitis on the dorsum of the wrist.

Adduction of the thumb

This is a common mechanism and occurs when catching a ball, opening up the MP joint of the thumb, spraining or rupturing the **ulnar collateral ligament** (*see* Figure 8.29), sometimes called '**skier's thumb**'.

Hyperextension of interphalangeal joint

Catching a large ball is a common mechanism, although there are many other sporting and work-related mechanisms. The everyday fall onto a hand is also very common. Any of these can result in a pure dislocation, or fracture dislocation/subluxation of the IP joint.

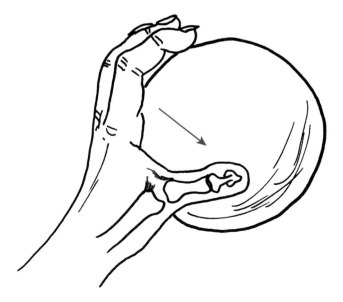

Figure 8.29 A sprain or tear of the ulnar (medial) collateral ligament, here catching a ball.

So many variations and combinations of forces may occur to injure a digit:

- Direct, or indirect blows.
- Avulsions.
- Twisting.

And with many it will have happened so quickly that the patient cannot tell you the MOI.

Direct force to the fingertips

Trapping fingers in doors and hitting with tools are prime examples, resulting in combinations of fractures and soft tissue trauma.

Dupuytren's contracture

This usually starts in later life and tends to run in families. The **palmar fascia** slowly starts to develop nodules and contracts, drawing at first the little finger down towards the palm and, if left to progress, the other fingers.

Our past Prime Minister, Baroness Thatcher, had this condition.

Osteoporosis

Osteoporosis tends to be worse in the following five places leading to common fractures:

1. Lower radius.
2. Neck of femur.
3. Upper humerus.
4. Pubic rami.
5. Vertebrae.

So, if there is an injury to one site, you must consider the danger to the others.

Bacterial infections

Infections are common, coming into the average A&E department daily. Most develop slowly over a couple of days, have a particular reason for being there, are easily managed and are self-limiting.

But a few are downright evil, rapidly damaging bone or spreading throughout the hand, damaging tissues, and on to the general circulation. Study them carefully so that you are not caught out, and always consider the possibility of associated diabetes.

Osteoarthritis

If this is thought to be a possible diagnosis, always enquire if there have been any fractures, or painful injuries, a while ago. Old fractures may have healed in a poor position leading to stress in the articular cartilage even years later.

OA in the hand is most common in the DIP joints. It is not the type of thing to be consulted about in an MIU or an ambulance; rather it starts with just developing stiffness of the fingers. This worsens over the years, becoming painful with the growth of nodules. Look at any room full of retired people and I guarantee that several will have the deformities to show you.

Rheumatoid arthritis

Whenever a pain is centred on a joint and arthritis is suspected, consider the possibility of a polyarthritis – not just RA, but gout and psoriasis as well. Sometimes at the very start of a condition, the pain will be fleeting, seeming to settle then flare up elsewhere until the classical pattern develops. An accurate history is so important.

Gout   ·

A family history may be elicited; well worth asking.

Sarcoidosis and reactive arthritis (Reiter's syndrome)

I want to mention these major conditions throughout the book so that they settle in your memory as something to consider when you are faced with a patient with joint pains that don't fit into a common pattern. In your role with minor conditions, you cannot be an expert at everything; but having just a little knowledge of other major conditions will be a tremendous advantage in forming a differential diagnosis.

Special pointer regarding burns

If a burn is deep or perhaps not an isolated accident, consider the possibility of a neuropathy being a contributory cause.

Section 3
Patient examination

Examination of the hand can be rather strange in that it sometimes gives great insight into conditions affecting the whole of the body rather than our musculoskeletal problems, and we must spend time looking at these points.

Meeting your patient

As with any part of the body, your examination starts as you go out to call the patient in to see you. Note how they hold themselves and the expression on their face. Ask yourself the following:

- Are both arms swinging, or is one held rigidly at the side?
- Is the affected hand hanging down, or elevated?
- Is the good hand supporting the other?
- Are they using the affected hand?
- Do they smile?
- Do they look tired or in pain?

Obviously your examination follows and varies, depending on the information gained from your questioning about history and MOI.

There is nothing wrong with holding, or touching and observing the hand while your patient talks; you choose what seems best for the individual occasion. There is no strict, preset order of history and examination – they blend.

Inspection

Remember **both hands must be seen**; also that for the majority of circumstances seeing the forearms up to the elbows is the ideal.

The general list of what you must look for when examining a patient can be found in Chapter 3 and by now it should be second nature to you. Here we look for the specifics applying to the hand, so you must now look for the following.

Musculoskeletal pointers

The position the hand or an individual finger is held in tells you a lot. Fingers straightened out mean that the patient cannot be in severe pain, because a painful joint will naturally assume a position of ease, which is usually slight flexion.

The thickness and roughness of skin will give you an indication as to whether the hand is used to heavy work or is engaged in more gentle pursuits.

Muscle wasting is especially noticeable in the thenar and hypothenar eminences and by hollowing of the spaces between the metacarpals.

Normal

Swelling of dorsum

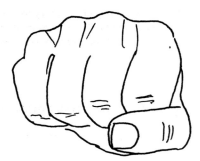
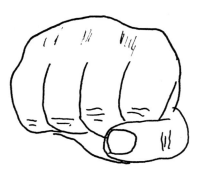

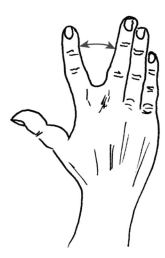

Figure 8.30 View of a normal fist, followed by the initial loss of the inter-metacarpal head 'valleys' in a dorsal swelling, and finally the bulging and abduction caused by a web space swelling.

Forms of swelling

Swelling from infection, inflammation or trauma mostly first shows on the dorsum because there is no strong fascia there, but it doesn't necessarily mean that the problem is dorsal.

Loss of the inter-metacarpal head 'valleys' may occur (*see* Figure 8.30) due to swelling.

Bulging web spaces with the fingers forced to spread apart can be seen if pus collects there, or there is inflammation or haematoma (*see* Figure 8.30).

Limitation of swelling into the fibrous divisions of digits is important to note.

Heberden's nodes at distal interphalangeal joints and Bouchard's nodes at proximal interphalangeal joints

Both Heberden's nodes (*see* Figure 8.31a) and Bouchard's nodes (*see* Figure 8.31b) are indicators of OA. Heberden's in particular are very common among the elderly population.

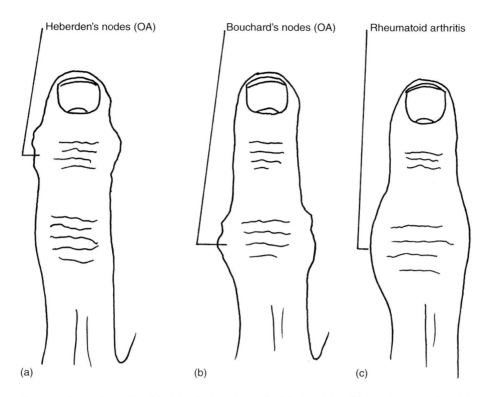

Heberden's nodes (OA)   Bouchard's nodes (OA)   Rheumatoid arthritis

(a)   (b)   (c)

Figure 8.31 Common finger deformities (a) Heberden's nodes, OA of the DIP joints (b) Bouchard's nodes, OA of the PIP joints (c) RA fusiform swelling of PIP joints.

Features common to rheumatoid arthritis of the hand

- Spindle fingers (fusiform swelling of the PIP joints) are typical of RA (*see* Figure 8.31c).
- Ulna deviation of MP joints.
- 'Z' deformity of thumb (IP joint hyperextension, MP joint flexion).
- Swan-neck deformity (DIP flexion and PIP hyperextension). This is sometimes, but not always, caused by damage to the FDS.
- Boutonniere deformity (PIP flexion and DIP extension). This is caused by an ED middle slip rupture, and can also be seen following trauma.

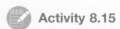 **Activity 8.15**   **Time: 5 minutes**

Can you cover up the list of RA features that you have just read and try to reproduce it in your notebook?
So often we read but, in our enthusiasm to progress, fail to learn.

If you missed more than one deformity, slow down a little, underline or highlight new points and go back to the text the following day to review your work.

A far more effective way to learn is to link the text with a patient whom you have seen. For instance, you meet a patient with advanced RA in the hands. When they have left, make a note in a book listing the joints affected and then, later, dig out this book and compare. By doing that you are:

- **seeing** the condition
- **writing** a note about it
- **reading** about it.

The more methods you use to learn, the easier facts will stay in your brain.

Ganglion

These rounded, cystic swellings of various sizes can sometimes be seen on the dorsal surfaces of the wrist. They increase in size slowly. On most occasions the patient has been to see their GP about it and been reassured.

Take every opportunity to palpate them and become familiar with their texture.

Gouty tophi

Although most common in the foot, gout may present to you in the fingers or wrist. There is a familial tendency, so ask your patient about their relatives.

Pallor of fingers

Any blanching or blueness of the fingers should be noted. **Raynaud's** phenomenon or, more rarely, **Buerger's** disease are possibilities and the patient will require referral for management .

Foreign bodies

When examining a wound of the hand or wrist, bear in mind the possibility of a tooth fragment being inside if it was caused by a punch.

'Hidden' tendon injury

When examining a wound on the posterior surface of the fingers or hand, the tendon may now have retracted into a different position from when it made contact, so that simple observation of an intact tendon at the wound site does not mean that there is no complete or partial injury present.

Subungual haematoma

A very common and terribly painful collection of blood under the nail, usually isolated but often associated with a fracture of the distal phalanx. If there is an associated fracture, you would have to think of it as a compound injury with all the associated dangers of infection.

Mallet deformity of fingers or thumb

This limp flexion of the distal phalanx of the digit, with the inability to extend it, is given this very apt title (*see* Figure 8.32). With a thin digit, it certainly does resemble a wooden mallet. If found in a thumb, consider RA and also ask if the patient has ever had a Colles fracture.

Rotation of the fingers

Unless you are used to managing hand injuries, rotation following a fracture is easily missed, but it is a vital deformity to notice and will need reduction for the patient to retain full use of the hand.

There are two methods of making any rotation obvious. The first is to ask the patient to make as much of a fist as possible; when this is done, **the centre line of each finger should approximate the scaphoid bone**. The second method is to **look at the fingertips end on** and rotation will show up if you look at the line of the nails (*see* Figure 8.33).

Dupuytren's contracture

Briefly mentioned in section 2 of this chapter, this is easily noticed by the rigid clawing of the fingers, tightening of the palmar fascia and nodular formation. Go on the internet to see a selection of images of the progression of the deformity over years. Once seen, never forgotten. However, remember that, as a 'minors' person, you will have the difficulty of considering this diagnosis at the very early stages, when problems are just starting and little is obvious.

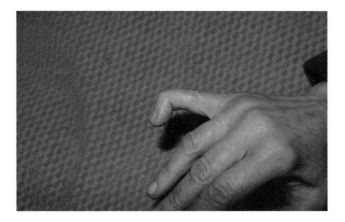

Figure 8.32 Mallet deformity.

 Activity 8.16   Time: **A quick question**

One of the things you must do as a student is to become more questioning; just reading is not the same as studying. As an example, at the end of the 'mallet deformity' paragraph. I suggest that you ask the patient if they have ever had a Colles fracture. If you questioned what I had written and started to try to find out why, very well done. However, if you just 'passed it over', perhaps you are trying to go too fast; slow down a little, enjoy the book more and do some more background work.

PS: Try looking up delayed rupture of EPL in section 5 of this chapter.

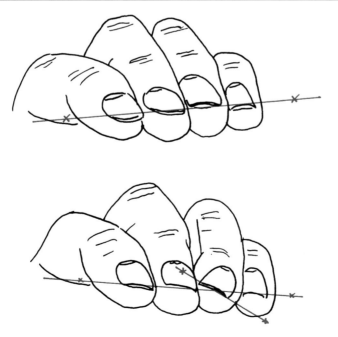

Figure 8.33 Rotation of fingers is easily noticed by looking at the nails end on.

Triggering of flexor tendons

The patient will explain to you that the finger 'sticks' or 'catches' while in the bent position, but they can then free it. Palpate the tendons in the palm; usually there will be a small nodule on the tendon where it is thickened.

Fungal infections

Deformed, crumbling, discoloured, or missing nails are commonly seen in fungal infections. The problem may have started on the toes, so examine them as well.

Volkmann's ischaemic contracture

This has been described and discussed in the previous chapter, but use this as revision. Can you describe the deformity?

Common fracture sites

Quickly observe and gently palpate all common trauma sites:

- Lower radius and ulna.
- Carpus.
- Radial styloid.
- Ulna styloid.
- Neck of fifth MC.
- CM joint of thumb.
- Ulnar collateral ligament MP joint of thumb.
- Anatomical snuff box.

Less common lumps and bumps

There are many conditions that present only very occasionally in the hand. I do **not** aim for you to be able to diagnose them with ease, but I feel that a brief background knowledge will be useful so that you can intelligently refer the patient for a definitive diagnosis.

 Activity 8.17   **Time: At least an hour**

Many thousands of pictures of all these conditions are available from Google Images. Breaking away from this book for a while and 'chasing' pictures up on the web is an excellent way of varying your learning for a while.
Take about 5 to 10 minutes to study each of the following conditions.

- Implantation dermoid.
- Glomus tumours.
- Mucous cyst.
- Osteoid osteoma.
- Chondromas.
- Soft tissue sarcomas.
- Metastatic tumours.
- Garrod's pads of PIP joints.
- Scleroderma and calcinosis.

I will not be mentioning them again in section 5.

Major illness pointers

Let's start this small section with an activity.

Activity 8.18　　　　　　　　　　　　　　　**Time: About a couple of hours**

To discuss the following major conditions and features individually is beyond the scope of this book. However, they are important and require about an hour of your time as background knowledge. You may have covered them previously if you have studied the general examination of patients. Give about 10 minutes to each feature.

- Clubbing.
- Splinter haemorrhages.
- Osler's nodes.
- Swelling of both hands.
- Cyanosis of the nail beds.
- Weakness of a hand and arm.
- Marfan's.
- Dry skin of myxoedema associated with thickening of the tissues.
- Deliberate self-harm to wrists.
- Flat to spoon shaped (koilonychia).
- White nails (leukonychia).
- Beau's lines, white transverse grooves.
- Dilated capillaries at the nail bed (systemic lupus erythematosus [SLE]).

Palpation

The two most essential basics are to feel the temperature of both hands and then assess the pulse.

Examination of the sensations to the fingers and hand come next (*see* Figures 8.34a-c). You must learn the key sensory areas by heart, but beware: slight variances occur.

The nodule of a trigger finger has already been mentioned.

Always give gentle increasing pressure into the anatomical snuff box; tenderness here does not mean that there is a fractured scaphoid, but it increases the likelihood significantly and makes an X-ray necessary.

Finding local tenderness throughout the fingers and hand obviously makes you suspicious of a fracture; but bruising and other soft tissue damage can also easily cause this. You should only become worried if longitudinal pressure along the fingers reproduces the pain (*see* Figure 8.35).

Crepitus at the **CM joint** is sometimes found with OA of the joint.

The ulnar styloid **fovea test** is carried out with the wrist deviated towards the radial side, and the operator places the tip of the thumb into the fovea between the ulnar styloid and the triquetrum. This is done on the unaffected side first and then the affected side; exquisite tenderness will show if there is a problem with the TFCC.

Range of movement

The exact order that you examine the range of joint movements is of no consequence. In fact, depending on the precise history of the injury or condition, only you can judge which movements will need examining at all in a given instance; it would be cruel to progress when a fracture is obvious.

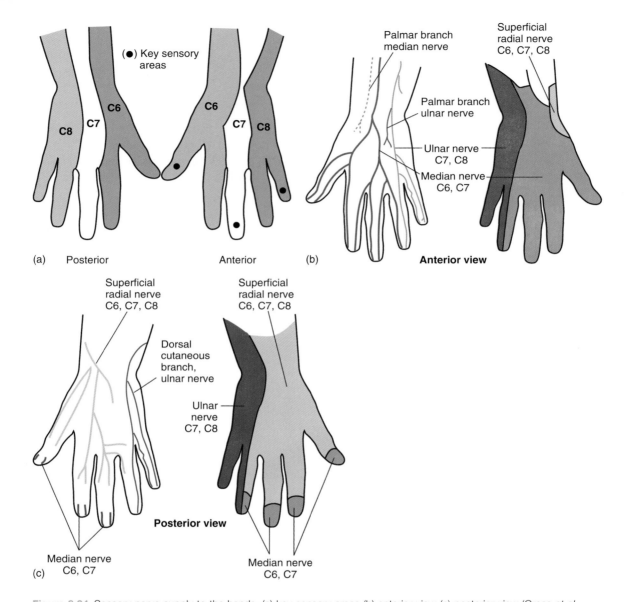

Figure 8.34 Sensory nerve supply to the hands: (a) key sensory areas (b) anterior view (c) posterior view (Gross *et al.*, 2009).

The basic three are:

1. Straighten out the fingers and thumb.
2. Bend the fingers and thumb.
3. Spread the fingers and thumb apart and then close.

But more is sometimes necessary, in which case choose from the following list:

- Form a complete fist; **all fingers should tuck up**; slight loss of flexion in just one can make the grip less effective. Assess the strength of the grip and compare with the other hand.

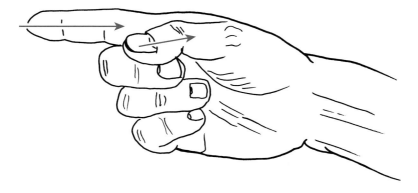

Figure 8.35 Pain on longitudinal pressure of the digits is very suggestive of fracture.

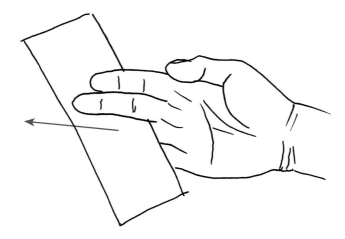

Figure 8.36 The strength of the interossei may be tested by placing a piece of paper between the patient's fingers and trying to pull it away.

- The strength of the interossei can be judged by placing a piece of paper between the fingers and asking the patient to stop you pulling it away (*see* Figure 8.36).
- The position of the hands in the praying position and its reverse (*see* Figure 8.37) will compare the flexion and extension of the wrist in both hands.

Examination of tendons

I now list some of the local major tendons. For wounds possibly associated with an injury to them, you should make the following detailed examinations, carefully isolating the individual digit you want to examine first.

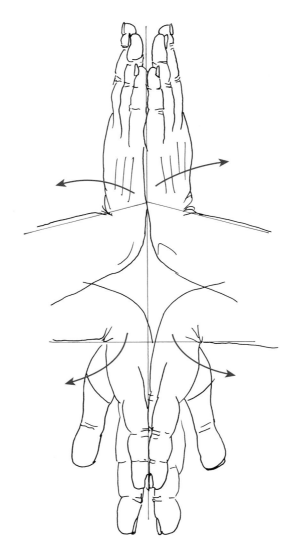

Figure 8.37 Demonstrating these two positions to the patient, then asking them to follow you, will show a comparison of dorsi and palmar flexion of the wrists on the left and right sides.

 Activity 8.19   **Time: About half an hour**

With all the muscle tendons to be discussed here, first try to recall the various origins and insertions to see how much you have remembered. Then, if necessary, revise the anatomy in section 1 before you progress.

The first two muscles have to be examined independently of one another, because there is so much overlap of function.

Flexor digitorum profundus

This is a muscle with divided tendons common to each of the digits, so it is unusual to see a patient who can flex a finger completely independently; move one finger and the others tend to also have some movement. There is also a further complication: because the tendon passes all the flexor joints of the fingers, hand and wrist, it will also have a secondary action on them as well as the primary action of flexing the distal phalanx (*see* Figure 8.18).

To test the primary action of this muscle, first eliminate the other finger movements by having the hand flat on a table with the palm uppermost. Then, while holding the unaffected fingers flat on surface, ask the patient to flex the distal phalanx while you are holding the proximal and middle phalanges still at the PIP joint.

Flexor digitorum sublimis (superficialis)

A similar situation to FDP occurs here, because the tendons are common to all the fingers. Have the hand in the same position and again eliminate the movements carried from the other fingers by holding them down, as you did when examining FDP previously. Now, ask the patient to flex the finger at the PIP joint with the DIP joint still extended. For this to show clearly, you may have to hold down the affected proximal phalanx and offer resistance over the anterior of the middle phalanx (*see* Figure 8.17).

Extensor digitorum

This is the main muscle for finger extension and also another muscle with tendons common to other fingers, to complicate matters. It is assisted by several other muscles (*see* Figure 8.16).

Extension is tested on a surface, with the forearm pronated and the palm supported with your hand flexing the MP joints slightly. The patient is asked to extend the fingers and resistance can be applied to the dorsum of the fingers with your other hand.

Flexor pollicis longus

Resist flexion against the volar of DP and ask the patient to try to flex the IP joint.

Extensor pollicis longus

The MP joint is held extended. Resist extension against DP.

Extensor pollicis brevis

Test the MP joint. Flex the MP joint. Resist extension against the dorsal proximal phalanx (PP).

Flexor pollicis brevis

Supinate. Extend and abduct thumb. Resisting against the volar surface of the PP, ask the patient to flex the thumb keeping the IP joint extended.

Factors affecting the range of movement

 Activity 8.20   **Time: 10 minutes**

Cover up my observations on this activity and then read on.
  Can you list the major factors that affect the range of movement of a joint?

Observations on Activity 8.20

The range of movement shown in any given joint may be due to several factors, including:

- pain
- swellings (blood, synovial fluid, oedema)
- soft tissue problems around joint
- skin contracture
- cartilage problems
- bone problems
- nerve involvement
- muscle, tendon or tendon sheath problems
- psychological factors.

By this stage of your study, I would have expected you to have thought of at least six of these general areas.

Catching, locking or triggering of a joint movement

The most common situation here is a condition called '**trigger finger**' when there is a swelling of the tendon inside its sheath, causing it to become locked and to require forceful release by the patient.

Finkelstein test

A final simple manoeuvre well worth learning is the **Finkelstein test**. Make a rather unusual fist with the thumb on the inside of the fingers and then place the wrist into ulnar deviation. If this causes severe pain, it is indicative of **De Quervain's** disease, a tenosynovitis in the wrist (*see* section 5).

   Use Checklist 8.1 to help you to remember your progress with examination.

Section 4
Minor musculoskeletal injuries

Fractures

Lower end of the radius and ulna

Of utmost importance for you here is that in the wrist and hand even slight differences in the position or direction of a fracture line can mean that the fracture behaves in a completely different way and may need different management.

   This book does not intend to cover all the many variations either in the lower radius and ulna or the remainder of the wrist and hand. However, what it does do is provide you with a sensible level of detail to effectively cover the vast majority of injuries you will meet.

Colles fracture

Definition

In general conversation, many use the term 'Colles fracture' to mean any of several varieties of fracture around the wrist. However, this is not accurate enough if you are diagnosing and prescribing treatment for injuries.

   It is satisfactory to talk in general terms of:

- a comminuted Colles
- an undisplaced Colles or
- a greenstick Colles.

Checklist 8.1 Record of progress

Physical examination of the wrist and hand

Examination	On self	Friend practice	Friend practice	Patient practice
Patient history, a variety				
Observation:				
Thenar				
Hypothenar				
Web spaces				
Nails, bed and cuticle				
Pulp space				
Dorsal inter MC spaces				
Boutonniere				
Swan neck				
Other contractures				
Ganglia, etc.				
All joint swellings				
Any rotational deformity				
Palpation:				
Anatomical snuff box and sphenoid				
Lunate and triquetrum				
Radial styloid				
Lister's tubercle				
Ulna styloid				
Base 1st MC				
Neck 5th MC				
All IP and MP joints				
Palmar fascia				
All bones				
All swellings				
1st MP joint, ulnar collateral ligament				
Crepitus				
Range of wrist movement:				
Flexion				
Extension				
Supination				
Pronation				
Radial deviation				
Ulnar deviation				
Plus all hand joint movements; test major tendons				
Sensations:				
Radial nerve				
Ulnar nerve				
Median nerve				
Circulation:				
To whole of hand and wrist. Temperature, pulse, colour.				
Specific tests:				
Fovea				
Praying and reverse				
Grip and fist				
Other:				
Antecubital and axillary nodes				
Finkelstein				

But, technically, for a fracture to be labelled a 'Colles fracture', there have to be several points that can seen on X-ray. They are as in Figure 8.38: fracture through the lower 1 inch (2.5 cm) of the radius with:

- impaction
- dorsal displacement
- dorsal tilting of the distal fragment
- radial deviation of the hand
- ulna styloid fracture.

The strong radial periosteum is torn on the palmar surface following injury, but on the dorsum it remains intact (*see* Figure 8.39).

The 'dinner fork' deformity, easily seen on a lateral viewing of the wrist and hand, is almost like a label saying that a Colles fracture exists. However, don't be complacent: on occasions I have been fooled simply by a large haematoma; always gently palpate as well, if it is appropriate.

Remember other injuries that may occur with a FOOSH; be meticulous about asking and examining, so that no secondary injuries are missed.

Initial management

Remove any rings (*see* Figure 8.40). Although often too late, when the patient first sees you is possibly the last chance before the swelling becomes too great and rings will need cutting off; document this if it is the case.

Suggest and coax the patient to have analgesia. Positioning is all important when making your patient comfortable and there is no 'one size fits all'. Everything depends on their level of pain and what feels best for them. Some possibilities are:

- lying on a trolley with the arm resting on their body, or pillows
- walking and sitting with their arm padded in a broad arm sling
- a temporary plaster of paris slab, held in place with a bandage.

Observation

Ensure that the circulation to the limb is intact (pulse, colour, warmth). With this fracture, an absent circulation to the fingers is very rare, although a little diminution is reasonably common.

Test and document the sensations of the radial, ulnar and median nerves, even though rarely damaged. Finally, despite deformity, you should be able to elicit a reduced level of finger movements (flexion, extension, abduction and adduction).

Give nothing to eat or drink until the person you are referring the patient to has seen them and decided if a reduction is necessary and, if so, the method. Omission here could seriously delay a patient's definitive management.

Post-reduction reviews (plaster checks)

The following general and specific points may also be used when a patient returns from a holiday and has not yet seen anyone in this country.

Many of the points mentioned here will apply equally to other fractures and dislocations around the hand and wrist.

General points

View the X-rays; as well as providing bone positions, they can sometimes show ridges of plaster that may be digging into the skin through padding.

Sort out specific problems and give necessary explanations. If needed, examine so that secondary injuries have not been missed elsewhere; pain from other injuries sometimes only develops later.

Ensure that movements, sensations and circulation of the limb distal to the injury is satisfactory.

Ask questions regarding pain; does its character, position and level fit in with what you would expect at this stage?

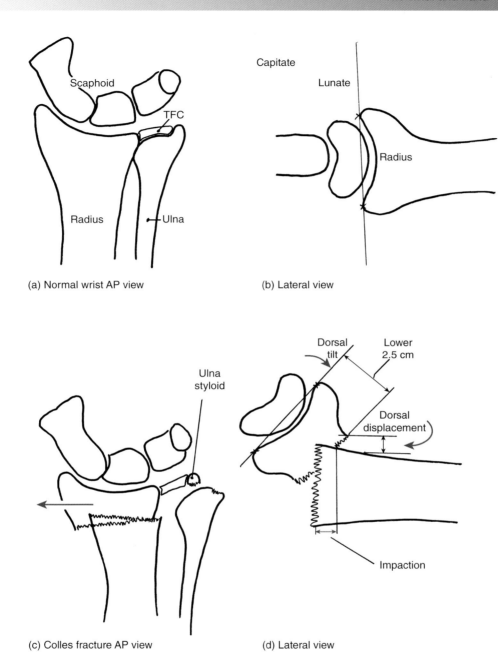

(a) Normal wrist AP view

(b) Lateral view

(c) Colles fracture AP view

(d) Lateral view

Figure 8.38 The recognition of a Colles fracture.

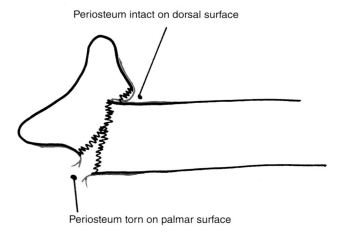

Periosteum intact on dorsal surface

Periosteum torn on palmar surface

Figure 8.39 Damage to the periosteum following a Colles fracture.

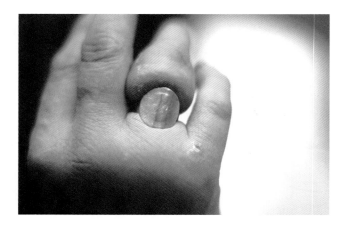

Figure 8.40 Remove rings from fingers as soon as possible.

Specific points regarding the plaster or device

- Look for **swelling**; can this be simply managed with instruction regarding elevation, movement and support, or does the device need adjustment?
- Look for **bruising**; often a patient doesn't expect the 'normal' post-reduction spread of blood and an explanation may give them immense relief.
- Ensure that both the **extent and strength** of the plaster is correct. Is there any damage, **cracks, sodden parts, dents** or **crumbling**?

Smith's fracture

This fracture is not seen often. It has an important place here because although looking like a Colles, if managed in the same way, it will be devastating to the patient. It must be recognised and managed differently.

Definition

The Smith's fracture is a fracture of the lower 2.5 cm of the radius, with anterior tilting and displacement: **the opposite of a Colles fracture**, hence the name 'a reverse Colles', used by some.

Initial management

Early management and observations are very similar to a Colles, the major difference comes with definitive care. Here the periosteum will be intact anteriorly and the distal fragment will need to be pushed posteriorly to regain the correct shape. The forearm will need to be held fully supinated by a full arm POP rather than the short plaster of a Colles, but often open reduction is necessary.

Barton's fracture

This is best thought of as another version of the Smith's fracture, when there is a fracture though the anterior articular surface of the radius. It is unstable and will need operative reduction and plating to prevent slipping.

 Activity 8.21   **Time: Approximately 1 hour**

Now detail the causes, patterns and management of Smith's and Barton's fractures.

As part of your study, you should also consider the rather interesting roles played by the periosteum of the radius during the reduction of both Colles and Smith's fractures.

Scaphoid fracture

The scaphoid fracture is the most common of the carpal fractures, occurring almost anywhere in the bone, but mostly seen at the weaker waist. In children, it is also the most common carpal fracture, but more common distally (Patel, Greydanus and Baker, 2009).

Diagnosis is the main problem; many fractures are clearly seen, but **a few are impossible to see on the usual set of scaphoid views**. If there is clinically a fracture present, but the X-ray appears normal, a routine would be to manage the wrist as a fracture and then repeat the X-ray in 2 weeks. By that time, either new bone growth will show, or reabsorption will have occurred at the fracture site. In either case, the fracture should then be visible (Stevenson, 2012).

The blood supply to the bone is of interest. It enters mostly distally and then spreads throughout the bone. If the distribution along the waist is spread out fairly evenly, all goes well if there is a fracture, with the proximal fragment still getting a reasonable amount of blood.

In some people, the majority of the blood vessels enter the bone distally, so, if fractured, the blood supply to the proximal fragment will be compromised (*see* Figure 8.7). When this occurs, it is called '**avascular necrosis**'; the bone deforms and crumbles, resulting in an arthritic wrist (OA). This is one very tiny bone but a great deal of trouble if it isn't looked after.

Management

Suspicion of the injury is the most important point, followed by effective immobilisation to give the fragments the best possible chance to heal. Opinions on the form of immobilisation vary considerably (Gow, 2000; Al-Nahhas, 2011). There is no one correct way of doing this: POP, brace each have their advocates. The aim is to place the wrist in a position that closes the surrounding bones inwards, holding the scaphoid very firmly (*see* Figure 8.41). The following usually apply:

- Wrist slightly extended.
- Radial deviation.
- Thumb MP abducted.

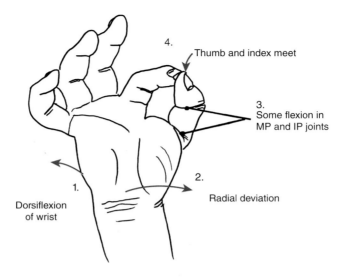

Figure 8.41 The hand and wrist in the position for immobilisation following a scaphoid fracture.

- MP joint slight flexion.
- IP joint slightly flexed, so that the pulp of the thumb will meet with the pulp of the middle finger.

Radial styloid fracture

The standard FOOSH applies, with the pressure mostly on the thenar eminence, although, if you wanted to impress students with your great age, you **could talk of car engine starting handles kicking back!!**

These fractures are commonly fissures or with little displacement. I have never known one to need reduction, just immobilisation in neutral for approximately 6 weeks.

Fractured ulna styloid

This is usually, but not always, part of a Colles or other lower radius fracture. If so, the ulna styloid is not considered in the reduction: it relocates without trouble at the same time as the radius. If this is occurring independently, a form of support is all that is required until pain subsides.

Any ulna styloid fracture indicates avulsion by the ulna collateral ligament complex as the ulnar border of the wrist is stressed.

Bennett's fracture subluxation

This is a small oblique fracture of the base of the thumb metacarpal, including the articular surface of the first CM joint (*see* Figure 8.42). There's usually some subluxation, or outright dislocation of the articular surfaces. The small fragment is 'left behind' and the remainder of the MC displaces radially and proximally.

Other varieties of fracture occur at the base or metaphysis and even a pure dislocation may occur. With children, greenstick varieties are common and the slight deviation of the angle of the cortex on X-ray may be difficult for the inexperienced to see.

The answer is just to see as many X-rays (with feedback) as you possibly can; it is only after extended practice that it becomes easier. The website associated with this book has a selection of my X-rays, along with diagnostic comments to help you get started.

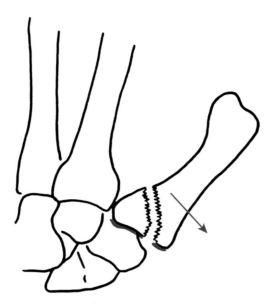

Figure 8.42 Bennett fracture.

With just clinical appearance, any of the previously mentioned injuries are easily confused with a scaphoid fracture. This is because the first CM joint is just 2 cm away and any haematoma easily tracks to fill the anatomical snuff box. However, palpation will find maximal tenderness distal to the scaphoid.

Management

This can range from an undisplaced variety of fracture having a POP applied with the thumb abducted; through to traction and pressure on the MC, then the plaster carefully moulded around the injury site; and, finally, through to open reduction and internal fixation. A great deal depends on the exact site, the displacement and the wishes of the patient.

Fractures of the metacarpals and phalanges

Fractured neck of little finger metacarpal

An isolated fracture of the **neck of the little finger MC** is the most common metacarpal injury. Many, even if considerably displaced, are treated conservatively with excellent functional results. Intervention criteria vary between surgeons Mackway-Jones (2000). Use your own local management guidelines. If at the next fracture clinic, colleagues disagree with your management, no harm will have been done.

Because opinions vary with this injury, it is worth routinely explaining this to the patient, so that they don't think that you have mismanaged them. Early explanation may save the patient much concern.

Remember it is important to ensure that you have not missed a **rotational deformity**. Often it is far from obvious from the direction the patient presents the finger to you. This is true of both metacarpal and phalangeal fractures.

 Activity 8.22   Time: **A quick question**

Which two observations will make a rotational deformity more easily seen? This was mentioned in section 3 of this chapter.

Observations on Activity 8.22:

First, asking the patient to try to make a fist, and, second, looking at the fingertips end on. If you remembered them, very good.

Further metacarpal fractures

Many other forms of MC fractures exist; most are isolated, but may be multiple. They usually have minimal or acceptable flexion displacement and are well splinted by the tissues either side. Swelling will be considerable and, if the patient is allowed home, will need the arm elevated high out of the sling to make the hand comfortable.

Phalangeal fractures

These are tiny, but occasionally troublesome; the management of some can become a challenging injury.

X-rays need to be enlarged and studied with much care. Trace out each IP joint to eliminate subluxations and dislocations; see if flake fractures involve the articular surface.

Management

Precise management of all the above fractures will vary, but some general rules apply. With both metacarpal and phalangeal fractures, the patient will find that the **position of most immediate comfort** is to have **all the joints slightly flexed**, as though holding a ball in the hand (*see* Figure 8.43a). This is ideal as a primary measure to make your patient comfortable, until seen in the fracture clinic. This flexion is also a good position if the surgeons do not expect the joints to regain movement, because, if the joints stiffen, the patient can still oppose with the thumb making the hand useful.

However, although comfortable, this position is not good for eventually regaining full movements. For this the '**position for function**' (*see* Figure 8.43b) is best, with the MP joint flexed to 90° and all the IP joints fully extended. This will keep all the MP and IP joint ligaments in tension so that **no contractures occur**.

Of course, this exact position is almost impossible to obtain: try it now on yourself. I have to press very firmly on my fingers to achieve it! In practice you get as near to it as you can without causing distress. Remember again to **explain to your patient why** the position is used.

As with many tiny fractures of the phalanges, **volar plate avulsion fractures** suffer from a large range of opinion as to the most satisfactory management (Body, 2005). Until randomised trials are designed, the best advice is to follow your local management guidelines.

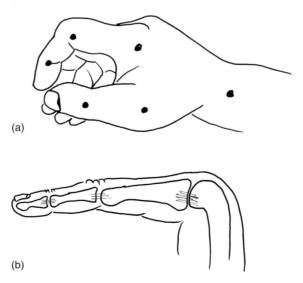

(a)

(b)

Figure 8.43 Hand positions: (a) for most comfort (b) for regaining function.

Dislocations of the hand and wrist

Several dislocations are seen at the wrist. None are common, all are major; in my whole lifetime I have only seen a few. Don't be fooled into thinking all is well because the hand does not look particularly deformed. Your suspicion should be aroused by a painful, swollen and tender hand and wrist, which has obviously suffered a severe force, and this should point you towards immediate X-ray. Only a couple of dislocations will be mentioned here.

Isolated dislocation of the lunate

This injury is best visualised on a lateral X-ray of the wrist, where the crescent of the lunate is clearly seen dislocated to the palmar surface (*see* Figure 8.44). It's **easily overlooked** and the only safe system is to **look for the crescent of the lunate fitting into the capitate** in every lateral wrist X-ray that you see. It will need reduction under general anaesthetic.

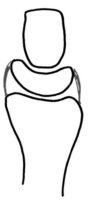

Anterior   Posterior

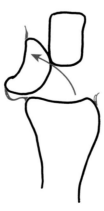

Figure 8.44 One form of dislocation of the lunate

Trans-scaphoid peri-lunate dislocation

This is more serious than the previous dislocation because the force has fractured through the waist of the scaphoid as well. The distal fragment of the scaphoid stays with all of the other carpal bones, while the proximal fragment and the lunate remain in their correct positions.

Activity 8.23   Time: **15 minutes**

Cover up the observations on this activity before you proceed.
  With either of these dislocations, can you think particularly of two complications that would be common? Write them down.

Observations on Activity 8.23

You should first think, how does the lunate get its blood supply? X-rays can be very misleading; seeing the bone swung around doesn't show you the possible damage to the attached blood vessels.

  Next, if the lunate dislocates anteriorly, it will obviously be pressing into the carpal tunnel. So, you should immediately be thinking of pressure on the **median nerve**. Can you remember the extent of the associated dermatome?

Activity 8.24   Time: **About half an hour**

Go to Google Images and look at X-rays of these dislocations. Enlarge the views and compare with normal.
  It is only by knowing the normal thoroughly that you will be able to routinely eliminate wrist dislocations in everyday life.

Soft tissue injuries

Ulnar collateral ligament

Damage to this ligament of the MP joint of the thumb can occur particularly in two ways.

  First, occupational: this is when a patient has to do a **wringing movement** on a frequent basis, putting frequent strain on the ligament over a prolonged time. This eventually causes attrition and the ligament gives way. **Gamekeeper's thumb** is a common title for this, because gamekeepers sometimes wring a bird's neck. Second, following an acute injury, when the thumb is wrenched and the ligament tears. An example of this would be catching a large ball that **hyperextends and abducts** the thumb. A tiny avulsion fracture sometimes occurs.

Diagnosis

With sprains and partial tears (often the most tender and painful on movement), stressing the ligament will produce pain, but the joint will not displace, whereas if completely torn it will easily displace to one side (sometimes without an appreciable increase in pain) (*see* Figure 8.29). Doubt may occur with an anxious patient, who may feel very uneasy, not wanting you to stress it at all.

Management

Incomplete tears will need immobilisation for 6 weeks with a splint or scaphoid type of POP. Complete tears will require repair. If at all in doubt, as always, refer the patient on to someone with more experience.

Triangular fibrocartilage problems

At this stage, go back and refresh your knowledge on wrist anatomy dealing with the TFCC before you go further.

Long-term or sudden acute stress to this complex can lead to continuing problems, varying from little more than a minor sprain to joint pain and instability.

 Activity 8.25   **Time: 10 minutes**

Go to Google Videos or YouTube now and put in 'ulnar fovea test'. You will find many short (2–5 minute) instructive videos on this excellent diagnostic test, and accompanying talks regarding TFCC problems. (But remember there is no peer review on the web!)

Looking at videos for a few minutes like this is an excellent way of having a break and change of scene from reading. At any stage of the book, if you start feeling that your mind is 'drifting', it is well worthwhile breaking off to do something like this. Short videos can be found for almost any condition.

Tendon lacerations

Wounds, burns and scalds are not discussed in this book because so much already exists on these specialities. However, just a few specifics are noted here.

Special points for you to **always** consider with this type of injury:

- Examine wounds **thoroughly** for any possibility of tendon damage.
- If a tendon is visible, it may not be in exactly the same position as when the injury occurred, so an **injury to the tendon may not be visible** to you.
- If you feel that the wound is superficial and that there is no damage to a tendon, still **always test for basic movements**.
- If you are **suspicious** regarding the quality of a movement, **refer**.
- **If suspicious of a glass foreign body, always X-ray**. Glass is usually suspected following pain on direct pressure, but can occasionally be 'cocooned' in a tiny haematoma, which minimises pain in the wound (*see* Figure 8.45).
- Don't be so focused on the wound that you do not **consider a small fracture**; listen carefully to the history.

Sprains to the wrist

As you understand already, there is an intricate system of ligaments throughout the carpus and wrist joints; all of them are easy prey to small-scale sprains. The main action of the practitioner is to rule out more serious conditions or injuries. This is done by careful examination and, if necessary, X-ray. The prime example of this is the scaphoid fracture, which is often initially thought to be a 'simple sprain'; **it must not be missed**. The consequences can sometimes be very severe, even destroying a person's career.

Damage to the nail bed

Nail-bed injuries are very common, especially the 'finger caught in a door' scenario. The possibility of a fracture of the distal phalanx should be considered, but judgement should be used: they do not all need X-ray.

Remarkably, it is rare for any long-term damage or infection to occur, although very acute pain often develops in the early stages with the formation of a **subungual haematoma**.

Management

The subungual haematoma is easily relieved, with either a special tailor-made trephining device or a flamed paper clip (*see* Figure 8.46a). Never use a sharp disposable needle: the point is too long, making it very likely that it will stick into

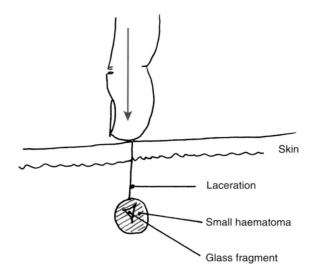

Figure 8.45 How a haematoma may sometimes prevent a glass foreign body giving pain on pressure.

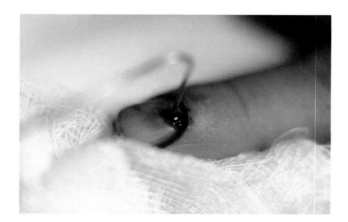

Figure 8.46a To release a subungual haematoma: a glowing red paper clip.

the nail bed. If the haematoma extends to the apex of the nail, trephining will not be necessary; the blood can just be released by inserting a blade through the skin under the nail (*see* Figure 8.46b). In all instances, the nail can be left on as protection, to fall away naturally in the weeks to come (Batrick, 2003).

With or without a haematoma, if the injury is compound, with the proximal part of the nail flipped on top of the skin, a different strategy is necessary. The proximal 'overlapped' part of the nail can either be cut off with scissors, or the nail can be manoeuvred back over the base of the nail.

Mallet deformity

Two conditions cause this deformity of the distal phalanx (*see* Figure 8.32). The first is an avulsion fracture of the base of the distal phalanx when a small flake of bone is pulled off by force applied to the ED tendon. The second is a similar

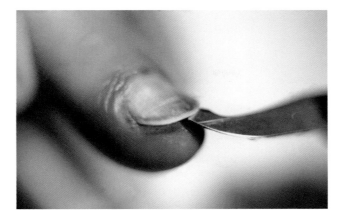

Figure 8.46b To release a subungual haematoma: a sharp blade, only used if the haematoma extends to the edge of the nail.

situation in which the tendon itself gives way instead. An X-ray is required to tell the conditions apart. Both are initially managed with some form of splint that keeps the distal phalanx in hyperextension for a few weeks. Very occasionally, operative repair is necessary later.

Section 5
Minor musculoskeletal conditions

Trigger finger

This condition can be congenital, but I am only mentioning the common acquired form occurring in later life. This is possibly a result of tendinitis or overuse of flexor tendons at the base of the fingers in the palm. Whatever the cause, it leads to a thickening of the tendon into a small nodule (Lundin, Eliasson and Aspenberg, 2012). This has difficulty sliding through the synovial sheath and the nodule becomes intermittently trapped. The patient manipulates it and the finger usually 'snaps' out straight again in seconds.

As the patient presents to you, there is nothing to be done except to explain to them what the condition is and refer them on to their GP for definitive management later. Your reassurance of this benign but alarming condition will be a great relief.

Soft tissue infections

Common to all infections I mention, you have to assess the progress. Ask yourself, is it:

- clearly **retained locally** with a surrounding area of erythema not increasing in size
- **spreading locally**, with the erythema increasing, but not passing fibrous boundaries
- **spreading throughout the hand** with cellulitis
- **lymphangitis** up the forearm
- **lymphangitis**, plus **lymphadenitis** at elbow or axilla
- also showing features of **spread to the general circulation**, with the patient feeling unwell, with raised temperature, etc.?

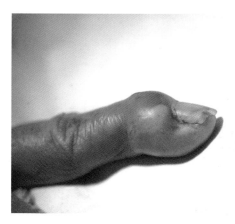

Figure 8.47 A paronychia.

Paronychia (Whitlow)

This is the most common of the hand infections. It can be visually stunning (*see* Figure 8.47), but starts in an insignificant way with minor redness around the nail fold.

It is caused by a minor break in the skin around the nail bed, sometimes habitual nail biting or an insignificant scratch from gardening.

Forms and features

Depending on the patient and the bacteria involved, a battle will ensue. Often the redness will settle down and disappear on its own with the patient never needing advice.

Alternatively, pus may start to form that can be difficult to see in the first few hours. If allowed to progress, the redness and pus will increase. But in all but the very worst cases the infection will stay confined by the fibrous septa between the distal and middle phalanges.

Tenderness is localised around the nail bed. Sometimes you are presented with a generally reddened distal phalanx and it is this maximal tenderness at the nail fold that is your most accurate diagnostic feature.

At any stage, antibiotics may be able to bring the infection under control, but those who attend any unit are usually at a stage that also requires the pus to be released for most pain relief and rapid settling of the condition (Shaw, 2005).

Patient advice

Stress to your patient how strict **elevation** of the limb will often be **as, or more effective, than analgesics**. This means walking around the house with the limb held up in the air, or, when sitting down, having it elevated on a cushion on the arm of a chair. Doing this will eliminate throbbing in the acute stages and get you more patient compliance than having it in a sling.

Ongoing management

Occasionally in health workers, a paronychia may be caused by the **herpes simplex virus**. If you are suspicious of this, it will not be for simple incision; refer your patient on.

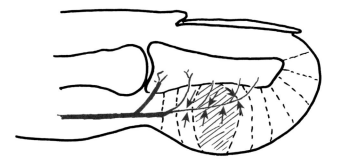

Figure 8.48 Lateral view of the blood supply to the terminal phalanx, the build-up of pus impeding the circulation in a pulp space infection.

Pulp space infection (Felon)

Compared with the paronychia, this is a far worse condition to have, a '**Pit-bull terrier' of infections**. It is usually caused by a seemingly trivial puncture wound to the pulp; in fact the causative injury is usually forgotten by the patient as the infection develops.

Clinical features

Tenderness in maximal over the pulp space, rather than the nail fold. The pulp is tense, sometimes dark 'congested' red. Don't expect to see the pus causing the pain.

The problem occurs because of the compartmentalisation of the pulp (section 1). With a worsening focus of infection, increased fluid and pus formation causes a pressure rise in one of these compartments (*see* Figure 8.48). Eventually interruption of the blood supply to parts of the distal phalanx occurs, sparing the base.

This mix of ischaemic tissues plus infection frequently results in osteomyelitis of the distal phalanx.

Initial management

Immediate referral to a senior doctor is important, rather than a junior who is new to such conditions and may not even know of the complication of osteomyelitis.

Ongoing hospital management

The secret of management is to recognise the formation of pus early, and to have it released before the pressure cuts off the blood supply to the bone. Obviously rest, elevation, analgesia, culture, sensitivity and antibiotics all have their place.

An excellent golden rule with a pulp space infection is the following:

GOLDEN RULE

With finger infections, if your patient has lost a night's sleep, then pus is likely to be present, requiring incision and drainage.

You should take in general pointers when assessing the patient's level of pain and discomfort. For example:

- Painful fingers are usually held flexed.
- Patients in pain don't walk with hands down by their side, or move their hand around a lot. The hand is kept high to ease the intense throbbing pain.
- They are frightened of you touching or moving it.

Apical pulp infection

Before we leave pulp space infections, I want to discuss this variety that has fewer complications.

 Activity 8.26   Time: **A quick question**

Why should a focus of infection at the apex (tip of the finger) be any different from the other pulp space infections? Write a brief comment and then look at my observations.

Observations on Activity 8.26

Now this is not too bad a condition. Because of its position at the apex, there are usually no fibrous septa dividing the pulp, and the digital arteries have long before gone into the distal phalanx, so there is no problem with osteomyelitis. The pus is easily evacuated thoroughly; in many instances, this can be done without an anaesthetic by decompression through a 'V' cut with scissors into the end of the nail.

Pyogenic tenosynovitis

This is a very unpleasant infection of the tendon sheath. Because of their extent (*see* section 1), the infection does not stay in one segment of the finger but spreads easily (and painfully) throughout the whole length.

Features

The following features should be carefully investigated:

- Flexion of the finger and **excruciating pain** if passive extension is attempted.
- Swelling/erythema extending through all the finger segments.
- Tenderness throughout the whole length of the finger.

The cause is usually a perforating puncture injury over the site of the sheath.

Initial management

Definitive management will not wait and requires immediate admission with hand surgeon advice.
Obviously rest of the part, elevation, analgesia, culture, sensitivity and antibiotics all have their place.

Deep palmar and web space infections

The palmar space infection is a deep-seated infection underneath the strong and unyielding palmar fascia. The cause is usually a puncture wound to the palm. Developing pus may stay in the palm, or commonly track distally to 'point' at the nearest web space, pushing the fingers apart (*see* Figure 8.30). This web space can also become directly infected from a wound in the web.

Clinical features

Once established, you are usually presented with **gross swelling on the dorsum** of the hand, but erythema is more evident on the palmar surface. There will be associated severe throbbing pain in the hand and tenderness in the palm.

Management

These conditions are discussed here for completeness because they are hardly minor. As rather deep-seated infections, they require expert and timely intervention, with admission and incision under GA.

As the abscess is developing, the features may not be as obvious, hence the SOS advice that I have asked you to give to all your patients. The golden rule must always be, to say with any infection:

GOLDEN RULE

If there are any problems that develop, and you are worried, return at any time.

Having to waiting in pain at home, possibly throughout the night, is unfair.

Beware of the '**collar-stud**' form of abscess. This is when pus forms both superficially and deeply. The inexperienced see and drain the superficial part of the abscess, not realising the **deeper pus below the palmar fascia** (*see* Figure 8.49).

Boils (furuncles) and carbuncles

On the dorsal surface of the skin of the digits are hairs – more obvious in males. We are prone to occasionally get boils (one head) or carbuncles (more than one head) originating in these hair follicles. The infection is usually caused by Staph. aureus.

Although boils and carbuncles can sometimes look alarming, the majority are self-contained, not spreading beyond the soft tissues of the finger segment in question and quickly settling without antibiotics when the pus is released.

Management

Most boils and carbuncles are easily dealt with in the community without the patient ever seeking professional help. Those attending usually have more severe forms that may need the pus evacuating, dressings and antibiotic cover.

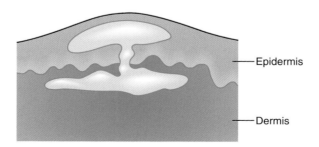

Epidermis

Dermis

Figure 8.49 'Collar stud' abscess (Duckworth and Blundell, 2010).

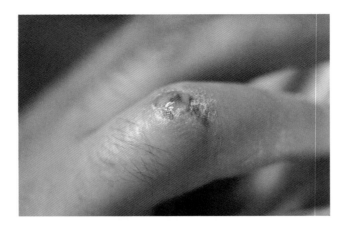

Figure 8.50 Septic arthritis of an IP joint.

Septic arthritis (pyogenic arthritis)

This is a very serious condition indeed and you need to be suspicious of the possibility of it. Be on the lookout for:

- infection centred over a joint
- history of puncture wound
- severe pain on joint movement
- infection that is not responding to treatment.

Early X-rays could show a foreign body, but will be negative for bone changes.

One example that I particularly remember was a patient being managed for an infected laceration over an IP joint, which was continuing to worsen after management for a week. Just the fact that **the usual course of treatment was having no effect** alerted me to the possibility of septic arthritis and I immediately referred the patient to a hand surgeon who confirmed the diagnosis (*see* Figure 8.50).

Never put off referral of a patient to someone more experienced if you have diagnostic doubts. The result will more often be negative but, so long as you can give an account of your reasoning (this book will help you), there is no shame. Knowledge and experience only build up over the years.

Fungal nail infections

Briefly mentioned under the section 3 of this chapter, fungal infections of the nails themselves are common. There tends to be a chronic presentation, with the condition having been there for months, steadily worsening.

Usually pain-free, the appearance can vary from yellowing, whitening, or browning of the nail, which will be fragmented, deformed or lifting off its bed.

Management

Reassurance that it is nothing serious is the main task, accompanied by health advice.

Signposting to the patient's GP is best so that they can decide on the worth of antifungal drugs and sometimes necessary prolonged treatment, both for the fingers and possibly affected toes.

Psoriasis

Thought of by most as simply a rash, commonly seen on the extensor surfaces of the elbows and knees, this is also a reasonably common cause of a poly-arthritis (Psoriatric arthritis). Usually this will not be too severe, most commonly affecting the DIP joints of the fingers and toes.

Orf

Just a passing mention is all that is necessary here. This infection, which is seen fairly often in country or farm dwellers, is quite unusual generally.

It presents as a rounded, raised, sometimes painful, red to blue pustule. It usually appears on the back of the hand and is common in those who have recently been in contact with sheep. It is caused by a virus and will heal in weeks if there is no secondary bacterial infection.

Once again, something that often doesn't need any active management from you, but your town-dweller patient returning from a country holiday will be eternally grateful for your knowledge and reassurance that they are not dying of bubonic plague!

Malignant melanoma

Any patient with a dark mark under a nail bed, especially one that you cannot recognise immediately as trivial, should be referred. This is so uncommon in this situation or elsewhere on the hands that I have never seen one, but they occur and should always be a possibility at the back of your mind.

Dupuytren's contracture

This is a crippling contracture of the **palmar fascia** (aponeurosis) occurring in middle age with a possible family history.

It starts insidiously with the little finger not able to extend completely, but it can progress over the years to draw all of the fingers into the palm.

Not a 'minors' problem, but rather a condition for orthopaedic or plastic referral for surgery in the future.

De Quervain's tenosynovitis

This condition is usually seen in middle age and is associated with a degree of overuse of the wrist and thumb. Often this is doing everyday tasks just a little more frequently – for instance, while doing some heavy DIY. The tendons of EPB and Abd. PL become thickened, with associated swelling of the wrist, and this prevents them from running smoothly inside their synovial sheath. To complicate the problem further, the sheaths are held down against the radius by fascia, making a tighter 'fit'.

RA is another common cause of this inflammation.

The patient presents with pain and tenderness over the tendons anteriorly as they run over the radial styloid, and crepitus can often be felt as the thumb is moved. Do you remember my mentioning **Finkelstein's test** in section 3? It's a useful diagnostic tool.

Management

Splinting of the thumb in slight extension and abduction should ease the discomfort considerably, along with rest and elevation of the part and anti-inflammatory drugs.

Local steroid injections or operations to ease constrictions are occasionally necessary.

Another similar condition sometimes occurs, when the tendons of ECRL and ECRB cross over the EPB and Abd. PL causing very similar features a few inches further up the forearm (**intersection syndrome**).

Sudeck's atrophy/Complex regional pain syndrome/Reflex sympathetic dystrophy syndrome/Shoulder-hand syndrome/

Quite what you call it, or its exact cause, I wouldn't care to say. And with anything that has this many names, it usually means that the experts in the field aren't all that sure either!

What I do know for sure is that reasonably commonly a condition can suddenly appear a few weeks following an injury like a fracture, usually near the wrist. Its course is prolonged with a 'burning' type of pain, swelling, shiny skin and discomfort, often severe, varying tremendously.

To make matters worse, there is no specific treatment except support, until it subsides. The mainstay is **timely** intensive physiotherapy.

One useless piece of information that may be of interest: Prince Charles had this condition following an arm fracture playing polo many years ago.

Delayed rupture of extensor pollicis longus

This well-recognised complication of a Colles fracture usually occurs some weeks after the injury. It is thought that it is possibly caused by friction at the site of the tendon passing over the fracture site, causing long-term damage to the fibres as well as weakness.

Management

This is by referral to orthopaedics; depending on the circumstances and the patient, it may require surgical repair.

Kienbock's disease

In this condition, and due to a vascular problem, the lunate bone necroses, collapses and deforms. This in turn later causes OA of the wrist, compounding the problem.

It occurs in late teens to young adults, has a slow onset but progresses, sometimes causing serious damage to the wrist joint. The exact cause is not known, but a short ulna is sometimes thought to be the instigator, stressing the bone.

Although the patient doesn't usually present for help until the disease has progressed for possibly months or more, you may be the first to be approached with the condition. You should consider it with any patient demonstrating pain or other features centred near the lunate.

Management for you is to be suspicious of it and get an initial X-ray.

 Activity 8.27   **Time:** **A short scenario for you, perhaps 15 minutes**

Cover up my observations on this activity and then read on.

The X-ray returns and shows changes that are consistent with Kienbock's. What could you tell the patient? Write down some ideas briefly.

Observations on Activity 8.27

Diagnosis is beyond our remit. However, an explanation to the patient could go along the lines of, 'I can see some arthritic changes, so I want to refer you. . .'

With that they will be relieved that a cause of their pain can be seen and that you are passing them on to a specialist; also they will have the word 'arthritis' to go home and wait with – not a load of fun, but not terrifying like the more sinister 'changes that need investigating.'

There is no completely right or wrong answer to this question. I feel it would be wrong to presume a definitive diagnosis from an X-ray alone; you or I would simply not see enough of this type of condition to become confident.

REFERENCES AND SUGGESTED READING

Al-Nahhas, S. (2011) Do Wrist Splints Need to Have Thumb Extensions when Immobilising Suspected Scaphoid Fractures, www.bestbets.org (accessed 24 May 2013).

Batrick, N. (2003) Treatment of Uncomplicated Subungual Haemotoma, www.bestbets.org (accessed 24 May 2013).

Body, R. (2005) Early Mobilisation for Volar Plate Avulsion fractures, www.bestbets.org (accessed 24 May 2013).

Duckworth, T. and Blundell, C.M. (2010) *Lecture Notes on Orthopaedics and Fractures*, 4th edn, Wiley Blackwell, Oxford.

Ellis, H. and Mahadevan, V. (2010) *Clinical Anatomy*, 12th edn, Wiley Blackwell, Oxford.

Gow, K. (2000) Immobilisation of Suspected Scaphoid Fractures, www.bestbets.org (accessed 24 May 2013).

Gross, J., Fetto, J. and Rosen, E. (2009) *Musculoskeletal Examination*, 3rd edn, Wiley Blackwell, Oxford.

Heaver, C., Goonetilleke, K.S., Ferguson, H. and Shiralkar, S. (2011) Hand-arm vibration syndrome: a common occupational hazard in industrialized countries. *Journal of Hand Surgery* (European volume), 36 (5), 354–363.

Mackway-Jones, K. (2000) Management of Fractures of the Neck of the Fifth Metacarpal, www.bestbets.org (accessed 24 May 2013).

Lundin, A.C., Eliasson, P. and Aspenberg P. (2012) Trigger finger and tendinosis. *Journal of Hand Surgery* (European volume), 37 (3), 233–236 .

Patel, D.R., Greydanus, D. and Baker, R. (2009) *Pediatric Practice Sports Medicine*, 1st edn, McGraw-Hill, New York.

Shaw, J. (2005) Incision and Drainage Preferable to Oral Antibiotics in Acute Paronychia Nail Infection, www.bestbets.org (accessed 24 May 2013).

Stevenson, J.D. (2012) Early CT for suspected occult scaphoid fractures. *Journal of Hand Surgery* (European edition), 37 (5), 447–451 .

Tortora, G.J. and Nielsen, M.T. (2012) *Principles of Human Anatomy*, 12th edn, Wiley Blackwell, Oxford.

Multiple choice questions

Before you start, take in the reasoning behind these MCQs, how to answer them and how to interpret the results, from the section at the end of Chapter 1.

1. **Regarding the sensory dermatomes of the hand:**
   A The median nerve supplies the pulp of the middle finger
   B The skin over the posterior of the index and middle MC is supplied by the radial nerve
   C The skin over the hypothenar eminence is supplied by the ulnar nerve
   D The above dermatomes never vary

2. **The flexor digitorum profundus tendon:**
   A Is supplied solely by the median nerve
   B Is inserted into the base of the distal phalanx
   C Has a synovial sheath
   D Is inserted into the shaft of the middle phalanx

3. **Heberden's or Bouchard's nodes are found solely in:**
   A RA
   B OA
   C Gout
   D The 30–50 year age group

4. **Specific complications of a Colles fracture include:**
   A Fat embolism
   B Mal union
   C Sudeck's atrophy
   D Myositis ossificans

5. **The scaphoid:**
   A Obtains its blood supply via its waist
   B Articulates with the lunate and trapezium
   C Articulates with the triquetrum and the triangular fibro cartilage
   D Has a proximal and distal pole

6. **A Bennett's fracture:**
   A Is oblique
   B Avoids the articular surface

   C   Involves the index finger MC
   D   Is associated with subluxation of the thumb MC from the trapezium

7.   **The TFCC:**

   A   Articulates with the pisiform on the lateral border of the wrist.
   B   Is only associated with minor sprains of the wrist.
   C   Attaches in part to the ulna styloid.
   D   Forms attachments to the lunate.

8.   **Which of the following are commonly caused by a FOOSH:**

   A   Barton's fracture
   B   Fractured distal phalanx
   C   Swan neck deformity
   D   Mallet deformity

9.   **A pulp space infection:**

   A   Is associated with Sudeck's atrophy
   B   Is a major cause of osteomyelitis
   C   Requires early recognition of pus formation
   D   Has maximal tenderness at the nail fold

10.   **Dislocation of the lunate:**

   A   May lead to ischemic necrosis
   B   Occurs with the concavity facing posteriorly
   C   Shows most clearly on an AP X-ray view
   D   May be a FOOSH injury

Answers are available at the end of the book. For an explanation of these answers and further resources visit the companion website at:

www.wiley.com/go/bradley/musculoskeletal

Part 3

The lower body

The lower back and hip

This is one of the smaller chapters for you, with far fewer injuries and conditions to study. That doesn't in any way detract from the need for you to study it in as much detail as you can. As elsewhere in this book, the golden rule must be as follows:

GOLDEN RULE

The only safe way to make a minor injury diagnosis is to eliminate the major causes of particular features.

Aim

To develop an in-depth understanding of the anatomy and physiology, history, examination and early management of minor musculoskeletal injuries and conditions of the lower back and hip.

Outcomes

That, by the end of this study, and all the associated activities and clinical experiences, you will be able to:

- demonstrate an in-depth knowledge of the anatomy and physiology of musculoskeletal structures around the lower back and hip
- take an effective history and examine patients presenting with lower back and hip problems, forming a differential diagnosis
- demonstrate an in-depth knowledge of minor musculoskeletal injuries and conditions of the lower back and hip
- apply these skills to the early management of patients, recognising any need for referral.

Managing Minor Musculoskeletal Injuries and Conditions, First Edition. David Bradley.
© 2014 John Wiley & Sons, Ltd. Published 2014 by John Wiley & Sons, Ltd.
Companion website: www.wiley.com/go/bradley/musculoskeletal

Section 1
Applied anatomy and physiology

As previously, we start with the skeleton and its joints and build on this with the soft tissues: muscles, fascia, bursae, etc.

Bones

Lumbar vertebrae

These bones are the 'dinosaurs' of the vertebral column, huge and chunky, made to carry much of the weight of the upper body. They are based on a ring of bone surrounding the spinal cord and cauda equina.

Parts that you need to remember are shown in Figure 9.1 and include the following:

- Spinous process.
- Transverse processes.
- Vertebral body.
- Pedicle.
- Articular processes (superior and inferior).
- Vertebral foramen (triangular in shape).

 Activity 9.1   Time: **Half an hour**

Further study will have to be done later, on the detail of the parts just listed. However, just for now, study the relationship of the abdominal aorta and posterior peritoneum to the vertebrae. This in particular is very 'majors' study. But remember, to be a good minor injury practitioner, you have to be able to eliminate major conditions first.

Intervertebral foramen

An intervertebral foramen is formed by the positioning of the hollows in the pedicles of the vertebrae immediately above and below. The foramina are approximately the diameter of a pencil and act as an opening for the passage of the spinal nerve. As in the cervical vertebrae, you will remember that they are numbered from the vertebrae forming the bottom half of the foramen, *see* Figure 5.2 in Chapter 5.

The major muscles controlled by nerves from specific root levels are as follows:

- L1 and L2: Psoas (flexes hip).
- L3: The quads (extend knee and patella reflex).
- L4: Tibialis anterior (dorsiflexes ankle and patella reflex).

 Activity 9.2   Time: **About an hour**

This is a brief overview of the lumbar plexus and in no way complete. At a suitable time, read further, including the associated construction of the spinal nerves. Finally, study the positioning of the intervertebral disc in relation to the vertebral foramen.

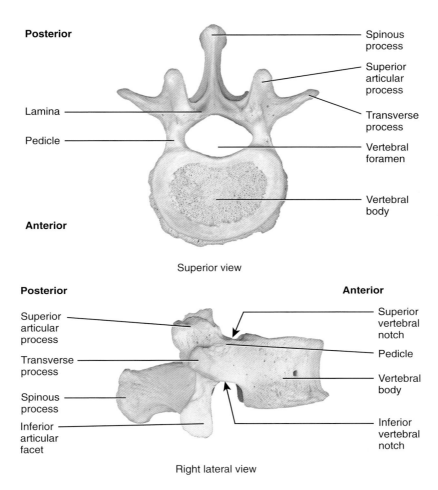

Posterior

Spinous process

Superior articular process

Lamina

Transverse process

Pedicle

Vertebral foramen

Vertebral body

Anterior

Superior view

Posterior

Anterior

Superior articular process

Superior vertebral notch

Transverse process

Pedicle

Spinous process

Vertebral body

Inferior articular facet

Inferior vertebral notch

Right lateral view

Figure 9.1 Lumbar vertebrae (Tortora and Nielsen, 2012). This material is reproduced with permission of John Wiley & Sons, Inc.

With age, osteophytic lipping may cause narrowing of an individual foramen or several foramina, causing compression to the nerve root at a particular level.

Facet joints

These tiny synovial joints are formed from the superior articular processes of a lower vertebra, with the inferior articular processes of an upper vertebra. Each of the joints, which are arranged vertically, is supported by its own small ligaments.

Sacrum

This is basically a triangular bone, concave anteriorly, which is formed by the fusion of the sacral vertebrae. It has massive articular surfaces either side for the iliac bones forming the sacro-iliac joints, and forms the posterior segment to complete the 'pelvic ring'.

Some of the root levels are:

- Level L5: Extensor hallucis longus (extends the big toe).
- Level S1: Gastrocnemius and soleus (plantar flex the ankle).

Coccyx

This is another triangular bone about the size of the distal phalanx of the thumb and formed from minute rudimentary vertebrae. It 'sits' on the end of the sacrum and forms attachments for pelvic muscles. It can be felt with a finger in the rectum (of clinical significance following a fall on the bottom)!

Intervertebral discs

These are situated between the vertebral bodies, formed from an inner (thick treacle) type of substance called the '**nucleus pulposus**' and surrounded by a fibro-cartilaginous outer layer – the **annulus fibrosus**. With age they can diminish in size, making the gap between the bodies narrowed.

Ligaments of the lumbar sacral spinal column

These are as follows (*see* Figure 5.7 in Chapter 5):

- Anterior longitudinal.
- Posterior longitudinal.
- Ligamentum flavum.
- Interspinous ligament.
- Supraspinous ligament.

They should be fairly fresh in your mind since studying the cervical vertebrae.

Pelvis

Become familiar with the following features shown in Figure 9.2:

- Two innominate bones:
  - Ilium.
  - Ischium.
- Pubis.
- Sacro-iliac joint.
- Acetabulum.
- Pubis symphysis.
- Pubic ramus.
- Pubic arch.
- Ischial tuberosity.
- Iliac crest.
- Pelvic brim.
- Obturator foramen.
- Anterior superior iliac spine.
- Anterior inferior iliac spine.
- Greater and lesser sciatic notch.

The 'pelvic ring' is formed by the two innominate bones with the sacrum.

Upper femur

The head forms approximately two-thirds of a complete sphere and has a small pit in the tip called the '**fovea-capitis**'. A ligament fits in there (**ligamentum teres**), through which blood vessels reach some of the top of the head. The majority of the blood supply to the head comes upwards through folds of the joint capsule running up the neck.

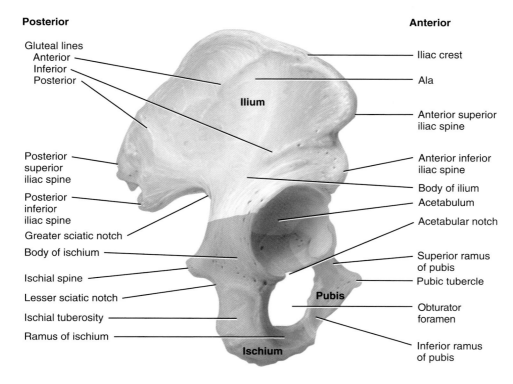

Posterior

Gluteal lines
  Anterior
  Inferior
  Posterior

Posterior
superior
iliac spine

Posterior
inferior
iliac spine

Greater sciatic notch

Body of ischium

Ischial spine

Lesser sciatic notch

Ischial tuberosity

Ramus of ischium

Ilium

Anterior

Iliac crest

Ala

Anterior superior
iliac spine

Anterior inferior
iliac spine

Body of ilium

Acetabulum

Acetabular notch

Superior ramus
of pubis

Pubic tubercle

Pubis

Obturator
foramen

Ischium

Inferior ramus
of pubis

Figure 9.2 Detailed lateral view of the right innominate bone (Tortora and Nielsen, 2012). This material is reproduced with permission of John Wiley & Sons, Inc.

The upper part of the neck is inside the joint capsule of the hip and does not have a layer of periosteum. The blood supply to the head is rather precarious to say the least. It comes from three sources:

1. Vessels running up the neck beneath the synovium into the head; these form the only significant supply and are frequently torn with fractures of the neck. They originate from the circumflex arteries surrounding the neck.
2. A few small vessels inside the bone of the neck.
3. Inside the ligamentum teres.

 Activity 9.3   **Time: 15 minutes**

Take a little time now to appreciate the extent and shape of the growing epiphysis that forms the head of the femur, the femoral capital epiphysis (some call it the 'upper femoral epiphysis'). Making a brief sketch (possibly just in the margin here) will help you appreciate a problem a little later in the chapter! Anything helps that gets you away from just reading about a topic.

Copy an image from a search engine like Google, or any anatomy and physiology book to hand.

Hip joint

The hip, a synovial ball and socket, is formed by the articulation of the head with the acetabulum. The 'cup' of the acetabulum is divided equally by the ilium, ischium and pubis. Inside, the hyaline cartilage forms a 'C' shape with a

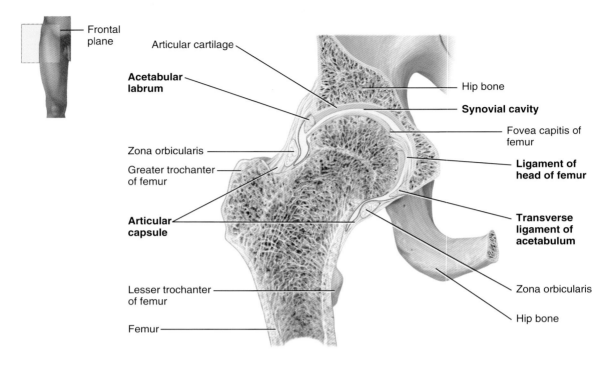

Frontal plane

Articular cartilage

Acetabular labrum

Zona orbicularis

Greater trochanter of femur

Articular capsule

Lesser trochanter of femur

Femur

Hip bone

Synovial cavity

Fovea capitis of femur

Ligament of head of femur

Transverse ligament of acetabulum

Zona orbicularis

Hip bone

Figure 9.3 Right hip joint, frontal section (Tortora and Nielsen, 2012). This material is reproduced with permission of John Wiley & Sons, Inc.

hollowing in the centre for the base of the **ligamentum teres**. The gap in the 'C', which is placed inferiorly, is called the '**acetabular notch**'; it allows blood vessels to enter the joint (*see* Figure 9.3).

Around the rim of the articular surface of the actetabulum is a ring of fibro-cartilage, the **acetabular labrum**, helping to deepen the socket.

The very strong capsule passes from the rim of the acetabulum to the neck of the femur.

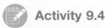 **Activity 9.4**   Time: **30 minutes**

Going by what occurs in other joints, what type of structures would strengthen this hip capsule? Write your answer, then follow with my observations.

Observations on Activity 9.4

The hip is strengthened by strong ligaments that blend into the capsule (*see* Figures 9.4a and 9.4b). They are the following:

- Iliofemoral (an upside down 'Y' shape), whose base is uppermost at the anterior inferior iliac spine, the ends to the extremes of the intertrochanteric line.
- Pubofemoral.
- Ischiofemoral.

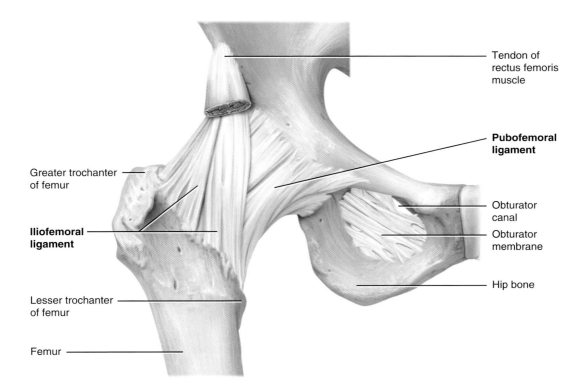

Figure 9.4a Right hip joint to show the capsule: anterior view (Tortora and Nielson, 2012). This material is reproduced with permission of John Wiley & Sons, Inc.

- Ligamentum teres, delta shaped, arising from the acetabular fossa and transverse acetabular ligament, and going to the fovea of the femoral head.

Several surrounding muscles also support the joint.

Major muscle groups

Near the hip

For now, learn the basics concerning the following groups. Later, possibly when you have finished studying the book, cover them again in detail.

Quadriceps femoris (quads) (extend the knee):

- Rectus femoris.
- Vastus lateralis.
- Vastus medialis.
- Vastus intermedius (*see* Figure 9.5).

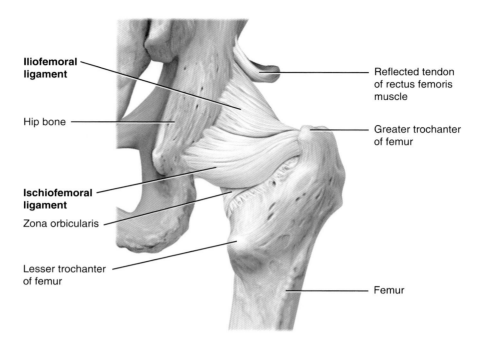

Figure 9.4b Right hip joint to show the capsule: posterior view (Tortora and Nielsen, 2012). This material is reproduced with permission of John Wiley & Sons, Inc.

Hamstrings (mostly flex the knee and extend the hip):

- Semi-membranosus.
- Semi-tendinosus.
- Biceps femoris (*see* Figure 9.6).

Glutei

- G. maximus (abducts and laterally rotates thigh).
- G. medius (abducts and medially rotates thigh).
- G. minimus (abducts and medially rotates thigh) (*see* Figure 9.7).

Hip adductors

- Adductor longus, brevis and magnus.
- Gracilis (*see* Figure 9.8).

Psoas (note silent 'P')

Flexes the thigh at the hip and flexes vertebrae. It has its origins mostly from the transverse processes of the lumbar vertebrae, joining with **iliacus** on the upper iliac fossa, to form the **iliopsoas**, inserting into the lesser trochanter of the femur (*see* Figure 9.9).

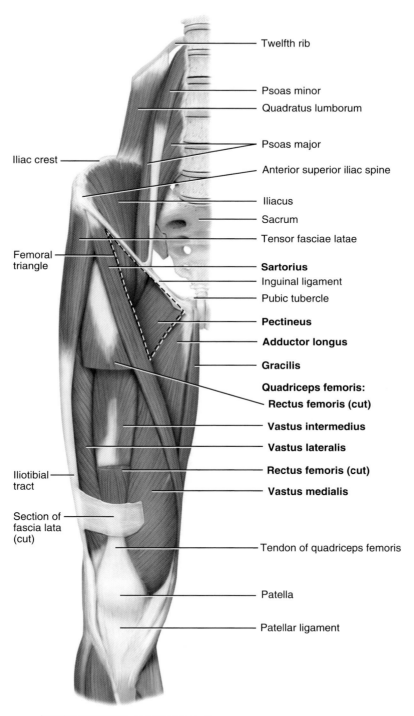

Twelfth rib

Psoas minor

Quadratus lumborum

Psoas major

Anterior superior iliac spine

Iliac crest

Iliacus

Sacrum

Tensor fasciae latae

Femoral triangle

Sartorius

Inguinal ligament

Pubic tubercle

Pectineus

Adductor longus

Gracilis

Quadriceps femoris:

Rectus femoris (cut)

Vastus intermedius

Vastus lateralis

Rectus femoris (cut)

Iliotibial tract

Vastus medialis

Section of fascia lata (cut)

Tendon of quadriceps femoris

Patella

Patellar ligament

Anterior superficial view (the femoral triangle is indicated by a dashed line)

Figure 9.5 Muscles of the thigh: anterior superficial view (the femoral triangle is indicated by a dashed line) (Tortora and Nielsen, 2012). This material is reproduced with permission of John Wiley & Sons, Inc.

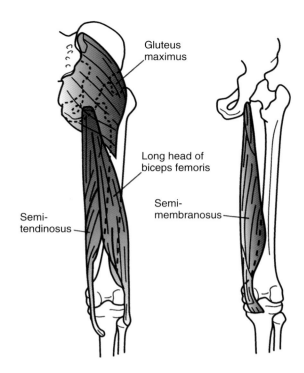

Figure 9.6 Extensors of the hip (Gross *et al.*, 2009).

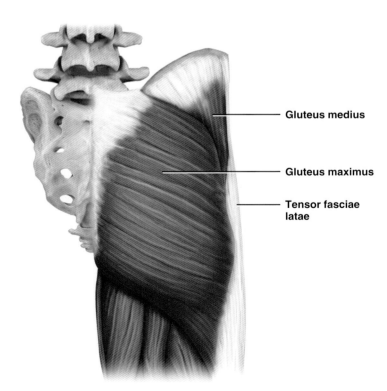

Figure 9.7 Muscles of the gluteal region: posterior superficial view (Tortora and Nielsen, 2012). This material is reproduced with permission of John Wiley & Sons, Inc.

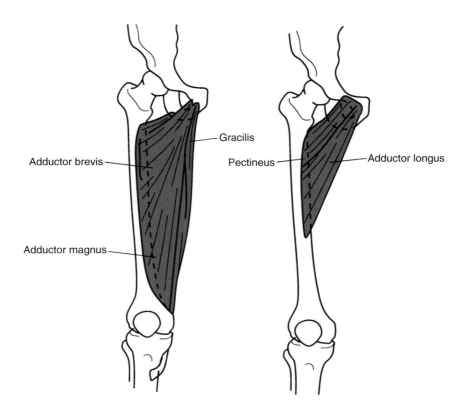

Figure 9.8 Hip adductors (Gross *et al.*, 2009).

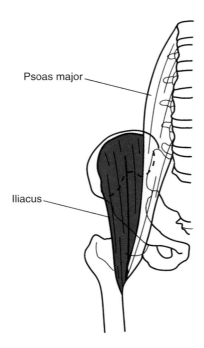

Figure 9.9 Flexors of the hip (Gross *et al.*, 2009).

Sartorius

This flexes the hip, and also adbucts and causes lateral rotation of the thigh.

Pyriformis

This originates from the anterior sacrum and inserts into the upper greater trochanter. The action is lateral rotation of the thigh.

In the lower back

- Latissimus dorsi.
- Erector spinae.
- Internal and external oblique.
- Quadratus lumborum.

Bursae

The **trochanteric bursa** is the most significant, situated directly over the greater trochanter, but others under the **psoas** and **obturator externus** tendons exist without causing as much trouble. Know of their general position now and look at the nearby structures that will increase pain if the bursa becomes inflamed (*see* Figure 9.10).

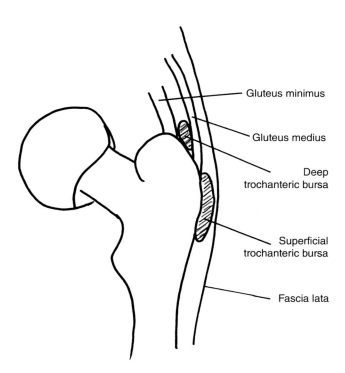

Gluteus minimus

Gluteus medius

Deep trochanteric bursa

Superficial trochanteric bursa

Fascia lata

Figure 9.10 Some bursae around the hip.

Fibrous tissue

Fascia latae (lata)

This shows on several of the illustrations nearby, especially Figure 9.5. It is an extensive sheet of strong fascia running down the outside of the thigh and dipping inwards dividing muscle groups. It starts at the iliac crest and inguinal ligament, and has many muscular attachments.

Iliotibial band or tract

This is a long and strong length of the fascia latae, passing downward over the bursa of the greater trochanter, down the outside of the thigh, finally curving inwards just at the level of the knee joint and inserting into the lateral aspect of the tibia near the tibial tuberosity. These are important structures for you to become aware of.

Section 2
History and mechanism of injury

A major point to stress in this section is the region's close proximity to the trunk and therefore the possibility of the origin of the clinical features being mistaken for musculoskeletal, when they are in fact referred from 'major surgical' areas.

In many situations, the onset and initial history of a major condition are exactly the same as those of a minor; referral for a senior opinion may therefore be the definitive route. Often your instinct will have to be your guide. Below are listed some mechanisms and history pointers that may assist decision making.

Lower back pain

Lifting an object by **bending the back**, instead of keeping the back straight and bending the knees, is the classical mechanism for both major as well as minor lower back injuries, and the main feature of the majority of 'health and safety' advice. Add to this an element of **rotation** – for instance, to pick something up from the side – and the danger of injury is considerably increased (*see* Figure 9.11).

Take every opportunity that you can to reinforce the dangers of bending and twisting to your patients. This may not help them too much over their current problem, but may save a disc prolapse in the future. Minds may be very open to your suggestions while they are in pain!

Red flags

Here are just **some** aspects of a patient's history that should make you extra cautious in your back pain diagnosis; expansion on this may be found in Simon (2011).

Although this listing is specific to patients with lower back pain, many of the principles can be applied elsewhere:

- A history of any **malignancy**. Even if many years ago, this could indicate new secondaries in the lumbar vertebrae or pelvic bones.
- **Osteoporosis**. This is especially common in **post-menopausal females** and should make you aware of the increased likelihood of fractures. You may have previously seen this at the upper humerus and the wrist.
- Back pain **for the first time** in the extremes of life. Anyone can get a simple lower back pain, but new first-time back pain in young children is uncommon and should be taken very seriously. Also, with elderly people, back pain is common, but is usually ongoing for years; if they have a **new** back pain for the first time, serious diagnoses should be more deeply considered.

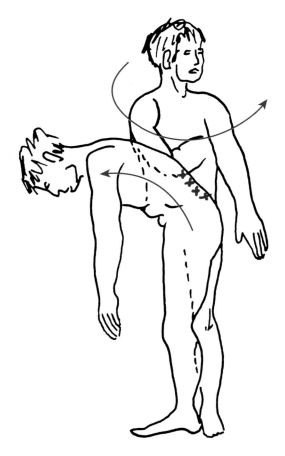

Figure 9.11 A dangerous lift, bending with rotation.

- A recent bladder or bowel problem. This could indicate a developing **cauda equina** syndrome. If you are not familiar with this syndrome, do not study it now: make a note in your diary for a later stage.
- General **new features suggestive of a serious general condition** – for instance, loss of appetite, progressive weight loss, night pain.

 Activity 9.5   **Time: A few minutes**

This activity is a little sneaky, but you have been warned in previous chapters. Cover up the list that you have just read and jot down the five red flags in your notebook.

Observations on Activity 9.5

It is so easy to simply read thinking that you have learnt. If the earlier list was completely new to you, perhaps forgetting one red flag is acceptable. Any more than that and you seriously need to do more highlighting, note taking or underlining of text to help memory. This is a **very** important list when trying to save a patient.

Multiple minor trauma

It is commonly thought that a single incident is the cause of a back injury such as a prolapsed lumbar disc. However, this is not the case. What usually happens is that multiple minor injuries occur to the part spread over possibly years. These are often hardly noticed by the patient. Eventually, the tissues give way, the disc prolapse occurs and the patient gets the acute features.

History of a lower back injury is often difficult to obtain, especially in elderly people. Minor strains are usually pain free within a week or two and memories fade, even in the young.

What to find out about your patient's back pain

- Site.
- Any radiation: hip or legs?
- Severity.
- Character of the pain.
- Easing and aggravating factors.
- Any pain at night?
- Any associations (i.e. paraesthesiae)?

Avulsion fractures of the pelvis

There will be a history of **violent muscle contraction**. The most likely causes are associated with sports in adolescents. This is because at this age there are more fragile apophyses that can more easily be pulled away from the bone. If the damage does not occur at this site, the tendon itself is very strong, but the muscle is weaker, so gives way at the junction with the tendon (*see* Figure 9.12). Here is a list of muscle origins likely to be affected:

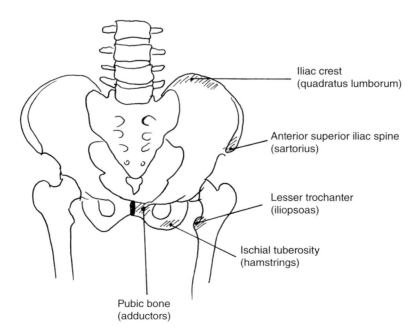

Figure 9.12 Avulsion fractures of the pelvis.

- Iliac crest: external and internal oblique, trunk rotation.
- Posterior iliac spine: erector spinae.
- Ischial tuberosity: hamstrings.
- Greater trochanter: gluteus maximus.
- Lesser trochanter: hip flexion with psoas, as in football.
- Anterior superior iliac spine: Sartorius (flexing knee).
- Anterior inferior iliac spine: quads (rectus femoris) (extending knee).

There will be sudden severe pain at the attachment area immediately following the injury.

Such fractures are unlikely but possible in adults and elderly people; you should always consider pathology.

The hip

Falls

Falls onto the side by an elderly patient are the most common cause of a fracture of the superior pubic ramus. This is obviously of more importance in post-menopausal women because of the increased risk of fracture.

Synovitis of the hip

The history may often disclose a recent bacterial or viral infection. The onset is sudden, with the patient not wanting to walk or even move the hip, but seeming otherwise well. This is unlike septic arthritis when they would appear toxic and ill.

Spondylolysis

Sports such as gymnastics, when a youngster has to do much hyperextension of the lumbar vertebrae, may produce repeated stress to the **pars interarticularis** area. This may eventually fracture causing a **spondylolysis** or **spondylolisthesis**, detailed later.

Strains of the adductor muscles

The football tackle is a major mechanism of these injuries.

Hamstring strains

These are commonly seen in sporting situations when the hamstrings are overstretched.

They can occur in many sports such as football with kicking, but hurdling is also a major one with massive stretching of the muscle, the hip fully flexed and the knee fully extended (*see* Figure 9.13).

They are more common in those who have not prepared for the activity.

Falling directly onto the bottom

This is a classical mechanism for fracturing the coccyx, or, if nothing shows on the X-ray, at least getting a very painful contusion around the bone.

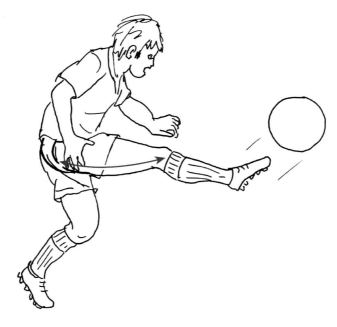

Figure 9.13 Hamstring strain.

Section 3
Patient examination

The initial 'call' to the patient from the waiting room to the examination cubicle is very useful here. Watch them closely, especially any problems they have arising from their chair and their gait into your cubicle.

Some of the major examination features for the lumbar spine and hip overlap, so it is best not to think of them in isolation. For instance, your examination of a patient presenting with lower back pain may start by putting the hip through a range of movements, to highlight possible problems originating there.

Examining a patient with lower back pain

Looking at the patient's back for the general shape and symmetry is important. Ask them to stand straight and see if the row of spinous processes is in a straight line. Sometimes a lateral curve (**scoliosis**) may be seen, sometimes associated with excessive protrusion of the ribs on one side.

Observe the normal curves, the slight forward curve (concave anteriorly) of the thoracic vertebrae (forming a gentle **kyphosis**) and the normal curve (concave posteriorly) of the lumbar vertebrae (**lordosis**).

Muscle wasting

If a condition has been going on for some time, a reliable indicator that something is preventing the patient from moving the part normally is muscle wasting. This should be noticeable even to the naked eye if you make it your routine to compare the size and shape of limbs. Muscle wasting is most easily seen in glutei and quadriceps.

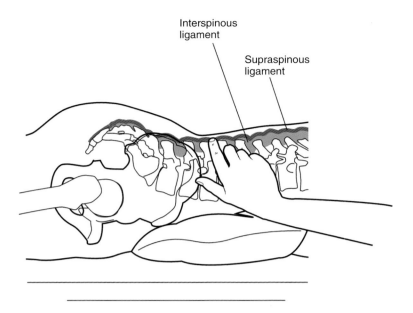

Figure 9.14 Palpating the major structures of the back (Gross *et al.*, 2009).

Unless you are lucky, measuring the length or circumference of the legs (looking for subtle differences) is rather a fruitless exercise. This is because, unless you do this often, you are unlikely to gain sufficient practice to be accurate. The same applies to many tests.

Observe the bulk and outline of the back, hamstring, quadriceps and calf muscles.

Palpation

Once you have asked about the general site of most discomfort, start by gently palpating the column of **spinous processes**, the **sacro-iliac joints** and the **iliac crests** (*see* Figure 9.14).

Following ordinary palpation, gentle percussion down the spinous processes with a fist, although sounding brutal, can be reassuring if negative and is completely painless in the majority of patients. However, if it causes pain, you should be suspicious of fractures or serious inflammatory disease.

Movements of the back

Ask the patient to bend gently forwards, **as much as is comfortable with the pain**, as if trying to touch their toes. As they do this, look at the spinous processes for any deviations.

Special tests

A good simple test to give you excellent and reliable information is **straight leg raising**. The essence of this is that, with the patient lying flat, each of the legs is raised in turn. The normal result is that the right and left can be raised equally without pain. If the patient has a disc lesion, pain and/or paraesthesiae will be caused in the back or down the leg on the affected side; this also limiting the amount that the leg can be raised.

A group of **muscle tests** will give the examiner precise information.

Activity 9.6   Time: **A few minutes**

Cover up the observations for this activity.

Earlier in the anatomy and physiology section, you already learnt some of the muscle tests that may be carried out to show problems at specific root levels. Can you think back now and say which deep tendon reflex and joint movement indicates a problem at L4 level?

Write them in your book; the repetition will help you remember.

Observations on Activity 9.6

It was knee jerk and dorsiflex the foot.

Ask the patient to draw up and push down their big toe. Resistance with your hands will demonstrate any weakness. The spinal level affected with weakness of big toe extension is L5.

Next try plantar flexion of the ankle with resistance. This, along with the ankle jerk, is from the S1 level.

Finally, the **dermatomes** of the leg are useful to know:

- Medial shin, L4.
- Lateral shin and dorsum of foot, L5.
- Lateral foot, S1.

Examining a patient with hip pain

Pain originating in the hip may:

- be felt in the groin
- be felt on the outside of the thigh
- radiate down the leg, even to the shin
- be felt in the knee.

and therefore may require examination of those parts.

Joint swelling

In most patients, swelling inside the hip joint is impossible to see, because of the vast amount of overlying soft tissues.

Bruising

Bruising following a fracture of the upper end of the femur is variable and there is an important point that you must be aware of. Fractures of the top of the neck (sub-capital and high trans-cervical) bleed mostly **into the capsule of the hip joint** and the blood is retained so that it doesn't often show on the surface of the skin even days later.

Basal fractures of the neck and trochanteric fractures are different. Because they are **extra-capsular**, the blood escapes into the surrounding tissue planes and rapidly shows on the surface.

Because of this, you cannot look at a hip and say, 'There is no bruising, so it is unlikely that there is a fracture.'

Palpation

Palpation of major landmarks is next. Choose a thin person when you first try; being able to literally see some of the bony prominences you are trying to palpate will make you feel more confident. Let's start with a simple activity.

Activity 9.7   Time: **About 10 minutes**

Try these now.

The ischial tuberosity

This is literally the lump of bone that you can feel in your bottom when you sit down on a chair, the lowest part of the pelvis.

The greater trochanter

This is the most lateral lump of bone that you can feel at the top of the thigh. Bringing the flat of your hand in from the side, it is underneath the first part of the body that it touches. A bursa is placed over it like a cap.

The adductor tendon

This is the third of the 'easy three' points for palpation at the hip. Place the flat of your hand at the top of the inside of your thigh, then forcibly adduct your leg against it, the tendon will stand out.

Hip movements

The following may be quickly and easily assessed, even by the inexperienced. The patient should be flat on their back.

- Flexion: the leg is raised or the knee is bent.
- Adduction: the knee is kept straight and the leg crossed over the midline.
- Abduction: the knee is kept straight and the leg swung outwards.
- Internal and external rotation: the foot is rolled inwards and outwards.
- Extension: the patient, lying on their side, extends their leg.

Trendelenberg test

This tests the effectiveness of the glutei muscles, which you will remember originate on the upper posterior ilium and insert mostly into the greater trochanter. Their task is essentially to abduct the thigh.

In the normal instance, if a patient is asked to stand on one leg (for instance, their left), these abductors on the left will contract, tilting the pelvis slightly down to the left and drawing the whole of the trunk over towards the left side. This in effect places the centre of gravity more onto the weight-bearing left side (*see* Figure 9.15a). This is easier seen from behind the patient, looking at the iliac crests.

This is the action when the test is normal or negative. When the test is positive (abnormal), the pelvis in this instance will tilt over to the patient's right side (*see* Figure 9.15b), and to compensate the spine will have to curve sideways to the affected side to keep the patient balanced.

There are several conditions that could cause this test to be positive, one of the most common being a very painful hip due to OA. Finally, be sure to make use of the examination list (Checklist 9.1).

Section 4
Minor musculoskeletal injuries

In this section I have artificially divided the injuries up into those basically of the back and vertebral column and then of the hip and thigh region.

Patient has a problem in their right hip

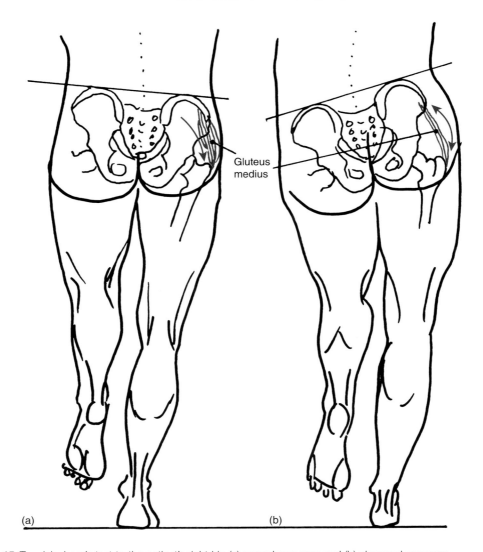

Figure 9.15 Trendelenberg's test to the patient's right hip (a) normal response and (b) abnormal response..

The back and vertebral column

Transverse process fracture

The danger to consider with this seemingly trivial fracture, is to think of it as a pure minor injury. The reason is that the small transverse process is the origin of and surrounded by muscle. So, a fracture here represents additional torn muscle and the possibility of significant haemorrhage.

Checklist 9.1 Record of progress

Physical examination of lower back and hip

Examination	On self	Friend practice	Friend practice	Patient practice
Patient history, a variety				
Observation:				
Scoliosis/lordosis				
Muscle wasting				
Posture				
Gait				
Palpation:				
Lumbar spine				
Spinous process				
Transverse process				
Sacro-iliac joints				
Iliac crest				
Lumbar muscles				
Hip				
Ischial tuberosity				
Greater trochanter				
Adductor tendon				
Herniae				
Range of movement:				
Lumbar spine				
Flexion				
Extension				
Lateral flexion, right and left				
Rotation, right and left				
Hip joint				
Flexion				
Extension				
Abduction				
Adduction				
External and internal rotation				
Sensations:				
Dermatomes				
L4, L5, S1				
Circulation:				
Compare right and left				
Specific tests:				
SLR				
Trendelenberg				
Knee jerk				
Ankle jerk				
Ankle dorsiflex				
Ankle plantarflex				
Big toe up				
Big toe down				
Other:				

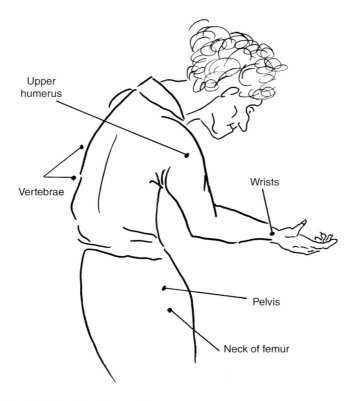

Figure 9.16 Common sites of fractures in osteoporosis.

Wedge compression fracture of the vertebral body

This is probably the most common lumbar fracture and is most certainly **not** a minor injury. These fractures commonly occur in patients with osteoporosis (*see* Figure 9.16), and in this situation the bone has several options. If the force applied is large, the body may completely crumble at once into the wedge shape. Alternatively, with lesser forces, it is possible for the bone to crumble in stages over months and years.

Features with the first option may be very severe, with the patient in absolute agony and unable to move. With the second option, features may be little more than a very bad back pain that they have experienced many times before.

Sprained or torn back muscles

By middle age I think that most people have experienced this condition: a heavy lift at the end of a tiring day when the back is exposed and weakened. The agonising pain, the week of stooping with the knees bent rather than the back, the slow recovery and, with a little luck, no further trouble.

Sacro-iliac strain

In this quite common condition, pain and tenderness will be centred around one of the two joints (*see* Figure 9.17).

The tiny ligaments forming the massive joint will have been partly stretched or torn. Resolution of the condition is far from a rapid affair, taking sometimes up to several months, but it will be eased with initial rest and analgesia. These may be followed by graduated exercises and other physiotherapy treatments.

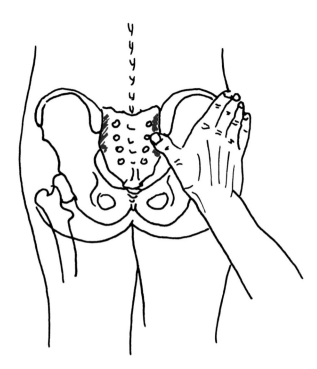

Figure 9.17 Palpating for tenderness with a sacro-iliac strain.

Fractured coccyx

This is a relatively minor fracture, but one that can cause considerable pain and discomfort. In the early stages, sitting without a cushion or air ring may be difficult. Reassurance, analgesia and advice are your best weapons. Diagnosis is suspected following the MOI and there will be extreme tenderness per rectum.

 Activity 9.8   **Time: A quick question**

What advice would the patient need following this injury, even if there is no fracture?

Observations on Activity 9.8

Constipation could be a very painful problem, especially in the first week. So they would benefit from your advice to **prevent** it occurring.

The hip and thigh region

Pelvic avulsions

There are several places around the pelvis where small, avulsion fractures occur (*see* Figure 9.12). These **apophyseal areas**, where tendons originate or insert into bone, are weaker structures and therefore more easily damaged. X-rays of these areas can be misleading if you are not familiar with paediatrics – with the various apophyses appearing usually around 13 years and fusing to the bone at about 20 years, advice will be required.

Management often consists of little more than rest, analgesia and referral.

Initially, these avulsion injuries can sometimes be difficult to differentiate from rather painful contusions where blows have occurred to the very superficial iliac crest.

Tendinitis

Tendinitis of muscle insertions, especially gluteus medius, occurs especially in women after running.

Bursitis

There are several small bursae around the hip and any may become inflamed after excessive activity, causing severe pain in the area and down the thigh.

Labral tears of the hip

These may occur after a major trauma to the hip joint.

Tears may produce locking, clicking, grinding or groin pain, especially with flexion and adduction.

Manipulations will cause discomfort and clicking; however such testing is not in the patient's best interest: leave it to those with experience to gain detailed information.

Hamstring strain and rupture

Damage usually occurs near to the **ischial tuberosity**.

All grades may be seen, from damage to just a few fibres through to a complete and agonising rupture, or avulsion of the apophysis of the ischium. However, most injuries are partial tears.

Management is with rest, ice, compression, elevation (RICE) and analgesia in the first instance, plus explanation and reassurance. Extensive detail can be found in Brukner and Khan (2012), including advice regarding the limited use of non-steroidal anti-inflammatory drugs (NSAIDs).

Slipped upper femoral epiphysis

Once again, slipped upper femoral epiphysis (SUFE) (or, as some call it, 'slipped femoral capital epiphysis' [SFCE]) is clearly a major condition, but I feel it important to include because minor variations can occur and possibly lead to confusion.

Figure 9.18 shows the normal and a SUFE.

The classical presentation is of an obese male child, early to mid-teens, complaining of sudden pain in the hip, often, but far from always, following some exertion.

Impacted sub-capital fractured neck of femur

This fracture is no minor injury, but once in a while it may present as one. It occurs if the compact bone of the femoral neck is rammed hard into the soft cancellous bone of the head (*see* Figure 9.19).

Over the years I have seen elderly patients with this fracture who amazingly were able to move their affected leg around and even hobble a few steps. X-rays may also be difficult to interpret, the fracture being difficult to recognise by the untrained eye. A lateral view is essential and may make all the difference.

Frightening, isn't it? A patient may still have a fractured neck of femur and be able to hobble. This highlights the importance of the decisions you have to make on a daily basis. Anyone can diagnose an obvious fracture, but you have to be quite knowledgeable and experienced to avoid this lurking trap!

Fissure fracture of the pubic bone

This is perhaps the most common of pelvic fractures, usually seen in elderly people. The wall of the bladder is immediately behind the pubis and therefore easily contused, sometimes giving the patient either frank or microscopic haematuria. It is seldom of importance.

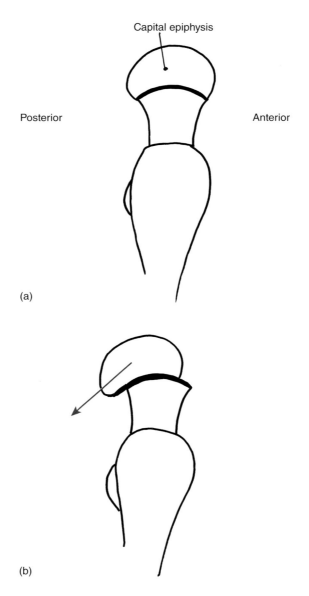

Capital epiphysis

Posterior

Anterior

(a)

(b)

Figure 9.18 Lateral views of the hip: (a) normal (b) a 'slipped' femoral capital epiphysis.

Osteoporosis should be considered as should fractures elsewhere (*see* Figure 9.16), especially in post-menopausal female patients.

Quadriceps injury

Tears usually occur near to the knee at the formation of the quadriceps tendon. They are therefore considered in the next chapter.

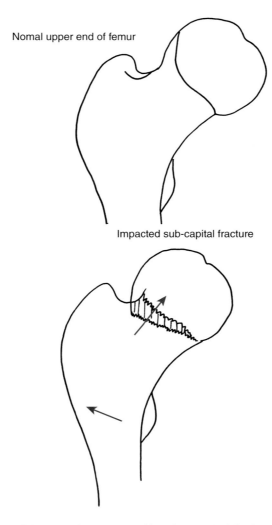

Nomal upper end of femur

Impacted sub-capital fracture

Figure 9.19 Normal anterior view of the upper femur, along with an impacted abduction sub-capital fracture.

Groin strain

This term is vague, but in common use. Generally it refers to pain at the adductor tendon and is caused by overstretching or tearing of the muscles that adduct the thigh.

 Activity 9.9   Time: **15 minutes**

Do you know the names of the muscles that adduct the thigh and are commonly injured in these strains? Write a couple down and then continue.

Observations on Activity 9.9

They are mostly the adductor longus, brevis, magnus and the gracilis. Sprain of the iliopsoas can also occur. It is extremely common, especially in amateur footballers following a tackle.

Section 5
Minor musculoskeletal conditions

The hip

Osteoarthritis

Osteoarthritis (OA) is perhaps the most common hip problem seen. It can present as fairly trivial hip pain in the early stages with only minimal joint changes showing on X-ray.

However, it can pass through all the ranges up to extreme levels of joint destruction, necessitating joint replacement.

 Activity 9.10   **Time: 15 minutes**

Whether your patient with OA is comparatively new to the condition or waiting for surgery, there are several things that you can offer them. Can you list a few?

Observations on Activity 9.10

Analgesia

To start, paracetamol or NSAIDs.

Walking aids

Stick, crutches, tripod or frame.

Warmth

Forms of heating pads.

Activity aids

Chair, beds.

Advice

- House design.
- Local authority help.
- Mobility, car, chair.
- Financial advice.

Herniae

Although unlikely to cause confusion, these should be considered with any pain around the hip and the patient questioned regarding past history.

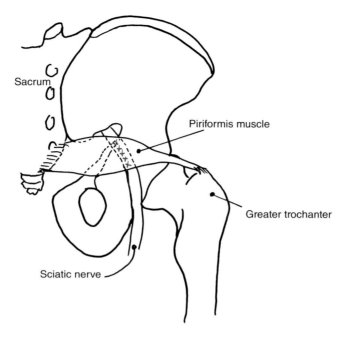

Figure 9.20 Piriformis syndrome, showing the relative positions of the sciatic nerve and the piriformis muscle.

Piriformis syndrome

This unpleasant condition causes a deep dull buttock pain and is sometimes associated with sciatic nerve compression (*see* Figure 9.20).

Patients are tender over the greater sciatic notch and pain may radiate down their leg.

If suspected, the management is to reassure regarding the possibility and refer them for senior assessment. If confirmed, the majority are managed non-operatively.

Snapping hip syndrome

This has several mechanisms and is defined as a palpable or audible snapping, or popping, near the hip. It is sometimes associated with pain over the greater trochanter, usually of slow onset following certain movements.

Cause is by the iliotibial band (ITB) rubbing over the trochanter, or the iliopsoas tendon against the **iliopectineal prominence**.

It is sometimes associated with irritation of the trochanteric bursa. Hyde and Gengenbach (2007) cover it in excellent detail with associated first-class illustrations.

Synovitis of the hip (irritable hip)

This is the most common cause of acute hip pain in children between approximately 3 and 10 years of age. The patient usually holds the hip in flexion, adduction and internal rotation, which coincidentally is the same position found in a posterior dislocation. They present with a **mild** illness and are not toxic.

Septic arthritis of the hip and osteomyelitis of the upper femur

The key to these conditions is to be aware of the possibility of them in the early stages of presentation. No 'Brownie' points here for thinking of them in the toxic patient screaming with pain.

Remember that the patient's hip pain may be referred to the knee and that early hip X-rays will show nothing.

The patient is usually a child up to approximately 4 years of age. They will have a high temperature, with associated features. Pain in the hip worsens with any movement. Immediate urgent referral is a must.

Perthe's disease (Legg-Calve-Perthe's disease)

Classical presentation is a boy up to approximately 10 years old with hip pain. In this condition, the femoral capital epiphysis deforms to a varying degree due to an imperfect blood supply, making walking increasingly difficult. The cause is unknown and, depending on age and progress, may require prolonged management and put an end to any major sporting activity. Although a major condition, **when presenting for the first time the features may seem quite insignificant**, so it should be in your mind when forming a diagnosis.

Congenital dislocation of hip

CDH is usually diagnosed in females following standard tests just after birth, but you should never presume that this has been done (the patient may be from a developing country), or that all is well. If a baby or toddler presents with a possible hip problem, always consider CDH.

In the newborn baby, for a hip joint to form correctly, the 'ball' of the femur and the 'cup' of the acetabulum need to be fitting accurately into one another. If they are not, even to a fairly minor degree, the joint may grow deformed.

Children may have what some term '**Clicky**' **hips** or more correctly '**Developmental dysplasia of the hip (DDH)**', when a specialised test for CDH is done (for example, **Ortolani's**) and is found to be positive. These tests are beyond the scope of the 'minors' professional – once again for no reason other than that they wouldn't be performed often enough for you to positively learn anything from them. However, comments on X-rays of this condition are to be found on this book's website.

An explanation for parents about your concern, and then referral, is all that is required of you.

Bursitis
Trochanteric bursitis

Lying directly over the greater trochanter is the trochanteric bursa; it is a common site for hip pain. Easily inflamed, not as easy to settle again, it may continue to hurt in a chronic form for many months or years.

Sometimes the bursitis occurs as a result of a direct blow (fall) onto the trochanter causing contusions, because it is so superficial. At other times excessive movement causes inflammation.

Iliopsoas bursitis

A similar condition, but not as common as the trochanteric bursa, this presents with severe pain in the groin and down the thigh.

Iliac apophysitis

This is an overuse traction injury; repetitive microtrauma is the cause.

There is a gradual onset of pain over the iliac crest, especially while running. This contrasts with rapid onset of an avulsion.

Management is with RICE.

Osteitis pubis

Consider this a possibility with any complaint of symphysis pubis pain.

There would be a slow onset of pain and tenderness, usually following an overuse mechanism. It can occur with many very active sports.

 Activity 9.11   Time: **30 minutes**

Cover up my observations and then list five extrinsic causes of hip pain.

Observations on Activity 9.11

I have listed seven for you, but there are others:

1. Sacro-iliac arthritis.
2. Psoas abscess or metastatic deposits in the lumbar spine.
3. Appendicitis.
4. Intra pelvic disease.
5. Femoral hernia.
6. Lymphadenopathy.
7. Radicular pain.

Lower back pain

The label 'lower back pain' sits rather dangerously in a book such as this. Certainly at one end of the scale, it may be caused by minor injuries or illnesses and last days only. However, at the other end of the scale, it is a crippling, devastating major problem that may ruin a person's career.

Patients with the more serious condition may become a legal minefield – a bit like the feared A&E problem of 'just a drunk' who dies of a head injury the following day.

 Activity 9.12   Time: **30 minutes**

In your own experience with what I have just said, how should the situation be approached?
Cover up my observations for this activity and write a few brief notes before you read on.

Observations on Activity 9.12

You are unlikely to be able to diagnose the definitive cause of your patient's pain. That would be a difficult enough task for a consultant without X-rays, scans and specialised tests. That is why the general, non-specific term 'lower back pain' has such widespread use. What you will probably be able to tell the patient is that, following their history and your limited examination, either:

- 'I can find nothing to indicate that you have a serious condition at the moment, so it is best that we manage your condition simply as non-specific lower back pain.' However, always add something like the following SOS, 'If you have any worsening pain and cannot get advice, return here at once.'

- Or 'I have found some changes that **may** indicate that you have X, Y or Z. For now we will take a specific course of action to ease things for you, and I will refer you to a colleague so that they can re-assess you.'

The only way to survive here is to consider every patient as an open book, and to have no preconceived ideas as to what is wrong with them. Follow the standard routine of a full history and MOI and an effective examination.

If, following examination, none of the features are found of the major conditions now described, it is safe to make the first of the two earlier statements. The most common scenario is a history of the patient making an inadvisable lift, straining (tearing) some of the lumbar muscle fibres such as those in the erector spinae group, oblique abdominals, etc. with localised back, sacro-iliac or buttock pain.

Lumbar degenerative disc disease

This is a common and serious cause of symptoms, with the full assessment and management of the condition well beyond your minors role. All your patients presenting with lower back or leg symptoms must be examined for this, and that is why I detail the features. Remember always that **minor conditions are diagnosed only after the elimination of likely majors**.

By young adulthood, degenerative changes could have occurred in the patient's disc, leaving them prone to herniation in later life (Skinner, 2006). Although trauma (i.e. poor lifting) could lead to a disc prolapse, these can certainly occur without any overt trauma.

The most frequent level for protrusion of the disc is L4–L5 and L5–S1. Pain is initially in the lower back while lifting; it then goes down the leg and is accompanied by numbness and weakness. Sometimes the leg pain occurs without the back pain.

 Activity 9.13   **Time: About 15 minutes**

Cover up my observations for this activity, then read on.

Earlier in this chapter you were told the clinical features that may be found with injuries at a particular root level. Can you remember them for the two most common levels of L5 and S1? Write them down to help you remember.

Observations on Activity 9.13

L5

- Weak extension, big toe.
- Sensation affected to the lateral shin and dorsum of foot.

S1

- Weak ankle plantar flexion.
- Weak ankle jerk.
- Sensations affected to lateral foot.

Mongolian blue spots

This is a form of birthmark sometimes found in the lumbar region. The blue/grey patches, which look like bruises, can be of varying sizes. They usually disappear before school age, but sometimes continue for years.

The main interest here is that they are not too common, so many professionals looking at them for the first time mistakenly think that they are a result of **non-accidental injury**.

Activity 9.14   Time: **10 minutes**

To become familiar with them, you can do no better then look at literally hundreds of pictures on Google Images or another search engine. Well worthwhile; why not have a break and look at them now?

Spondylolysis and spondylolisthesis

Spondylolysis is where a stress fracture or defect occurs in part of the lumbar vertebrae called the 'pars interarticularis' (near the facet joints). In spondylolisthesis, movement occurs at this site allowing the upper vertebrae to slide over the lower (*see* Figure 9.21).

The most likely levels for this are at L4/5 and L5/S1. It occurs in both children and adults. Features can be from non-existent and just discovered by chance at X-ray through degrees of back pain to neurological deficits; that is why I have given some detail about it in a 'minors' book. Brukner and Khan (2012) cover the two conditions well, including further clear illustrations.

Spinal stenosis

This is a narrowing of the spinal canal or vertebral foramen. Degeneration is the cause of the condition due to one or several of the following:

- Disc herniation.
- Facet joint arthritis.
- Hypertrophy of the ligamentum flavum.

Patients have pain in their leg/s that is worse when they are standing or walking. Being bent forwards a little sometimes tends to ease symptoms, as when walking uphill. **Another major condition, but it may start with seemingly trivial features**.

This now leaves many conditions that have lumbar pain as part of their clinical features. Depending on your previous experience, some of these conditions will be familiar to you, but few students will have met them all.

Activity 9.15   Time: **Several hours**

It is important that with all your 'minor' patients these conditions are somewhere in the back of your mind. So study the list below; it is not exhaustive, but perhaps 15 minutes on each will considerably help your diagnostic confidence.

- Osteoid osteoma.
- Multiple myeloma.
- Nephritis.
- Pyelonephritis.
- Kidney tumours.
- Ureteric colic.
- The range of malignant tumours, especially head of pancreas.
- TB and osteomyelitis of spinal column.
- Leaking abdominal aortic aneurysm (AAA).
- Abscesses:
  - pilonoidal
  - nodes in groin
  - cellulitis.

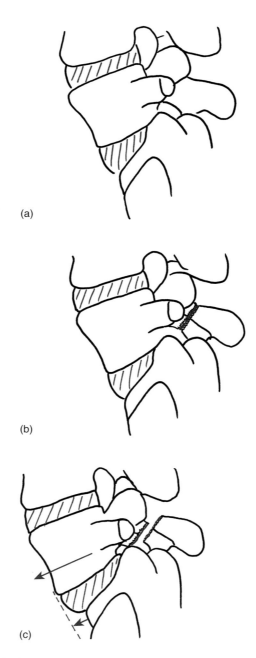

(a)

(b)

(c)

Figure 9.21 Left lateral views of the lumbo-sacral junction: (a) normal (b) spondylolysis (c) spondylolisthesis.

REFERENCES AND SUGGESTED READING

Brukner, P. and Khan, K. (2012) *Clinical Sports Medicine*, 4th edn, McGraw-Hill, Sydney.

Gross. J., Fetto, J. and Rosen, E. (2009) *Musculoskeletal Examination*, 3rd edn, Wiley Blackwell, Oxford.

Hyde T.E. and Gengenbach, M.S. (2007) *Conservative Management of Sports Injuries*, 2nd edn, Jones and Bartlett, Sudbury.

Simon R.R. (2011) *Emergency Orthopaedics*, 6th edn, McGraw-Hill, New York.

Skinner H.B. (2006) *Current Diagnosis and Treatment in Orthopaedics*, 4th edn, McGraw-Hill, New York.

Tortora, G.J. and Nielsen M.T. (2012) *Principles of Human Anatomy*, 12th edn, Wiley Blackwell, Oxford.

Multiple choice questions

Before you start, take in the reasoning behind these MCQs, how to answer them and how to interpret the results, from the section at the end of Chapter 1.

1. **Which of the following may be associated with groin strain?**

    A Adductor longus, gracilis

    B Sartorius

    C Pain at the adductor tendon

    D Quadriceps

2. **The trochanteric bursa:**

    A Is removed during a hip replacement operation

    B Is the only one on the outer side of the hip

    C Is frequently a site of lateral hip pain, bursitis

    D Is in close proximity to the iliotibial band

3. **For a male child with hip pain, the following should be considered:**

    A Slipped upper femoral epiphysis

    B CDH or DDH

    C Perthe's disease

    D Synovitis

4. **Which of the following statements are true?**

    A A patient with a fractured neck of femur will not be able to weight bear or walk

    B Strain of the iliotibial band causes knee pain

    C The capsule of the hip joint is relatively weak

    D With synovitis of the hip, your patient will be toxic and obviously ill

5. **The Trendelenberg test:**

    A Is a measure of the integrity of the hip joint

    B Is never positive with OA of the hip

    C Will indicate a problem with hip adductors

    D Will be positive when normal

6. **Which of the following would point to a disc prolapse specifically at level L4?**

    A Paraesthesiae medial side of shin

    B Ankle dorsiflexion weakened

    C Knee jerk diminished

    D Back pain

7. With an acute strain of the muscles in the lower back:

   A The SLR test will produce pain on both sides
   B There is a likelihood of limited flexion of the lumbar vertebrae
   C Percussion of the lumbar vertebrae will produce severe pain
   D The knee jerk reflexes will be unaffected

8. Spondylolisthesis:

   A Occurs following a defect in the vertebral body
   B Usually presents with severe neurological features
   C Commonly occurs at level L2
   D Is associated with a sign on X-ray called 'decapitation of the terrier'.

9. In the lumbar vertebral column:

   A The spinal cord becomes the cauda equina usually at level L1–2
   B The sacro-iliac joints allow no movement in the normal adult, except during pregnancy
   C The latissimus dorsi muscles are deep to the erector spinae group
   D The facet joints are orientated horizontally

10. Which of the following may be associated with hip pain?

    A Pyelonephritis
    B Mongolian blue spots
    C Enlarged lymph nodes in the groin
    D Perthe's disease

Answers are available at the end of the book. For an explanation of these answers and further resources visit the companion website at:

www.wiley.com/go/bradley/musculoskeletal

The knee and leg

Aim

To develop an in-depth understanding of the anatomy and physiology, history, examination and early management of minor musculoskeletal injuries and conditions of and around the knee and leg.

Outcomes

That, by the end of this study, and all the associated activities and clinical experiences, you will be able to:

- demonstrate an in-depth knowledge of the anatomy and physiology of musculoskeletal structures around the knee and leg
- take an effective history and examine patients presenting with knee and leg problems, forming a differential diagnosis
- demonstrate an in-depth knowledge of minor musculoskeletal injuries and conditions of the knee and leg
- apply these skills to the early management of patients, recognising any need for referral.

Section 1
Applied anatomy and physiology

Another complex but interesting joint; I will give you only the points required for your understanding. The remaining facts can be put to one side or covered at a later date as your need or interest arises.

Bones

- The lower end of the femur.
- The upper tibia.
- The patella.
- The upper fibula.

Managing Minor Musculoskeletal Injuries and Conditions, First Edition. David Bradley.
© 2014 John Wiley & Sons, Ltd. Published 2014 by John Wiley & Sons, Ltd.
Companion website: www.wiley.com/go/bradley/musculoskeletal

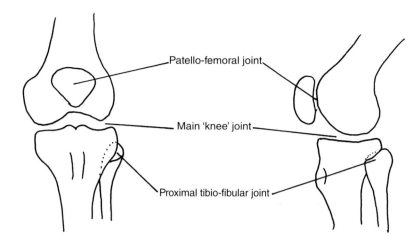

Figure 10.1 Three joints that comprise the knee.

These form three joints (*see* Figure 10.1):

1. The **main knee joint**, between the femoral condyles and the tibial plateau. Although initially thought of as a pure hinge joint, it does have an extra 'trick' of cleverly gliding and rotating slightly to maximise the joint's stability and effectiveness.
2. The **patello-femoral joint** between the femoral condyles and the posterior surface of the patella; this communicates freely with the main knee joint. Both are freely moving synovial joints with **hyaline cartilage**.
3. Finally, a tiny joint at the side of the knee, which in most people doesn't communicate with the main joint; it's the **proximal tibiofibular joint**, between the head of the fibula and the lateral border of the tibia. With this there is articular cartilage between the joint surfaces, but the bones are held firmly together and have very minimal (mm) gliding movement. For our practical purposes, they can be thought of as fixed.

Here are various terms that you need to learn by heart, before you read further. Start with the lower femur:

- Medial condyle.
- Lateral condyle.
- Medial epicondyle.
- Lateral epicondyle.
- Intercondylar notch.
- Patellar surface of femur.
- Articular cartilage.
- Adductor tubercle.

 Activity 10.1   **Time: 30 minutes**

Could you name all the terms listed on a blank drawing?

Another way to help the names of the parts of bone to stay in your mind is to try your hand at drawing them.

For the non-artists among you, earlier in the book I showed you how to do this by building on simple shapes. Have a try now, based on my examples in Figure 10.2.

Don't expect to make an excellent job of this the first time, but persist in your efforts. Students who are learning from you will feel so much happier with your various explanations if you can make the occasional sketch, like me drawing on a whiteboard.

Why is it important to learn all these parts of the bones? Is this detail really necessary?

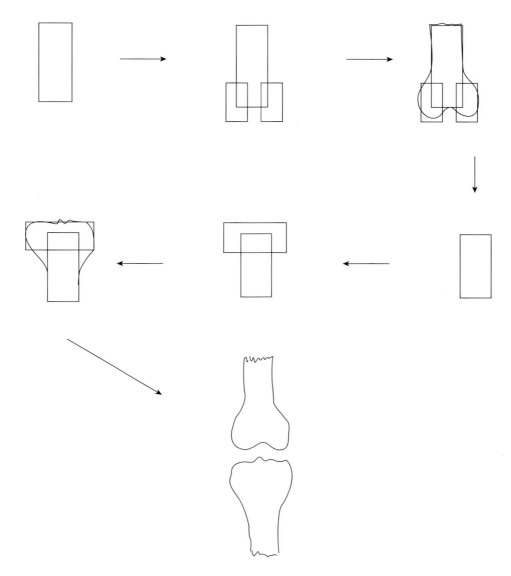

Figure 10.2 How to make a rough drawing of the knee.

Observations on Activity 10.1

As well as being useful landmarks during examination, knowing these parts enables you to use a 'shorthand' while writing notes and explaining to another professional. The majority of these projections on bones are places where muscles and other soft tissues are attached. Tenderness on or near any of them can inform you of damage to the associated soft tissues.

Activity 10.2   Time: **30 minutes**

Continue now with the remaining bones from the following list, trying to identify all the parts.

If your artistic attempts are failing miserably (and don't feel low about that – we can't all be Monet), just try tracing!

- Tibial plateau.
- Lateral tibial condyle.
- Medial tibial condyle.
- Tibial tubercle.
- Intercondylar eminence.
- Fibular styloid process.

- Head of fibula.
- Articular cartilage.
- Gerdy's tubercle.
- Superior tibiofibular joint.
- Head of fibula.

Articular cartilage

The articular surfaces of the bones are covered in hyaline cartilage. Why not shade the surfaces in to make it clearer and help it to become fixed in your mind. Including seemingly simple actions into your learning, such as this shading, really pays dividends.

Now that this basic 'scaffolding' of the knee is complete, it's an excellent time to have a break so that you do not become stale.

Soft tissues

Explanations are more difficult here because you can see the bones as very separate structures, very clearly defined. With the soft tissues in and surrounding the knee, they often blend into one another, so to talk of them in isolation and for you to visualise them, can be difficult.

Joint capsule

Illustrations of the capsule alone are difficult to find, the reason being that so much other tissue is around it and blended into it. Basically it consists of fibrous tissue for support, lined with synovial tissue to provide the synovial fluid (*see* Figure 10.3). Anteriorly, because of the patella, it is deficient. Otherwise the extent of the capsule is not quite as you would expect, because, as well as surrounding the articular surfaces, it branches off into some of the nearby bursae. These are synovial fluid-filled sacks that act as cushioning. Also look at the extent of the capsule significantly above the patella. Usually flattened and not able to be felt, see in later chapters what happens following some trauma.

 Activity 10.3   Time: **5 minutes**

Figures 10.3 and 10.4 are very complex illustrations, so why not try to build up your own simplified AP and lateral views of the capsule by photocopying the simple drawings in Figure 10.1 and adding the capsule and its strengthening structures.

It will only take a few minutes, but will really help you retain the information.

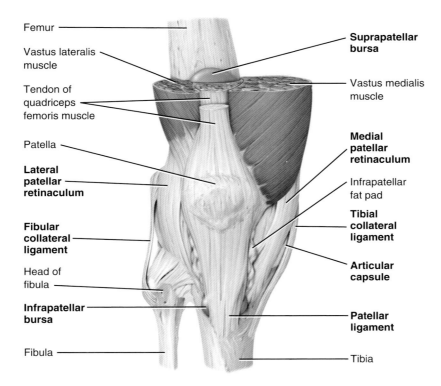

Femur

Vastus lateralis
muscle

Tendon of
quadriceps
femoris muscle

Patella

**Lateral
patellar
retinaculum**

**Fibular
collateral
ligament**

Head of
fibula

**Infrapatellar
bursa**

Fibula

**Suprapatellar
bursa**

Vastus medialis
muscle

**Medial
patellar
retinaculum**

Infrapatellar
fat pad

**Tibial
collateral
ligament**

**Articular
capsule**

**Patellar
ligament**

Tibia

Figure 10.3 The joint capsule, anterior view (Tortora and Nielsen, 2012). This material is reproduced with permission of John Wiley & Sons, Inc.

Although satisfactory, these layers of the capsule are not the toughest of structures. We also need to talk of the accompanying ligaments and some of the nearby muscles and tendons, which add necessary strength.

For now, do your best to learn about the soft tissues from this book alone. It is just enough for you to thoroughly understand what is going on, without confusing you.

Almost part of the outer layers of the capsule are the short **capsular ligaments**. These run from the lower femur to the upper tibia and attach to the menisci.

The first of the major outside strengthener groups is called the '**collateral ligaments**' (*see* Figures 10.3 and 10.4); they are positioned on either side of the knee and are named:

- the lateral collateral ligament (LCL) or fibular collateral ligament
- the medial collateral ligament (MCL) or tibial collateral ligament.

You may find that even these are subdivided and given different names by different authors – something you'll have to live with I'm afraid. This is especially true if you read an American text or one written for a particular type of specialist.

These two ligaments help to prevent the bones moving from side to side with varus and valgus forces. An important point is that they are not just attached to the bones immediately above and below the joint, but in some instances several centimetres from the joint line.

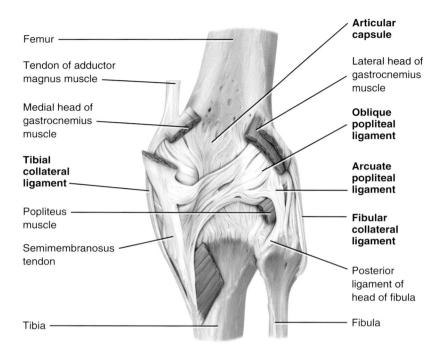

Femur

Tendon of adductor
magnus muscle

Medial head of
gastrocnemius
muscle

**Tibial
collateral
ligament**

Popliteus
muscle

Semimembranosus
tendon

Tibia

Articular
capsule

Lateral head of
gastrocnemius
muscle

**Oblique
popliteal
ligament**

**Arcuate
popliteal
ligament**

**Fibular
collateral
ligament**

Posterior
ligament of
head of fibula

Fibula

Figure 10.4 The joint capsule, posterior view (Tortora and Nielsen, 2012). This material is reproduced with permission of John Wiley & Sons, Inc.

 Activity 10.4   Time: **A quick question**

Remember that the ligaments are not just attached to the bones immediately above and below the joint, but in some instances several centimeters from the joint line.
  Why do you consider the above to be an important point?

Observations on Activity 10.4

If they are injured, **the associated tenderness could be anywhere along the length of the ligament**, not necessarily in the centre over the joint line, where you may have expected tenderness.

Lateral collateral ligament

Also sometimes called the '**fibular collateral ligament**', this runs from the lateral surface of the femoral condyle, past the joint line to the head of the fibula. Although it is certainly an individual structure, it can be thought of as one of a group of structures that strengthens this lateral aspect of the joint.
  Deep to the LCL is the lateral **capsular** ligament, which may be subdivided into several other structures. Of these I would like you to know the tendon of the **biceps femoris** muscle (one of the hamstrings group in the back of the thigh); this surrounds the LCL and also inserts into the head of the fibula, offering support to the joint. Also anteriorly, a large sheet of very strong fascia called the '**fascia lata**' (FL) (sounds like a strong coffee!), or '**iliotibial band**', covers both and inserts into the upper tibia at the roughened prominence on the tibia called '**Gerdy's tubercle**'.

Activity 10.5   **Time: 15 minutes**

I am listing here a few common anatomical terms:

- anatomical position
- valgus
- varus
- medial
- lateral.

There is a great danger that the less experienced among you have not considered the exact meaning of these for many years. Use an anatomical text or web source now and look them up if you are not completely sure. Don't be embarrassed about revision of points like this. An excellent test of your understanding is to explain a term to a junior; to teach effectively you must have a high level of understanding.

Medial collateral ligament

On the opposite side of the knee is the **medial (or tibial) collateral ligament**. As with the lateral structures, it is not just a simple band on its own, but a grouping of structures, each adding to the support of the joint.

Deep to it is the **medial capsular ligament**, which, unlike its partner on the lateral aspect, attaches very firmly to the medial meniscus, making the meniscus more liable to injury. Note the positioning of the **semimembranosus** adding support.

Cruciate ligaments

These two structures (the anterior and posterior) are about the width of a little finger, approximately 3–4 cm in length, and are situated deep inside the knee joint between the femoral condyles. Each runs from the upper surface of the tibia to the intercondylar area of the femur, crossing one another, hence the name (*see* Figures 10.5 and 10.6).

Their major job is to prevent anterior and posterior movement of the tibia in relation to the femur.

Although positioned deep inside the capsule of the knee joint, neither are bathed in synovial fluid. This is because the synovium is wrapped around them, in a similar way to the contents of the peritoneum. If torn they will bleed and because the outer joint capsule is intact preventing the blood from escaping from the joint cavity, the injury will rapidly produce a tense haemarthrosis.

Menisci

The medial and lateral semi-lunar cartilages (menisci) are of different sizes, the lateral being smaller and more rounded. Both are firmly attached to the circumference of the tibial plateau by part of the capsule called the '**coronary ligaments**' and are joined together anteriorly by a **transverse ligament**. The menisci act to deepen the fairly flat tibial plateau, making it better suited to the rounded femoral condyles. They are not essential components, but the knee works far more effectively with them.

Being cartilaginous, they are mostly avascular structures, but have a little blood supply on their outer margins.

With flexing and extending the knee, both cartilages move a fraction over the upper surface of the tibia, but, as mentioned previously, the medial cartilage is more firmly attached than the lateral and is therefore more easily damaged.

Extensor apparatus

Perhaps the most straightforward and well known of the knee mechanisms, this apparatus is the collection of structures that enables us to straighten out our leg or raise the straightened leg off the ground. There are five components altogether (*see* Figure 10.7), from above down:

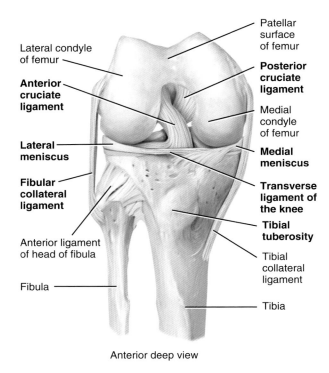

Patellar
surface
of femur

Lateral condyle
of femur

**Posterior
cruciate
ligament**

**Anterior
cruciate
ligament**

Medial
condyle
of femur

Lateral
meniscus

**Medial
meniscus**

**Fibular
collateral
ligament**

**Transverse
ligament of
the knee**

**Tibial
tuberosity**

Anterior ligament
of head of fibula

Tibial
collateral
ligament

Fibula

Tibia

Anterior deep view

Figure 10.5 Cruciate ligaments (Tortora and Nielsen, 2012). This material is reproduced with permission of John Wiley & Sons, Inc.

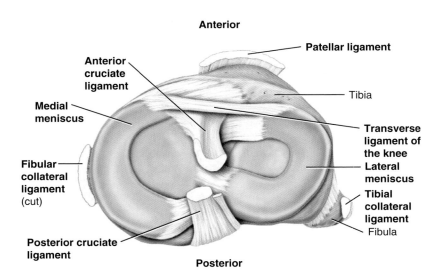

Anterior

**Anterior
cruciate
ligament**

Patellar ligament

Tibia

**Medial
meniscus**

**Transverse
ligament of
the knee**

**Fibular
collateral
ligament
(cut)**

**Lateral
meniscus**

**Tibial
collateral
ligament**

Fibula

**Posterior cruciate
ligament**

Posterior

Figure 10.6 Superior view of menisci (Tortora and Nielsen, 2012). This material is reproduced with permission of John Wiley & Sons, Inc.

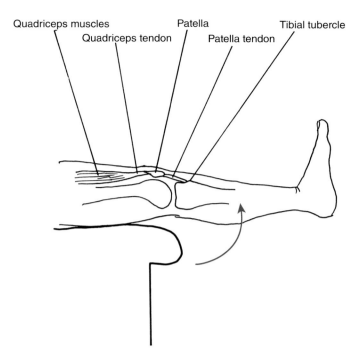

Figure 10.7 The extensor apparatus, straight leg raising.

1. Quadriceps muscles.
2. Quadriceps tendon.
3. Patella.
4. Patella tendon.
5. Tibial tubercle.

Posterior of the knee

If you look at the posterior surface of a knee (and few people do), you can see a lateral and a medial bundle of muscle and tendons; these are all part of the famous hamstrings at the back of the thigh (*see* Figure 10.8).

The medial bundle consists of the **semimembranosus** and the **semitendinosus**. The lateral is the **biceps femoris**.

Between these, the joint capsule is strengthened by the many tendons. The short popliteus muscle crosses the back of the knee from its tibial origin medially, running inside the joint capsule to the lateral meniscus and upwards to the femur.

Do you know the name of the large muscle in Figure 10.8 shown in the calf, with a medial and lateral origin above the knee?

Fat pads

Pads of fat occur at the knee and are most noticeable below the patella.

Bursae

Surrounding the knee are many bursae. Their positions should be noted so that you can easily recognise their swelling and other features of inflammation (*see* Figure 10.9).

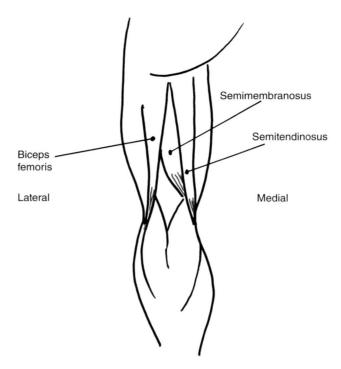

Semimembranosus

Semitendinosus

Biceps
femoris

Lateral   Medial

Figure 10.8 A posterior surface view of the knee, showing some of the muscles.

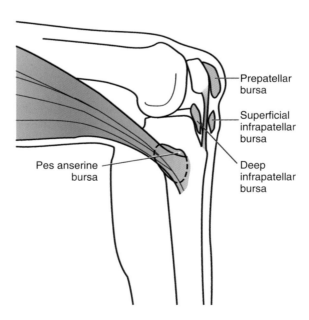

Prepatellar
bursa

Superficial
infrapatellar
bursa

Pes anserine
bursa

Deep
infrapatellar
bursa

Figure 10.9 Bursae around the knee (Gross *et al.*, 2009).

The most important are the following:

- Supra-patellar.
- Pre-patellar.
- Infra-patellar, subcutaneous and deep.
- Pes anserine.
- Semimembranosus.

Section 2
History and mechanism of injury

By now you should be familiar with the large amount of space I give to the history and MOI; obtaining this knowledge is **the** major stage in your patient's management.

The importance of detailed questioning

It is important when listening to your patient's history that you ask enough detail of what happened to be able to visualise the situation yourself. Only then will you be able to form a clear idea of the injury sustained or the build-up to a condition. Consider the following scenario, this time based on a paramedic practitioner:

Paramedic (P): 'How did this happen?'
Footballer (F): 'I fell over.'
P: 'What were you doing?'
F: 'I was running for the ball and was tackled.'

 Activity 10.6 Time: **A quick question**

Is any more questioning of the patient required for an MOI, or is this enough for the average ENP or ECP?

Observations on Activity 10.6

Well, it would be okay for the ordinary paramedic who will be taking the patient directly to A&E, or the nurse initially receiving the patient in A&E, but it is far too little detail if you want to even start to form a diagnosis.

As you know, some patients are what are called 'poor historians', meaning that to get more out of them will be difficult or impossible.

Let me take the earlier conversation a little further now and show you how carefully increased questioning can open up so many possibilities:

P: 'Fine, but can you describe **exactly** how it happened?'
F: 'Yeh! As I was running, this chap came in to tackle me from the right side. I twisted to the left, I think my right foot stuck in the ground and I felt this sudden pain in the knee.
P: 'Anything else? For instance, did you hear anything?'
F: 'Funny you should say that. I think I heard it "pop", but it was just immediately so painful.'
P: 'Nothing else?'
F: 'Couldn't continue with the game!'

So, with just a little 'nudge' we have far more information and are well on the way to the formation in our brains, of a short list of possible diagnoses.

This list of initial possibilities, your **differential diagnosis**, is then used to inform the examination of your patient, the subject of our next section.

A few minutes on references

I now want to try to interest you in references. It sounds a little 'dry', but just bear with me: the more senior among you will already understand the importance.

Activity 10.7   Time: **30 minutes**

As a student, it is the ideal for you to get used to reading around a subject. Just to read this chapter about knees will not make you the most knowledgeable nurse or paramedic in the world, but, if it encourages you to take every opportunity to read and ask further questions, it will have done a good job.

I am pointing you to a reference of a piece of work written by a doctor in Liverpool who came across a problem knee patient (Emms, 2002).

Go to the 'References and suggested reading' section towards the end of this chapter. There you will see all the information you require to find this reference. I was able to download and print it out from the internet in minutes; it makes fascinating reading.

Throughout this book, be on the lookout for such useful references; they are interesting and should help you with further study.

Examples of MOIs

Now we will cover some of the more common ways of injuring a knee and how knee conditions may present. By remembering these, you may be able to recognise common presentations simply by listening to your patients as they provide the history. They are not in a particular order.

Direct impact over the front of the patella

A classical presentation here is the driver or front passenger of a vehicle in a head-on collision. Obviously high-speed impact can telescope the fascia towards the legs, trapping them. However, even lesser forces, with seat belts in use, plus modern cars and safety foam on the surfaces, can cause an impact of knees against the dashboard (*see* Figure 10.10), especially if the driver is short and needs the seat close to the wheel to reach the pedals.

As well as injuries to the obvious superficial tissues, the major pathology to expect is a fractured patella.

Activity 10.8   Time: **10 minutes**

Before we leave this first example of an MOI to the knee, I would like you to consider two questions:

1. What else may cause a direct blow over the front of the patella?
2. We have already mentioned damage to the skin and soft tissues near to the patella, but, if the force applied to the leg is large enough, where will it go and what other structures may be damaged?

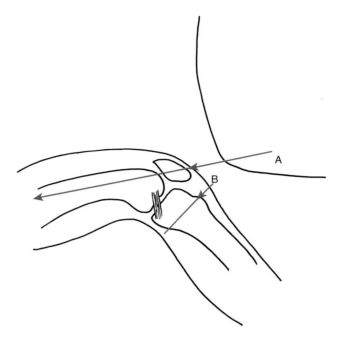

Figure 10.10 Direct impact to the knee in a car. Arrow 'A' shows the force hitting the patella, then travelling up the femur. Arrow 'B' shows the force hitting below the patella, forcing the tibia backwards.

Observations on Activity 10.8

1. A few examples could be:
   - playing hockey
   - a direct kick in football
   - pedestrian hit by car.
2. This is the topic of the next section.

Injuries to associate with direct impact to the patella

This mechanism is a little easier for the on-scene paramedic to appreciate. If the force is large enough, it can continue along the line in Figure 10.10, following arrow 'A', fracturing the femur, or even pushing the femur posteriorly, dislocating the hip joint.

If the femur is fractured, there will be the characteristic position of the leg with shortening and external rotation. However, if there is a posterior dislocation of the hip, there will be flexion of the hip and knee plus shortening and internal rotation (*see* Figure 10.11).

Frontal impact near to the tibial tubercle

This is fairly similar to the mechanism just mentioned with the knee flexed, but the impact is just a little lower down. Here the force of impact misses the patella and femur, but instead pushes the upper end of the tibia posteriorly (*see* the arrow 'B' in Figure 10.10), easily tearing the posterior cruciate ligament (PCL).

A strong muscular contraction

Another situation to result in injuries to the knee is to have an unexpectedly very strong contraction of the quadriceps. This can occur when trying to kick a ball that is missed, or going downstairs and missing a step (*see* Figure 10.12).

Posterior dislocation of the hip

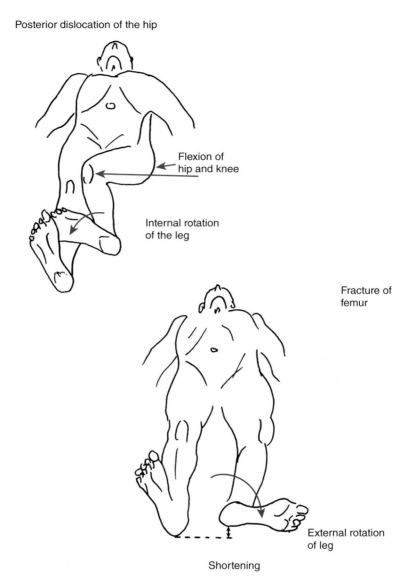

Flexion of hip and knee

Internal rotation of the leg

Fracture of femur

External rotation of leg

Shortening

Figure 10.11 The classical positions that a leg is found in, with a posterior dislocation of the hip and also a fractured femur.

With this force, any part of the extensor mechanism of the knee can be damaged, for instance:

- Torn quadriceps.
- Torn quadriceps tendon.
- Transverse fracture of the patella.
- Torn patella tendon.
- Avulsion fracture of the tibial tubercle.

Before going further, let's consider factors that may have a bearing on what damage occurs to any of our patients.

Activity 10.9   Time: **15 minutes**

A set force is applied to a patient's knee. What factors surrounding the incident have any influence of what damage is done? List those you can think of in your notebook, then check your answers with the observations on this activity.

Observations on Activity 10.9

- Direction of the force, what angle was it?
- Duration of the force.
- Strength of the patient's tissues.
- Do they have any illnesses to complicate matters?
- Are they on any drugs?
- Were they wearing any protection?
- Was the ground soft or hard?

Each of these factors could make differences to the end result. Each has to be in your mind as you are asking questions.

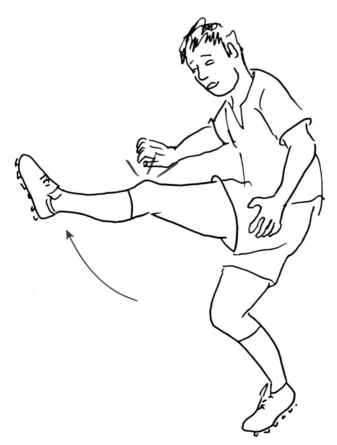

Figure 10.12 A strong muscular contraction may fracture the patella.

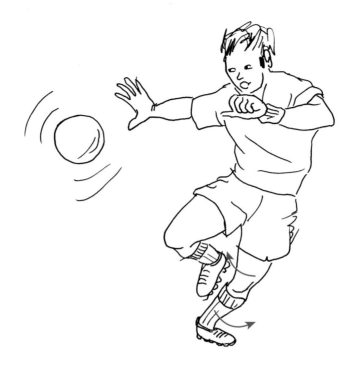

Figure 10.13 Another classical mechanism: the body weight on the limb, the foot firmly on the ground, slight flexion of the knee and then rotation.

A sporting twist

Here is another classical mechanism that is essential for you to learn. Try to have a mental picture of the possible situations. It could be a young man tackled on a football field, a dad chasing his small child in the garden, or perhaps an elderly man stumbling in the park while walking his dog:

- The body weight is on one leg.
- The foot of that leg is fixed on the ground momentarily.
- The knee is in slight flexion.
- The body rotates toward the midline on the leg, or, to put it another way, the tibia externally rotates on the femur (*see* Figure 10.13).

As this happens, the femur grinds (rotates) on the firmly fixed tibial plateau.

There are several injuries that commonly occur with this situation and exactly what damage does occur depends on the direction of the twist and factors we discussed in the last activity. Here are the individual possibilities:

- Tears of the menisci.
- Tears of the anterior cruciate ligament (ACL).
- Tears of the collateral ligaments.

Imagine the femoral condyles against the tibial plateau as being like a chemist's mortar and pestle, but it is the menisci that are being 'ground' in this instance.

Sometimes the wrenching is so severe that all three structures are damaged at the same time; it all depends on the factors listed earlier. Just the type of footwear (studs on boots, for instance) can keep the foot rigid and increase torsional stresses.

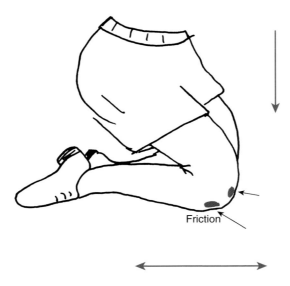

Downwards force

weight of body

Friction

Figure 10.14 Mechanism causing forms of bursitis in the knees.

Lateral dislocation of the patella

A twisting mechanism while weight bearing is usual and with recurrent dislocations the patient is often said to have been 'simply walking'.

Although there is sometimes no abnormal background, it is often associated with an incorrect alignment of the patella, especially in women. A more shallow lateral condyle of the femur is also sometimes seen.

Friction; 'rubbing' trauma to the front of the knee

This is a well-known and quite common mechanism for a patient to get a bursitis around the knee. The patient kneeling a lot, and shifting around over the floor on their knees, causes a great deal of friction. They continue for too long, until a particular task is complete and their knees then 'revolt' (*see* Figure 10.14, and also Figure 10.9).

Over the years this condition has been given fanciful titles such as 'housemaid's knee', 'clergyman's knee' and 'carpet fitter's knee'. However, I have never seen any of these people attending with bursitis! The exact positioning of the angle of the knee will determine which of the bursae (prepatellar or infrapatellar) are affected.

The more frequent and recent use of knee protectors for those in industry and the serious DIY trade will probably mean that we shall see still fewer in the future.

Overuse (accumulative) injury

These have been mentioned in many previous chapters, were a patient may not realise that what they have done is the cause of their problem.

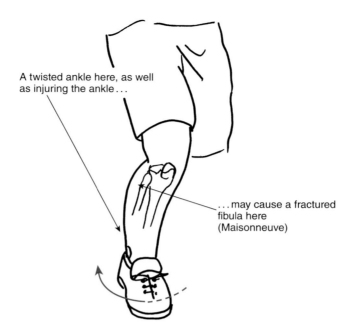

A twisted ankle here, as well as injuring the ankle...

...may cause a fractured fibula here (Maisonneuve)

Figure 10.15 The mechanism for a Maisonneuve fracture.

Twisting the ankle

No I haven't made a mistake – twisting their ankle can give your patient a fracture at the knee as well as an ankle injury (*see* Figure 10.15).

Any severe external rotation force to the ankle gives the possibility of the twisting force carrying on up the fibula shaft, fracturing anywhere up to and including the fibular neck (**Maisonneuve fracture**). It's not every day that you learn a little French as well as trauma is it?! Maybe a golden rule would help you here:

GOLDEN RULE

With all ankle injuries, expose and examine the knee as well.

Force to the lateral aspect of the leg

A blow to the lateral aspect of the leg around the knee causes the tibia to be forced into valgus. This valgus force stresses the soft tissues on the **medial side** of the same limb, often tearing the MCL. Fractures of the lateral tibial condyle may also occur with a concentrated severe force, as the femoral condyle is pushed into the upper tibia. This will be detailed later. So, initially the nurse/paramedic will see mud, swelling or bruising, grazing or laceration to the site of impact on the lateral side, but the medial side of the limb will be where most of the damage could have been done (*see* Figure 10.16).

A side rugby tackle or football foul would be common sporting ways to get this set of injuries, or a pedestrian hit by a car.

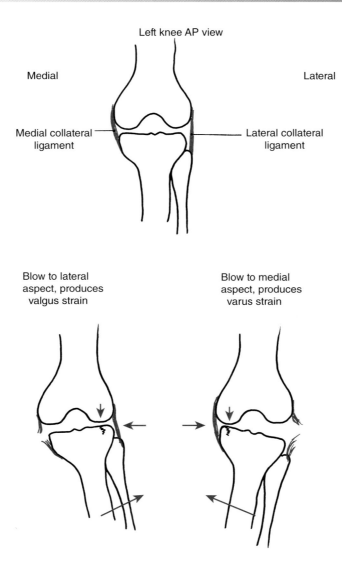

Figure 10.16 The mechanisms of damage following both valgus and varus stress to the knee.

Force to the medial aspect of the leg

This force to the medial aspect of the leg near to the knee is obviously more difficult to get, making the associated injuries less common. It will cause a mirror image to the previous trauma, with a varus stress to the tibia, resulting in damage to the lateral soft tissues, especially the LCL. More severe impact may cause fractures of the medial condyle of the tibial plateau, to be discussed later (*see* Figure 10.16).

Once again, sporting tackles are a major cause, with direct RTCs a hot follow-on.

Forced hyperextension

Here the major injury to consider is damage to the ACL. The hyperextension can occur with blows from behind (*see* Figure 10.17).

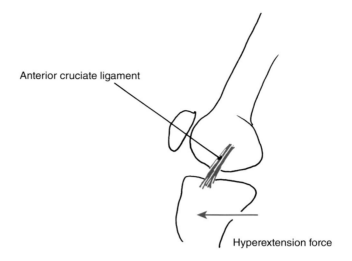

Anterior cruciate ligament

Hyperextension force

Figure 10.17 Mid sagittal view. Forced hyperextension of the knee can damage the ACL.

 Activity 10.10   **Time: A quick question**

We have just considered many different forms of trauma that may affect the knee, but for each of them what else do we have to consider that may well be of equal importance?

Observations on Activity 10.10

With all the mechanisms mentioned in this section, do not fall into the dangerous habit of just considering the trauma to the knee. Remember again that we are dealing with a whole patient, who, because of the force detailed earlier, will also have fallen over. If they have fallen, the majority will have put at least one hand out to try to save themselves. This leads you to ask about the common injuries associated with a FOOSH. Also consider the head receiving another common associated injury; always enquire.

Illness presentations and patterns of disease

Usually conditions will present to you in a reasonably uniform way, but they may demonstrate tremendous variety. An example of this mentioned to you previously is sarcoidosis.

Just to home in on the area that the patient tells you about – for instance, knee pains – and not to ask about general feelings will lead you astray in the history 'puzzle'. Always give yourself the best possible chance by considering the patient as a whole and asking about other problems, examining as necessary.

Septic arthritis and osteomyelitis

Both these conditions may occur through blood infection from a septic focus elsewhere, with osteomyelitis of the upper tibia being a known presentation in young males around 10 years of age.

Primary malignant tumours around the knee

I doubt if you will see one in your lifetime, so we are not to spend time on them except to say that they occur, and, because of that fact, keep the possibility in the recesses of your mind as a very slim possibility.

Activity 10.11   **Time: 10 minutes**

Use the internet to look up primary malignant tumours that can occur at the knee; under no account spend longer – it is just not necessary: this is background study for completeness.

Gout

This is a form of adult arthritis, due to faulty purine metabolism, and is usually seen in the 50-plus age group.

Although by far the most common presentation is at the 1st metatarso-phalangeal joint, it is also able to present elsewhere.

The first onset is often 'out of blue' so difficult to diagnose in the knee.

Small firm lumps may occur at the various joint sites, called '**trophi**'. Pain and the local features of inflammation are often severe, causing great distress.

Historically those with gout have been portrayed as over-indulgent eaters. This is not the case, although the omission of certain foods rich in purine is required.

Rheumatoid arthritis

RA showing in the knee is part of the generalised disease and features should be looked for in other joints. For a patient developing the disease for the first time, the classical presentation is of a young to middle-aged female developing pain, stiffness and inflammatory features in several joints.

Although it can show in a knee first, more usually the small joints of the hand (PIP and MCP) are affected and will take the patient to their GP.

Well you have now completed another important section. Well done. From now on with every patient you care for, try to get a clear understanding of the MOI and history.

Section 3
Patient examination

Gaining practical skills in examining a knee will take time. Don't expect to read this section and then make an excellent job of examining the next patient whom you see. The ideal is to work alongside a mentor, gaining instant feedback on a daily basis. But, if you are learning on your own, you can still become remarkably effective at examining if you follow this text, practise **and don't cut corners**.

'While I'm here, could I ask you about . . . ?'

Quite a heading, eh?! But, although a patient asking you this can sometimes be an annoyance, think of it another way. As I have said before, they trust you enough and feel safe asking you to help – **quite an honour** really. It's not their fault that our health services are so multifaceted that patients are confused as to who it is right or wrong to ask.

Every knee examination that you ever perform will vary in some way. You would be a poor professional if you blindly followed a set scheme. Examinations should vary with the patient, their character, what has happened to them, the discomfort they are in, their level of anxiousness, the surroundings, etc.

An excellent routine

You must decide how you want to start. One way is by touching medial and lateral aspects of the lower leg while asking the patient if they can feel your touch and if it feels normal (sensations). At the same time, you would be looking at the colour of the limb and judging the temperature (circulation). Finally, you would ask them to plantar flex and dorsiflex the foot (movements).

By doing these checks, in seconds you will have found or eliminated major damage to:

- blood vessels
- sensory nerves
- motor nerves
- major muscle groups.

There can be few situations where you get such a payback of vital information.

Observation

For the experienced, watching your patient walk in to see you gives valuable information. Make use of the circumstance, especially noting their gait.

Your first experience of examination could be to keep your hands to yourself and simply LOOK and take in what you see. So many practitioners go straight in with their hands and this may sometimes unnerve or even frighten the patient.

I have seen so many conditions missed over the years, purely because the professional concerned didn't examine the patient thoroughly enough. Then, along comes a consultant who attends to an often basic point like undressing the patient adequately and all is disclosed.

In Chapter 3, after activity 3.7, I listed items that you should look for in all areas. I would like you to revise this; by now a good 90% or more should be memorised.

Some initial legal thoughts

Unless your Trust has previously assessed you as competent at detailed aspects of examination, no one can legitimately turn around to you and say, 'Why didn't you examine that joint properly? All that can be expected is the relatively superficial observations of the standard emergency nurse or paramedic.

But this also means that **you must not go beyond your limits of knowledge, skill and experience** while making decisions about a knee, based on what you find.

For example, it is not good enough that you read this chapter, go away and examine a patient's knee in detail, deciding that they do not need referral to a doctor. To avoid claims of negligence being made against you, decisions regarding your remit must have been clearly made by a manager beforehand.

 Activity 10.12   Time: **30 minutes**

I would like you to read a chapter in a book. Look in the 'References and suggested reading' section towards the end of this chapter, for Corfield, Granne and Latimer-Sayer (2009). Read Chapter 6 on 'Negligence: The legal standard of care', pp. 22–25, by I. Granne and L. Corfield.

Similar information can also be found on many websites; try Googling '**The Bolam test 1957**' and '**Wilsher and Essex 1986**'.

You probably know by now that the website associated with this book has some legal/ethical test scenarios for you. This could be an ideal time to try them out.

A frequently asked question from both nursing and paramedic professionals is, '**How much of an examination of my patient should I make?**' The trouble is, the answer varies with each patient. You just have to stick to a routine of taking an accurate history, so that you know of the range of possible diagnoses, and then follow on with an appropriate examination level that comes with experience.

Try this activity.

 Activity 10.13　　　　　　　　　　　　　　　　**Time: About 30 minutes**

Let's suppose you are doing a session at a walk-in centre. Consider these two patients:

1. You are about to examine a 12-year-old boy with a painful knee, wearing jeans, who has started to limp on his left leg the previous day. There is no history of injury, although he always plays a lot of football.
   Just on this information alone, what would be the extent of your examination?
2. You are to examine a 60-year-old patient who has type 2 diabetes. She has some pain and discomfort behind her left knee.

   Once again, just on this information alone, what would be the extent of your examination?

Observations on Activity 10.13

1. The 12-year-old boy
   Jeans, shoes and socks off so that the whole of both legs can be seen and compared. There could be enlarged glands in the groin from a septic focus somewhere that 'mum' doesn't know about. Always palpate if thought necessary. All the joints in both legs may have to be put through a range of movement. From there you will have to keep an open mind and build on what you find.
2. The 60-year-old woman
   Because of the diabetes, I would certainly ask if I could see both feet. No connection with the knee at all, but diabetic foot problems are common and patients don't always come before it's too late, so grasp the opportunity!

I would also want to look at the 'good' knee for similar problems (for example, arthritis, cysts).

Palpation

Your first experience of 'hands on' examination must be to palpate the various bony prominences and 'get to know your way around' the knee. Do this by following my activity boxes below. Take your time and complete them thoroughly; after each one initial your record of progress form (Checklist 10.1). To gain confidence, palpate your own knees first; best to do this when the family are out of the house – otherwise they may think you just a little strange!

If new to it, you will be a little unsure of the structures. All our lumps and bumps vary slightly in size, position and padding of fat and muscle. The answer is sometimes to try a different joint, but often the only answer is the advice of a senior colleague. This is one reason why I have previously asked you to try to find a mentor.

While learning knee examination, an excellent way is to use patients who have no knee problem for example.

You are managing a patient with a wrist injury and while assessing them you will always ask about injuries elsewhere in the body. So, instead of just the briefest of looks at the other limbs, if time permits, ask them if you may examine the knee in a little more depth. Literally a minute spent palpating a couple of landmarks or performing one particular test is little extra stress for the patient and gives you great experience. Everyone is happy: you gain experience and the patient has a little more thorough examination than usual, feeling that you have **taken more of an interest in them**.

Checklist 10.1 Record of progress

Physical examination of the knee and leg

Examination	On self	Friend practice	Friend practice	Patient practice
Patient history, a variety				
Observation				
Palpation:				
Patella				
Tibial tubercle				
Patella tendon				
Quads muscle				
Quads tendon				
Femoral condyles				
Joint spaces				
Fibula head				
and neck				
Medial ligaments				
Lateral ligaments				
Range of movement:				
Flexion				
Extension				
Distal movements				
Sensations				
Circulation				
Specific tests:				
SLR				
Valgus stress				
Varus stress				
Patellar tap				
Apprehension				
ACL/PCL				
Gait				
Other:				

Activity 10.14   **Time: 10 minutes**

With the knee fully extended, palpate the outline of the patella. Notice that if you hold it either side between two fingers, with a relaxed patient, it will move painlessly to and fro laterally by about a centimetre (*see* Figure 10.18). However, if they tense the leg (contracting the quadriceps muscles and tightening the quadriceps tendon), the patella will become rigid and not move at all.

Always warn the patient about whatever movement you are about to do. Some who have previously had lateral dislocations of the patella, or have conditions of the patello-femoral joint, may feel apprehensive, or be in pain as you do this. Some call this the 'apprehension test'.

 Activity 10.15   **Time: 5 minutes**

Find the tibial tubercle, the often large lump of bone in the midline of the limb, at the anterior of the knee, about 2 cm below the joint line (*see* Figure 10.19). This is usually more prominent in men (knobbly knee contests) than the shapelier legs of women.

In the adult, they can usually be seen at 20 paces, so no need for too much congratulation here!

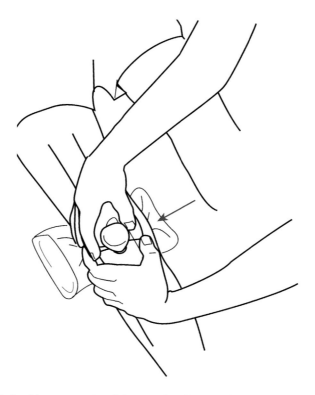

Figure 10.18 Patella side-to-side movement and the apprehension test (Gross *et al.*, 2009).

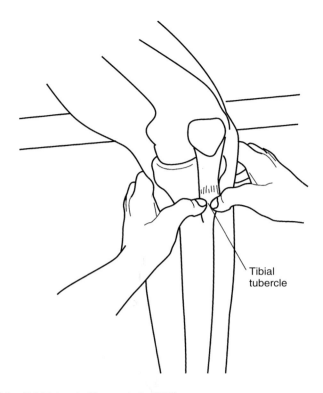

Tibial
tubercle

Figure 10.19 Palpation of the tibial tubercle (Gross *et al.*, 2009).

Before you get much further with handling friends, colleagues and patients, it would be best if we briefly spoke of the subject of consent.

Previously both nurses and paramedics have simply got on with their management of patients, possibly with a passing comment to the patient, such as 'Let's splint this for you now; it will make it feel much better'. However, both professions now have extended roles and in many instances are expected to perform a far greater range of tasks. A detailed knee examination is such a task and, although in many instances 'consent by implication' is still satisfactory, it is best practice to get into the habit of formally asking every patient if you may examine them. A few simple words of your own choosing, such as 'I need to examine your knee now; is that all right?' are all that are necessary for most.

I feel that is far enough to go with the subject of consent for the purposes of this book, but later it will be more appropriate to read further. The book's website will be a help to you as well.

Extensor mechanism

This is a group of structures that together act to extend the knee. The testing of their effectiveness is simplicity itself and a grand place to start.

The ability to extend the knee proves there is no **complete** disruption of all the five components of the extensor apparatus that you have been told of previously in Section 1 of this chapter.

However, your patient may still have a partial lesion; you have to make a judgement as to how 'brave' they being – a balance between your getting the information you require and not putting them through too much discomfort.

Activity 10.16   **Time: 10 minutes**

Next I want you to palpate some soft tissues for the first time.

- Start by feeling distal to the patella for the patella tendon with your index finger and thumb (*see* Figure 10.20). Asking the patient to tense and relax their quads muscles makes this tendon more obvious.
- Now try palpating the quadriceps tendon immediately above the patella; once again tensing of the quadriceps will help to make it tight and therefore more palpable.
- On now with the patient's ability to extend the knee from the sitting position, or straight leg raising (SLR) from the lying position (*see* Figure 10.7).
- This imminently straightforward test gives you very useful information regarding the extensor mechanism of the knee. Ask the patient to raise their heel off the ground, maybe supporting some of their weight at first.

 Activity 10.17   **Time: 15 minutes**

Now, from anterior to posterior, trace the massive curves of the medial and lateral femoral condyles, ending in the medial and lateral joint spaces (*see* Figure 10.21). These joint spaces are a little more difficult to find.

    This is no joke and I know that I am repeating myself, but, if you are learning without the aid of a mentor at your side, it's so important when you are first learning palpation of joints that you use thin people. Never even think of examining a 'chubby' knee until you are confident of finding a joint space easily every time; if you don't heed my words, you will find that depression and inadequacy will surely follow you!

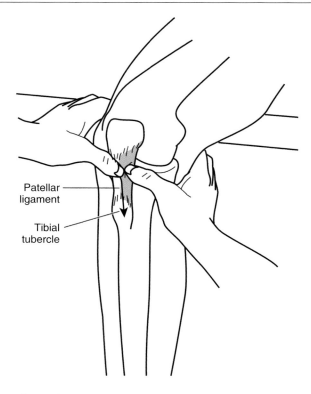

Figure 10.20 Palpation of the patellar tendon (ligament) (Gross *et al.*, 2009).

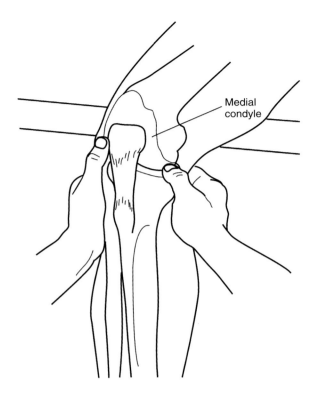

Medial
condyle

Figure 10.21 Palpation of the femoral condyles and joint spaces (Gross *et al.*, 2009).

Fibula

The head and neck of the fibula are the next landmarks and usually quite easy to find. Most importantly, the **common peroneal nerve** (also called the **'lateral popliteal nerve'**) winds around the neck on the outside of the knee (*see* Figure 10.22) and is rather exposed. This nerve supplies sensory distribution to the outer side of the lower leg and foot, and is motor to the muscles in the anterior compartment of the lower leg that extends the toes and ankle.

Any bruising, swelling or tenderness over this site should instantly attract your attention and the need for further motor and sensory testing.

Medial collateral ligament (or tibial collateral ligament)

For this and its partner, the lateral ligament, you should revise the extent by looking again at your notes in section 1 of this chapter. When I first tried to find these soft tissues, I would have pictures at my side while palpating, to make things clear.

It is important that, with some of the soft tissues, they either **cannot be felt as distinct structures** or are often at best a 'suggestion' of a structure.

Note that you are only feeling this structure because it passes over a hollow (the joint line) and that it has quite a large extent both above and below the joint line. The tenderness associated with a strain or rupture may be anywhere along its length; this applies to the lateral side as well.

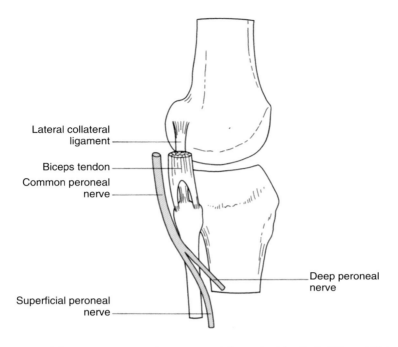

Figure 10.22 The passage of the common peroneal nerve around the neck of the fibula (Ellis and Mahadevan, 2010).

 Activity 10.18　　　　　　　　　　　　　　　　　**Time: 5 minutes**

The medial collateral ligament

With the knee flexed a few degrees, use your finger to trace the medial joint line from anterior to posterior from the hollow at the medial border of the patella.

After a few centimetres, the joint line is less obvious as the MCL passes over it – no massively obvious band, but a far more subtle obliteration (*see* Figure 10.23).

If this is still not obvious to you on a thin patient, you will have to ask a senior colleague for help.

 Activity 10.19　　　　　　　　　　　　　　　　　**Time: 5 minutes**

Valgus stress the medial collateral ligament

This is quite an easy test to perform and then add to your repertoire.

Holding the lower half of the leg with one hand, the other presses the outside of the leg by the knee causing a valgus stress (*see* Figure 10.16). If the MCL is completely ruptured, there will be a noticeable 'give' when stressed, compared with the normal feel.

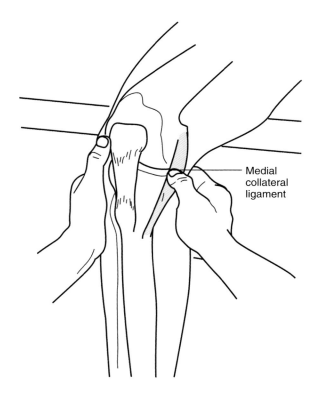

Medial collateral ligament

Figure 10.23 Palpation of the medial collateral ligament and joint line (Gross *et al.*, 2009).

Lateral collateral ligament (or fibular collateral ligament)

Here we have a much easier job because the ligament has a far more cord type of structure, rather than the flattened strap of the MCL. It is made easier too because it is inserted directly into the obvious head of the fibula: all very superficial structures.

 Activity 10.20   Time: **5 minutes**

The lateral collateral ligament

One rather clever way of making the LCL 'stand out' for initial practice like this is as follows. To feel it in your right leg, sit with your right leg crossed over your left, so that your right foot rests on top of your left knee (sounds like something out of a Christmas game, doesn't it?) (*see* Figure 10.24).

Now start the palpation of the joint space at the hollow on the lateral side of the patella and move your finger posteriorly. After about 3 cm there will be a clear obstruction; that will be the lateral ligament. Great, isn't it? Also note that is goes to the fibula head.

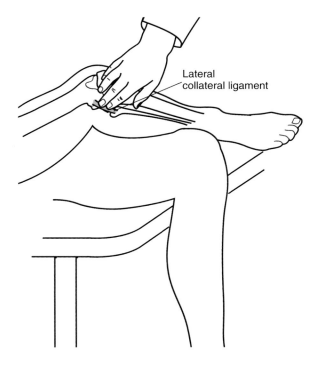

Lateral
collateral ligament

Figure 10.24 Palpation of the lateral collateral ligament (Gross *et al*., 2009).

 Activity 10.21   **Time: 5 minutes**

Testing the integrity of the lateral collateral ligament

This, like the test for the MCL is quite simple to perform.

Holding on to the lower leg and ankle with one hand, produce a varus stress against the outside of the slightly flexed knee. This will stress the LCL producing pain at first, plus, if it is disrupted, excessive movement. Pain will be more severe with a partial tear.

Range of joint movement

There are two ways of recognising joint movement: when the patient does it for you (**active** movement) and when the patient relaxes and you try to put the limb through a range of movement for them (**passive** movement).

An in-between is **assisted** movement, where the patient has the ability, but lacks the confidence or strength, or is in too much pain, to do it on their own. Here you take up some or all of the weight of the distal leg and see how far it will flex or extend.

Each way has its place. The patient usually tries to accomplish the full range of active movements first and, if they cannot, you then assist. Remember to be as gentle as possible, looking at the patient's face for signs of fear.

Generally speaking, if the knee can be put through a range of movement passively without much pain, but the pain is distressing if done actively, it obviously points to a problem based in the muscle or tendon.

While considering knee movements, it is worth mentioning the term '**locking**'. To the ordinary person, you would think that locking meant that a part would not move at all (locked in position). However, just to confuse you, in orthopaedics the term has a special meaning with regard to the knee that is not obvious, but is one that you will have to learn to avoid confusion.

Put simply, a locking knee means that the patient is unable to completely extend it. They can usually flex it; it's just the extension that is the problem. Locking is usually found in a patient with a meniscus tear. It can be just a few degrees short of complete extension (and therefore difficult to notice) or, more unusually, the knee may not be able to get further than a right angle.

Don't use the term when talking with patients –it will lead to confusion.

Testing the integrity of the cruciate ligaments

 Activity 10.22   Time: **10 minutes**

Anterior/posterior drawer test

This is just one simple method of deciding if these ligaments have been torn (*see* Figure 10.25a and 10.25b).

Your patient lies down with the affected knee flexed to about a right angle. The operator sits on the side of the couch facing the patient. The patient's toes are wedged under the operator's bottom. The upper tibia is firmly held between both hands, with the thumbs either side of the tibial tubercle on the joint line. The leg is then pushed backwards and pulled forwards. In the normal knee only a millimetre of movement can be felt, but, if either cruciate is damaged, significant movement is felt.

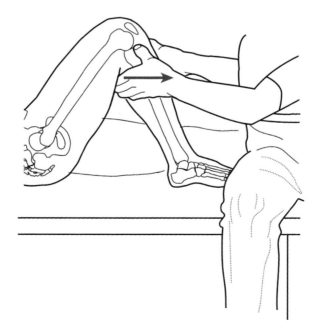

Figure 10.25a Drawer test, for the cruciate ligaments: anterior (Gross *et al.*, 2009).

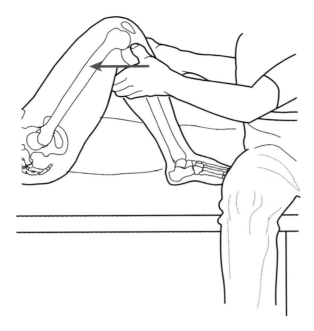

Figure 10.25b Drawer test, for the cruciate ligaments: posterior (Gross *et al.*, 2009).

Examination of swellings around the knee

As well as the need to palpate various cysts and bursae around the knee, there is one specific test that I would like you to become familiar with: it's the patella tap test and it points to there being a significant collection of fluid in the knee joint itself.

 Activity 10.23   **Time: 10 minutes**

The patella tap test

The patient lies with the knee extended. One of the operator's open hands rests on the thigh above the patella and is pressed firmly downwards and distally. This forces any fluid in the joint capsule distally, out of the pouch of the capsule proximal to the patella, and raises the patella off the femoral condyles. Two fingers of the other hand then press down on the patella and it can be felt to tap against the femoral condyles (*see* Figure 10.26).

Ottawa knee rules

A very important activity for you next – it must not be missed because of its great implications for your future clinical practice.

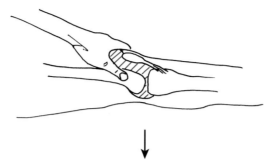

1. Squeeze more fluid underneath the patella

2. Press on the patella 'tapping' it onto femur

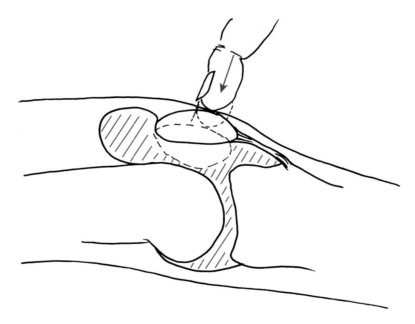

Figure 10.26 The patella tap test.

 Activity 10.24   **Time: 30 minutes**

The Ottawa knee rules

I would like you to go on the internet, into Google or another search engine, and put in 'Ottawa knee rules'. There are many sites that state these rules and discuss them as well; they are very important to know. Alternatively if you want some variation, YouTube have some short videos that are fine.

  Also read Bryony (2012).

  Write some notes, or take some print-outs. Maybe discuss their worth with one of the senior doctors you meet.

The dangers of other books

You may have noticed the large number of physical examination books on the library shelves these days. Most are excellent, but there is a danger that you should be aware of. This is that **most are primarily written for doctors or medical students in hospital**. To get as wide a readership as possible, all branches of the professions are provided for and just about every test imaginable is covered. In some ways this is good. However, for the average paramedic, ECP or ENP, this is too much information and in the end it becomes difficult to realise which tests need to be carried out routinely. Over the years, I can remember many instances of students coming to me wanting to discuss tests that I had never even heard of and I dread to think what 'tortures' some have put their patients through in attempts to be as thorough as instructed in a book they have been reading.

Also for paramedics and ECPs, the environment in which they work is often not suitable for such detailed examinations because of influences such as the following:

- **Privacy**, either out in the street or with several relatives present in a room at home.
- Temperature, even indoors **may be cold** in winter.
- **Lighting** for the paramedic may be very variable.
- **Little available time**; in difficult situations you just cannot hang around.
- **Initial severe pain** of injury; many tests are too painful to be attempted soon following an injury.
- **Lack of skilled assistance** and analgesia for undressing is the norm out of hospital.
- **De-skilling** with infrequent use.

Very detailed examination books just do not consider these points, making it very difficult for the non-medical practitioner to balance what is required.

A prime example when considering the knee would be the **McMurray test**. This would be used in hospital, mostly by orthopaedic specialists, to help when clinically deciding if a patient had a meniscus tear. You basically grind the upper end of the tibia on the femoral condyles, and it takes skill in interpretation. Can you just imagine the unnecessary pain you would put your acute patient through?

To overcome some of these dangers, perhaps this is a good place for a golden rule:

GOLDEN RULE

When considering a specific diagnostic test, only perform it if the result may change your clinical course of action, or is necessary for referral.

In Checklist 10.1, try to keep up your listing of the aspects of knee examination that you have covered clinically.

Section 4
Minor musculoskeletal injuries

Before covering the contents of this section, you should remember that the basic assumption is that you are dealing with a 'minors' type of patient. Someone who has walked or hobbled in to see you in a unit, or that you have gone out to see as an ECP on a green call.

Some of the bony injuries to be detailed are usually found following the application of major forces to the body. In these instances, never, ever, think of the patient as having just the one presenting injury. Always **manage the force applied to the body**, not just the obvious result.

So, with a MOI of a powerful football tackle in mind, rather than a high-speed RTC or 20-foot fall off a roof, read through the following text for a fair introduction to injuries around the knee.

Fractures of the patella

These are often seen associated with a dashboard impact, but a sporting kick or strong quadriceps contraction can have a similar effect. There are several main varieties (*see* Figure 10.27) and, with the patella being enclosed in a strong retinaculum, the extensor mechanism can sometimes remain intact, making an SLR still possible although painful. Signposts bringing your attention to the fracture can be overlying bruising, haematoma, graze or laceration.

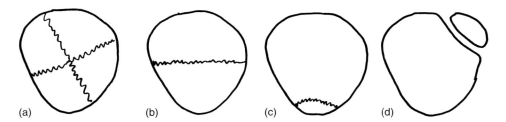

(a)   (b)   (c)   (d)

Figure 10.27 Main designs of patella fracture: (a) stellate (star-shaped) (b) transverse (c) avulsion fracture of the inferior pole (d) not a fracture at all, but a fairly common variation where the patella has an accessory centre of ossification. It is called a 'bipartite patella'.

If the MOI was a high-speed RTC impact, this should lead you on to also consider an associated dislocated hip on the same side, as mentioned in Section 2 of this chapter.

The posterior (articular) surface of the patella is continuous with the joint capsule, so any fracture with cortical damage here will bleed into the joint, sometimes forming a tense haemarthrosis (*see* Figure 10.28).

Initial management

The leg is usually most comfortable immobilised in extension. Along with the array of specialised temporary splints available, don't forget the benefits of the simple yet effective pillow.

The immediate comfort of needle drainage of the haemarthrosis will be very welcome.

Open reduction will be required for transverse fractures, and removal of the patella if the articular surface is badly damaged, so as to prevent early OA years later.

Bipartite patella

In most people, the patella forms from one centre of ossification, but occasionally more than one is found (as with Andy Murray). This causes no particular problem in the majority, with just some irregularity on palpation, but, if the person needs a knee X-ray, the deformity can show up and seem similar to a fracture, sometimes causing confusion. The senior professional should, however, be aware of this variation and be able to reassure the patient (*see* Figure 10.27d).

Dislocated patella

Clinical features

Lateral displacement of the patella is usually obvious, unless the patient has very fat knees, in which case the fat can to some extent hide the deformity and leave you faced with something less obvious (*see* Figure 10.29). The knee is usually presented to you in a flexed position, with the patient reluctant to move from this.

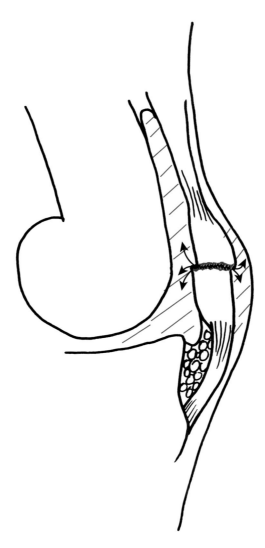

Figure 10.28 How a fracture of the patella may cause a haemarthrosis.

Even if the condition is recurrent, which is common, there is often considerable pain and discomfort. Patients with recurrent dislocations usually realise immediately what has happened and tell you straight away that 'it has come out again'.

If you are unsure of the diagnosis immediately, comparison with the 'good' knee and some gentle palpation should quickly make it clear. An X-ray would only be considered pre-reduction if the history was unusual, tending towards a severe force and the possibility of an associated fracture nearby.

It would be incorrect to say that the patella always dislocates laterally, but that is the only form that I have ever seen.

Remember what you learnt earlier about the extensor mechanism, how rigid the patella became when the quads were contracting and how you could wobble it from side to side when relaxed. Here is an important point to consider: as you are immobilising your patient, the patella has every chance of spontaneously relocating, especially under the influence of analgesia. With this dislocation and a tensed patient, the extensor mechanism is shortened. With the leg extended, the patient relaxes the extensor structures increasing their length.

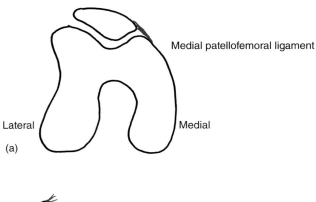

Medial patellofemoral ligament

Lateral   Medial

(a)

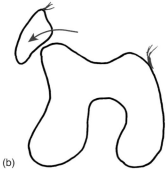

(b)

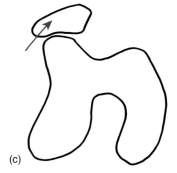

(c)

Figure 10.29 The patella femoral joint: (a) normal 'skyline' view (b) lateral dislocation (c) direction of pressure for reduction, if used simultaneously with extension of the knee.

Formal reduction

I have never seen a simple dislocated patella that required a general anaesthetic to be reduced. Most reduce spontaneously before even reaching professional help. Those that arrive still dislocated in A&E are easily reduced with the assistance of a sedative and/or analgesia. Difficulty beyond that is usually because of inexperience of the professional. The major points to consider are:

- pain relief and fear
- talking the patient through relaxation of the quadriceps

- assisting them to a degree of **extension of the knee; this alone is often enough to allow it to spontaneously relocate**
- pressure on the lateral border of the patella, pushing towards the midline (*see* Figure 10.29c).

Once reduced, the knee will then require examining. The form of immobilisation following reduction varies locally (Thomas, 2001).

Almost all these injuries are simple and initially no further consideration is required. However, in a very small proportion of patients, fractures of either the femoral condyle or the patella can occur. I have never seen a dislocation combined with ACL rupture, but you must still be alert to the possibility.

Dislocated knee

This is a dire orthopaedic emergency that I have only seen a couple of times in my life and will only give a brief mention here. It is associated with massive force as seen in major trauma such as RTCs, rather than sporting injuries. ATLS protocols are usually the primary name of the game here. Never treat an injured area in isolation: always consider the patient as a whole.

Finally, do not call a dislocated patella 'a dislocated knee'– it can cause much confusion, especially to another professional over the phone.

Fractures of the tibial plateau

An important application of the tibial anatomy is that the plateau is formed of an inner 'honeycomb' of cancellous bone within a thin outer layer of compact bone and articulcular cartilage. This makes it light and strong, but has the disadvantage that once breached it crumbles easily, deforming the joint surface.

Associated with this damage will usually be a haematoma into the soft tissues and a haemarthrosis.

More detail of these injuries is not necessary here, because such fractures will need orthopaedic referral for assessment of combined bone and ligament trauma and, in many instances, open fixation for further management. The seriousness of these injuries is usually obvious immediately by just looking at the knee, followed by minimal palpation.

Supracondylar and intercondylar fractures of the femur

A brief mention here of these major injuries, for completeness only; and for the terrible time when they arrive by mistake in an MIU.

Once stable, the **circulation distal to the injury is the priority**.

Before we leave these fractures, just sometimes following a fracture of the femur, bone-forming cells escape into the haematoma involving the large muscle groups such as the quadriceps. When this happens, bone forms in the muscle belly, therefore restricting knee movement. This is called '**myositis ossificans**' and could be a 'walk-in problem' for you.

Neck of fibula

Fractures of the upper end and neck of the fibula can commonly be associated with injuries to the ankle. It is important that, at this stage of your education, you get into the habit of always palpating the full length of the fibula following ankle injuries and, similarly, if the upper fibula is injured, enquire regarding pain in the ankle. X-rays on the book's website will help you with this injury.

Clinical features

Often the pain and discomfort of other associated injuries makes the patient trivialise the problem at the upper fibula, at least initially. That is why a thorough examination is so important. They have not had a direct blow over the fractured area and rotational forces carry on up the fibula, so you do not initially expect an injury there. Swelling and discolouration can be very minimal at first, especially for the paramedic who tends to see most injuries far sooner than their hospital-based colleagues.

Initial management

This would be closely involved with the usual associated ankle injury; for instance, resting in a splint or raised on a pillow with analgesia until ready for reduction.

 Activity 10.25   Time: **A quick question**

The fibula is such a delicate bone, tucked away and, unlike its partner the tibia, not carrying any of the body weight to the ankle. So, why bother giving it so much 'floor space'?

Observations on Activity 10.25

Well, it has rather a close relationship with a local nerve supplying the muscles of the lower leg. The track of the common peroneal nerve (lateral popliteal nerve) takes it winding around the neck of the fibula (remember Figure 10.22), before branching out to the muscles of the anterior leg.

If the fibula fractures, sharp ends of bone or simply haematoma can easily damage the nerve. This is motor to the extensor muscles of the leg that extend the toes and dorsiflex the foot. In more simple language, the patient may get degrees of numbness and paraesthesiae, plus weakened extension of toes and foot, or a drop foot if damage is severe.

Fractured tibial tubercle

This is usually an avulsion fracture of the knee's extensor mechanism, with the tubercle being pulled off during forceful extension of the knee, during sports.

Minor soft tissue injuries

Medial collateral ligaments

These ligaments, which may also be called the 'tibial collateral ligaments', support the knee medially.

Forms of injury

The possibilities for injury are:

- strain
- partial rupture
- complete rupture
- complete rupture plus damage to other structures such as:
  - medial meniscus
  - ACL.

All depends on the amount of force applied to the joint.

Clinical features

Your patient's pain will be centred over the site of the ligament with associated overlying tenderness. The pain on valgus strain would be worse if there was just a partial tear, pulling on the damaged tissues, because a complete lesion would just allow the joint space to open out.

Expect any associated skin trauma to be on the lateral surface of the knee as the valgus force was applied, with just minimal swelling on the medial surface. Of course you would have to add additional features with associated meniscus and ACL problems.

Initial management

Until the diagnosis is confirmed, the injury will be managed with initial support on pillow or splint. Partial lesions will be managed immobilised in extension with a cylinder.

Complete lesions will be for repair.

The lateral collateral ligaments

The amount of damage to these LCL and other structures in the complex depends (as with the MCL) on the amount of force applied to the limb. If very severe, all could be torn through, the force then passing through the centre of the knee itself tearing the cruciates, but more detail of these later.

Because these lateral ligaments are not attached to the lateral menisci, the menisci are usually sparred with a varus force to the joint, the usual mechanism for these injuries.

Clinical features

The varus force impact will leave any impact skin trauma on the medial surface of the knee (*see* Figure 10.16). This is an important point for clinicians to consider: **force applied on one part of the limb producing the opportunity for significant damage to soft tissues on another**. Any professional can understand a direct impact causing, for instance, a fracture locally, but a higher level of knowledge and understanding is required for the continuing force and damage to be appreciated.

 Activity 10.26   **Time: 15 minutes**

You are working in an MIU and suspect that your patient has damage to a collateral ligament. How may your depth of examination vary from that of a doctor, or, indeed, should there be any difference?

In your rough shorthand, list the points you have thought of and only then read my observations.

Observations on Activity 10.26

Well, this activity should have brought up quite a few thoughts and no quick 'one statement answers all' situation exists. To reach a decision, you have to consider several aspects.

The first of these is your exact role. The role of practitioners with the same title varies throughout the UK. An ENP, ECP or advanced paramedic may be expected to fit differently into existing systems. You have probably realised this, seeing how difficult it would be to move to similar jobs around the country.

Generally you have to **decide if you are employed to find that a situation is abnormal, or to reach a definitive diagnosis and then manage it**. You will find that you are expected to reach a definitive diagnosis in some circumstances, but also know when to stop when your findings start pointing in another direction. The thought must always be, and we have already considered this as a previous golden rule: when considering a specific diagnostic test, **only perform it if the result may change your clinical course of action**.

Don't put patients through unnecessary examinations just because you know how to perform them. I was always taught the worth of what is called '**masterly inactivity**'.

Different levels of experience are important. A GP standing in, doing a session, may well have many years of orthopaedic experience and be far better than you at interpreting a clinical test.

The availability of referral may vary from a fracture clinic on site to a different hospital and a few days' wait. This would mean that one practitioner may have to 'go further' with an examination than another.

After that brief diversion, back to our LCL now. One rather interesting way in which they vary from the MCLs is that you have to remember that **the common peroneal nerve winds around the head of the fibula** on this same lateral side and may also be injured by the force causing the varus strain. So in every instance ask and examine your patient for abnormal sensations to the outer leg and dorsum of foot, plus dorsiflexion of the toes and foot.

Initial management

This is similar to MCL care, with strains simply requiring a form of temporary support and rest, then referring on of the more serious conditions.

Perhaps we should have a word of warning here, and not just for LCL injuries. These soft tissue injuries to the knee can so easily lead you to danger. Always be on your guard because **they are notoriously difficult to be certain about immediately following injury and without advanced techniques such as scans**. Because of this, it will save you future embarrassment to **always leave your patient with the understanding that, if anything goes wrong, or they have further problems with their knee, they should always return SOS**.

Cruciate ligaments

Hidden away in the centre of the knee, 'holding it all together', are the cruciate ligaments (CL), crossing over one another like intertwined fingers. They are immensely strong, yet still vulnerable, so you must study them in some detail.

Damage to them is commonly associated with other injuries such as torn collateral ligaments and meniscus tears. This is because the MOIs are similar and damage to a cruciate ligament allows the forces to continue further into the knee with the resultant damage (*see* Figure 10.30).

Because of the synovial tissue wrapped around the ligaments, tears will result in a haemarthrosis coming on rapidly and often being quite tense.

Pain will be situated deep inside the joint with possible tenderness anteriorly on a flexed knee.

In the acute knee, active movements will be severely limited, although, if there are no accompanying meniscal injuries, passive movement should be good, depending on the extent of haemarthrosis.

Overall **an ACL tear is far more common than the posterior**. Valgus or varus forces are likely to tear both, whereas other mechanisms will have ACL- or PCL-specific results.

Clinical features

Although incomplete tears occur, **that level of diagnosis is beyond the remit of non-medical practitioners**; we recognise the likely CL problem and refer our patient on for a definitive diagnosis. As an example of this, one of the characteristics of this condition is that the patient sometimes say that **they heard a 'popping' sound** at the time of injury. To me, this fact alone points me along the course of referral to a more senior practitioner. **In my opinion, it is bad practice to perform any further test on a patient, possibly with a haemarthrosis and anxious**.

Sometimes your patient will present with a previous history suggestive of a CL injury, often weeks beforehand. They trivialised it at the time, because they want to do little more than walk around and have simply struggled on with their lives.

Here their problems would be a lack of stability, **the knee 'giving way' and letting them down**, with straightforward walking being okay, but any turns (weight on the problem knee and twisting) not being safe. In this type of knee, **not acutely injured**, no haemarthrosis, the anterior draw test would be very acceptable to the patient and provide you with important information.

Remember that a patient with a tear of one of these ligaments may still be able to walk in weight bearing; never consider non-weight bearing as an essential for a significant injury.

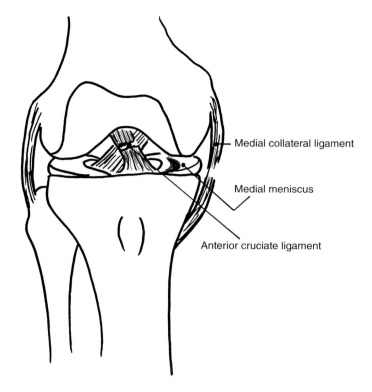

Figure 10.30 Patterns of injury to knee structures.

Initial management

Initial support and immobilisation, followed by needle aspiration of the haemarthrosis and compression, will make the patient much more comfortable while awaiting definitive repair. It's all down to the availability of surgery.

The delayed discovery of this condition does not preclude repair, but is not ideal for the patient's comfort and long-term recovery. An inactive knee weakens more, leading to more instability and protracted recovery.

Menisci

These are not now thought of as 'cartilage' despite the older term 'semilunar cartilages', but rather as very substantial soft tissues like hardened tendons. If unsure, revise your anatomy of them now in section 1.

Forms of damage

There are several possible variations of a tear (*see* Figure 10.31). The menisci (especially the lateral) have the ability to move out of the way of damage a little, but eventually, if the force is great enough, they will tear. A variant called a 'discoid' meniscus is worthy of further study, although uncommon (Patel, Greydanus and Baker, 2009).

Clinical features

The clinical features depend very much on the position and extent of the damage.

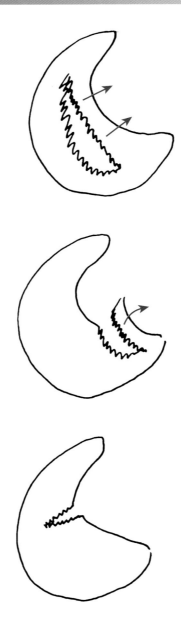

Figure 10.31 Some forms of meniscus tears.

 Activity 10.27   **Time: A quick thought**

Can you think of an observation that you should always make as a routine part of any knee examination?
   Clue: it gives you an overall indication of the patient's discomfort/severity of problem.

Observations on Activity 10.27

Within a week of disuse, the quadriceps muscles will have become noticeably weaker and you will see wasting if you compare with the other side. This should become one of your standard points to consider with any examination. It doesn't point to a specific condition, but it does say that this knee is troubling the patient so much that they are hardly using it. Having a tape measure handy to measure the diameters of both thighs can help to demonstrate lesser degrees of wasting.

Anyway, back to the acute stage. When thinking of the diagnosis, it is useful to list, and learn by heart, the following features:

- Classic MOI.
- Usually male adult.
- Inability to continue with the activity at time of injury.
- Pain at the joint line.
- Joint effusion.
- Lack of full extension (locking).

None of them on their own suggest that this patient has a meniscus tear, but placed together they are good pointers.

The effusion caused by an inflamed synovium comes on slowly and may not be present at all when first seen by a paramedic. In fact, as I have said before, this lack of swelling is a constant problem that paramedics have throughout the whole sphere of diagnosing injury and illness, and is one not always appreciated by other professionals.

Paramedics see most patients so early on in the progression of their condition that they often have to be far more careful in their examination and 'reading' of a situation.

 Activity 10.28   Time: **A short diversion story**

This aspect was highlighted to me in my early days as an A&E charge nurse. The then 'ambulance drivers' (well it was a long time ago) would bring patients in to me following an RTC, in established clinical shock, without any pre-warning of their arrival.

I would complain and they would say, '. . .honest, Dave, he was stable at the scene, just a little pale. . .' At first I wouldn't believe them, but then a worldly-wise consultant explained how conditions, especially haemorrhage, progress with time and how much more difficult the assessment was for those at the initial scene. A lesson well learnt that has helped me to appreciate trauma progression many times since then.

Initial management

Initially if the effusion is severe, it may be aspirated for the patient's comfort. If the patient is a professional footballer, they would then immediately have some form of repair done. However, with lesser mortals like us, we would be referred to a clinic and have some form of wait for definitive care, unless of course the locking is substantial, when something would have to be done immediately.

The quadriceps and extensor mechanism

Earlier you looked at the detail of the extensor mechanism; if you need a recap, go back now and refresh your knowledge. Here we are to consider injuries to each part in turn, starting with the bulk of the quadriceps muscles themselves and then working distally.

Forms of injury

For the body of the muscle to become torn, we are in the realm of sports injury, or perhaps we should say people of all ages, shapes, sizes and levels of fitness trying to do some activity they are not used to.

Basically the actual tear can vary considerably from the overstretching of a few muscle fibres through to a complete tear with massive haematoma formation.

Clinical features

The main feature is intense pain at the time of injury in the anterior of the thigh, followed by further intense pain on any attempt to extend or flex the knee. The thigh will be tense and tender because of a protective spasm of the muscles and far more so with a massive injury because of the possible tamponade, due to haematoma formation (compartment syndrome).

Walking will be all but impossible, the patient having to stop the activity they were doing and get carried.

Initial management

The majority of tears are of only moderate size and can heal by themselves in time. The age-old initial management of RICE applies here. The patient will require immediate rest in bed and would be more comfortable if the whole leg was raised on several pillows.

Ice packs, laid over the most painful area, are next. They should not be placed directly on the skin, but rather with a towel intervening to prevent skin damage. Replacement should occur about every hour at first and then the packs re-applied a few times a day.

After a few days, when starting to gently mobilise, an elasticated type of support will offer compression, helping to prevent further bleeding. Severe tears will require a stick or crutches to allow phased weight bearing. As time progresses, exercise should increase, to regain normality.

Throughout, suitable analgesia will assist.

Quadriceps tendon

Inferiorly the muscle bellies fuse to form the quadriceps tendon, inserting into the upper pole of the patella. This is a frequent place for complete tears to occur.

Especially with thinner people, it is clear enough for you to be able to place your finger in to feel the rift; compare both sides if in doubt. With this injury, the patient will be completely unable to weight bear or extend the knee. Theatre is the only option.

Patella tendon

When the patella tendon tears, the patella rides high up on the femur, caused by the pull of the quadriceps. As with the torn quadriceps tendon mentioned earlier, there will be local tenderness and a little swelling, but the main feature will be the inability to extend the knee or weight bear.

Another form of this injury is seen just below, where, instead of tearing through the tendon, the pull of the quadriceps avulses the tibial tubercle.

Hamstrings

Just as the quadriceps can receive trauma, usually during sports, so the massive hamstring group at the back of the thigh are frequently injured. Tears can once again range from the trivial through to massive tears.

The muscles involved are the:

- semimembranosus
- semitendinosus
- biceps femoris.

They all have their origin attached to part of the pelvis with a fantastic name, the ischial tuberosity. This lump of bone, although buried deep in your bottom, is very easy to feel.

Fascia lata

The final soft tissue to mention is the FL. This is a thick sheet of fascia spread out over the lateral surface of the thigh, forming a thick, tendon-like structure (called the 'iliotibial band') inserting into the upper tibia just below the knee joint.

Like any of the soft tissues, it can be overstretched and irritated causing much pain, swelling and discomfort in the knee over the lateral side.

Whether you call this an injury or a condition is open to debate, but it leads you well into the next section.

Section 5
Minor musculoskeletal conditions

Chondromalacia patellae

This affects far more females than males, probably because of the very different female anatomy of the hips and thighs. The wider female hips make a larger angle with the femur and patella at the knee. Because of this, the patella will not ride as accurately between the articular surfaces of the femoral condyles, producing irregular wear and eventually pathology.

Over recent years, chondromalacia patellae (CP) has become a rather 'umbrella' term for any condition producing pain around or under the patella, similar to people talking of a fractured neck of femur. I personally see no harm in this, especially for non-professional use; it seems a rather good general term to help a patient understand the condition. However, for accuracy, some want the term reserved for those patients in whom it can be demonstrated that there is actual damage to the cartilage of the patello-femoral joint.

Types of condition

There is variety here, ranging from symptoms with no discernable cartilage damage at arthroscopy through to severe OA changes in the patello-femoral joint.

Obviously damage to the cartilage will be more common when the joint is subjected to excessive amounts of wear and tear, as in accomplished sports people.

Clinical features

The common presentation is with **anterior knee pain**, felt either under or around the patella. This will be worse on movement and also leave residual pain even at rest. Tenderness will be found on palpation around the margins of the patella, as well as on pressure against the condylar surfaces.

Attempting to move the patella sideways, especially laterally, will produce at least apprehension (the apprehension test) or frank pain.

Feelings of outright crepitus may occur, or, more frequently, a 'popping' or other sounds.

Initial management

This consists of analgesics and anti-inflammatory drugs, developing to physiotherapy and specialist referral and advice.

Because the presentation is rarely too acute, your advice is perhaps the most important element to help the patient. Understanding what is wrong is a big step forward and you should never underestimate the effect of this on your patient.

Operative measures can be taken later, varying from alteration of the insertion of tendons, to arthroscopic 'clearing up' of the joint, to muscle adjustments.

Patella tendinitis

Clinical features

This condition is common with specific sports, which have given it varying colloquial names (jumper's knee, etc.). However, it boils down to overuse, putting the tendon under excessive stress, either over time, or with forceful concentrated effort by the athlete.

Pain at the tendon is the striking feature, associated with the other standard inflammatory features of localised swelling, redness, heat, limited movement, tendon thickening, etc.

Initial management

Stopping the source of the stress to the tendon is the obvious first measure, so advice to the patient regarding cutting down the activity is important. This could vary from your advising an elderly patient to take things more easily to the need for detailed history taking by a sports expert regarding the patient's training activities (way beyond our everyday remit). This may sound a little excessive, but sometimes the footwear, warming up, timing of workouts, etc. can have a significant effect for the patient, to whom their health and sporting activity can mean everything in life.

Next comes analgesia and anti-inflammatory agents, followed by immediate ease with RICE actions and physiotherapy.

Rheumatoid arthritis

This is a generalised autoimmune disease that shows in specified and widespread sites in the soft tissues surrounding joints and spreads into the joints themselves. Females are predominantly affected, often starting in the early twenties or thirties.

Osteoarthritis of the knee

Factors that predispose to the formation of OA in the knee are:

- **meniscus injury**, possibly many years before
- previous **arthritis of a hip**, putting excessive stress on a knee
- previous **fracture in the knee** (for example, tibial plateau) not able to be accurately reduced
- something like many **years of strenuous sports** like running, causing damage
- **fracture or orthopaedic disease almost anywhere in the same leg**, altering alignment of knee articulation – for instance, fractured neck of femur, or Perthe's disease.

Clinical features

Bearing in mind all the variety you have considered, the **typical** presentation for you to have in your mind is as follows:

- Patient, middle-aged to elderly.
- Often know that they already have some form of arthritis, or are very suspicious of it.
- Knee pain, described frequently as:
  - like intense toothache
  - a continual throbbing ache
  - sometimes sharp and radiating both up and down the leg
  - all the above, worse when weight bearing (sounds miserable, doesn't it?)
- Swelling of the synovium surrounding the joint.
- Sometimes genu varum or genu valgum deformity depending on the exact site of most of the bone changes.

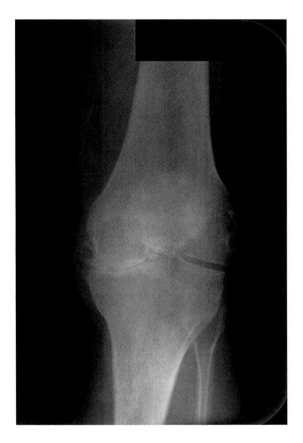

Figure 10.32 X-ray changes associated with OA of the knee.

X-ray changes

For the ENP, ECP or advanced paramedic, the detailed interpretation of X-rays is beyond our remit. However, to be able to recognise the basic changes associated with OA of the knee is of great value (*see* Figure 10.32). The website associated with this book also gives you explained examples and exercises.

The following changes occur as the disease progresses, but at a different stage and rate in every patient, depending on their tissues and their lifestyles:

- **Narrowing of the joint space**, plus its eventual **elimination** as the various cartilages are progressively destroyed.
- The bone between the two articular surfaces slowly come into contact causing what is called '**eburnation**', a whitening on the X-ray.
- The **bone deforms** (collapses).
- Around the margins of the joint, little outgrowths of bone appear (**lipping**) and enlarge with time (**osteophyte formation**).
- The bone surrounding the joint becomes less dense, less white on the X-ray (**osteoporosis**) and **cysts** are sometimes seen.

Once you have looked for these on a few knee X-rays, they will become second nature to you; practice makes perfect.

Activity 10.29   **Time: 5 minutes**

Have you been studying or just reading? Can you list the five X-ray changes that you have just read?
If not, perhaps you need another break from study.

Initial management

OA of the knee on its own is unlikely to be a primary reason for calling an ambulance or attending an A&E department. However, injury to a knee with existing OA is a common situation and you have to give due consideration to the pre-existing pain and discomfort that the patient will be experiencing. Any injuries on or near to these existing delicate and tender tissues may present you with a diagnostic minefield. The answer: examine thoroughly, make your judgement and, if in any doubt, refer.

For the patient who has an exacerbation of OA features without other problems, advice regarding pain, anti-inflammatory drugs, rest, elevation and warmth all have their place. Some who have never used a stick may need to use one for a while, or, if already using a stick, crutches may provide more temporary relief.

Septic arthritis of the knee

Sometimes also called '**pyogenic arthritis**' or '**infective arthritis**', this is a very different proposition from the OA just discussed. The situation here is that the joint capsule has either been punctured with the introduction of bacteria into the joint, or the bacteria have reached the joint capsule via the bloodstream – this often in young children a few days after an infection elsewhere.

Clinical features

With adults, there will usually be a clear history of puncture wound to the knee in the past 24 hours or so, **if you ask about it**. Local features include:

- increasing pain in the joint, especially on weight bearing
- increased skin temperature over the joint as well as a general pyrexia
- associated general symptoms of an infection
- erythema of the overlying tissues
- tense swelling of the joint
- limitation of all movements.

Management is immediate referral.

Acute osteomyelitis

A common site for this infection is the end of the metaphysis at the proximal tibia, due to the slower passage of blood through vessels in this area (*see* Figure 10.33).

The infection is usually from a focus in another part of the body; the bacteria are blood borne, lodge and multiply in the site. Occasionally there is a history of a previous penetrating injury as the source of bacteria. Have acute osteomyelitis in your mind as a possible diagnosis in any children aged about 10 to 12 years, presenting with any of the following features:

- Site of infection.
- Increasing severe pain.

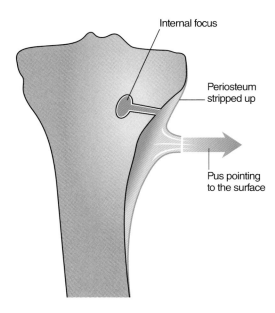

Internal focus

Periosteum
stripped up

Pus pointing
to the surface

Figure 10.33 Acute osteomyelitis of the tibia (Duckworth and Blundell, 2010).

- Swelling.
- Tenderness.
- Redness.
- Diminished walking, limping.
- Local heat and a pyrexia.
- Features associated with a pyrexia.

Immediate management

- Referral of the patient immediately.
- Admission.
- Blood culture.
- Theatre.
- Antibiotics.

Bursitis

Review the sites of bursae from section 1 if you are a little unsure, and also the MOIs in section 2.

Types of condition

The condition may be caused by a direct infection from a puncture wound over the bursa, or by spread of bacteria through the blood supply.

The pre-patellar or infra-patella bursae are the most commonly affected, but others around the knee are occasionally seen.

Clinical features

The standard features of inflammation apply here; there will be local:

- pain
- swelling of the bursa itself and also of the surrounding soft tissues
- limitation of function
- increased local heat
- erythema.

Initial management

Pre-patellar bursitis is an example. Stop all unnecessary walking. Next, when the patient is sitting down, suggest raising the leg comfortably on some kind of stool. Finally, pain relief and maybe anti-inflammatory drugs can be used.

With this treatment, few occurrences will give trouble for long and most should rapidly start to settle and the excess fluid reabsorb.

If you have a patient who is not responding, the measure of the patient's assessment of their own inactivity and/or the initial diagnosis needs consideration.

Cysts around the knee

The popliteal fossa at the posterior of the knee is a common place to find cysts, often called '**Baker's cysts**'. These are sometimes continuous with the capsule of the knee joint and, although they may stay a given size as when first discovered, they commonly slowly increase with time, like a balloon being inflated with synovial fluid.

They occur because of no particular reason or may develop as the lining of the joint is affected by disease – for instance, commonly following OA.

Clinical features

Some patients are frightened, or at least anxious, when feeling a lump for the first time.

The cysts may be painful, sometimes considerably so, especially if they spontaneously burst, releasing the fluid into the soft tissues. Alternatively, cysts can become infected, with all the associated features of infection that you already know well.

As they enlarge, they may cause considerable discomfort while walking.

Initial management

Immediate reassurance of an anxious patient is the first priority; the second is simply referral.

Osgood Schlatter's disease

This condition is called an '**apophysitis**'. This means that there is an ongoing strain of the tissues of the **tibial tubercle** where the patella tendon is inserted into bone. This pulls on the area, causing the laying down of new bone and inflammation (*see* Figure 10.34). As in most conditions, there are varieties that show just a few problems, going through the range to quite severe pain.

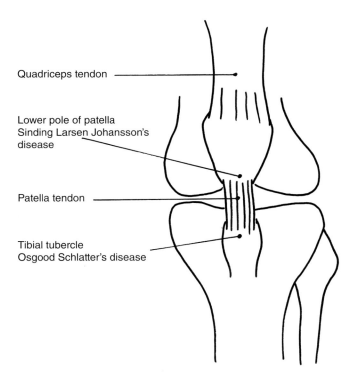

Figure 10.34 Sites of Osgood Schlatter's and Sinding-Larsen disease

Clinical features

- Usually occurs in pre-teenage boys, especially those who are at their height of football enjoyment, like in a school team.
- Pain at the tibial tubercle is the standard presentation, with parents often minimising it thinking it is just 'growing pains'.
- There will be a firm swelling with tenderness over the tibial tubercle.
- There will be limitation of movement, and the patient will often be limping or at least unable to run and play the game as he could.

Immediate management

Obviously there will be a range here, starting with explanation, reassurance and simple advice before referral. The ongoing specialist care for those with a more severe form of the condition would usually consist of immobilisation in a form of cast followed by physiotherapy.

Sinding Larsen Johansson's disease

This is another condition, very similar to Osgood Schlatter's, but of the lower pole of the patella/patella tendon junction (*see* Figure 10.34). Similar age groups, presentations and management apply.

Problems following the common total knee replacement surgery

This is a very common and effective operation for gross OA of the knee, giving the patient a new lease of life and mobility. The vast majority of patients have an excellent result that continues for years. However, there is a very small proportion who run into problems.

Infection

The worst imaginable is the evil of infection following an otherwise good result from the operation. Always bear this in mind as a possibility if the patient complains of sudden and worsening pain in the joint, and do not expect to be presented with all the classical features: **they may be subtle at first**.

Loosening

Joints do not last for ever; they have a life span. At the time of writing, the average patient can expect 10–15 years of use from the operation, but this does not occur with all patients and loosening of the joints' bond to the bone can certainly occur earlier in some unfortunate ones. As with infection, this initially presents as progressive unexplained pain in and around the knee. The patient will start to limp and have restriction of movement and swelling.

 Activity 10.30   **Time: 10 minutes for each condition**

I would like you to study just a little about the following conditions, but keep to the 10 minutes:

- Plica syndrome.
- Iliotibial band syndrome.
- Discoid meniscus.
- Pelligrini steidas.
- Osteochondritis dissecans.

    As a senior professional you should know of their existence, but it is not necessary for you to study them in detail at this stage.

REFERENCES AND SUGGESTED READING

Bryony, P. (2012) Predicting the need for knee radiography in the emergency department: Ottawa or Pittsburg rule? *Emergency Medicine Journal*, 29: 77–78.

Corfield, L., Granne, I. and Latimer-Sayer, W. (2009) *ABC of Medical Law*, BMJ Books, London.

Ellis, H. and Mahadevan, V. (2010) *Clinical Anatomy*, 12th edn, Wiley Blackwell, Oxford.

Emms, N.W. (2002) Hip pathology can masquerade as knee pain in adults, *Age and Ageing*, 31: 67–69.

Gross, J.M., Fetto, J. and Rosen, E. (2009) *Musculoskeletal Examination*, 3rd edn, Wiley Blackwell, Oxford.

Patel, D.R., Greydanus, D. and Baker, R. (2009) *Pediatric Practice Sports Medicine*, 1st edn, McGraw-Hill, New York.

Thomas, M. (2001) Cricket Pad Splint is Better than Plaster Cylinder for First Patellar Dislocation, www.bestbets.org (accessed 24 May 2013).

Tortora. G.J. and Nielsen, M.T. (2012) *Principles of Human Anatomy*, 12th edn, Wiley Blackwell, Oxford.

Multiple choice questions

Before you start, take in the reasoning behind these MCQs, how to answer them and how to interpret the results, from the section at the end of Chapter 1.

1. **With a meniscus injury, the patient will usually give a history of:**

   A A direct blow to the knee
   B A hyperextension injury
   C OA of the joint previously
   D Pain in the patella tendon

2. **With a valgus force applied to the knee, you would expect to find:**

   A Damage to the lateral collateral ligaments
   B Damage to the medial collateral ligaments
   C Damage to the patella tendon
   D Fractures of the lateral tibial condyle

3. **Doing excessive kneeling could lead to the following conditions:**

   A Haemarthrosis
   B Pre-patellar bursitis
   C Infra-patellar bursitis
   D Discoid meniscus

4. **The anterior cruciate ligament is:**

   A Only damaged by a hyperextension injury
   B Sometimes damaged by a hyperextension injury
   C There to prevent posterior movement of the tibia on the femoral condyles
   D Most often damaged by a rotational force

5. **An effusion into the knee joint:**

   A May produce swelling above the patella
   B May be confirmed using a patella tap test
   C May first show as obliteration of hollows either side of the patella
   D May produce features seen on X-ray

6. **Active straight leg raising:**

   A Tests the extensor mechanism
   B Is impossible following a fractured patella
   C Requires intact peroneal tendons
   D Cannot be done with Osgood Schlatter's disease

7. **Which of the following should always be done when assessing a knee joint?**

   A The patella tap test
   B The McMurray test
   C An examination of the knee on the 'good' side
   D A goniometer reading

8. **A fracture of the neck of the fibula:**

   A May damage the lateral popliteal nerve
   B May damage the common peroneal nerve

    C   May cause a drop foot

    D   May be a Maisonneuve fracture

9.   A fractured patella may be associated with:

    A   Pre-patellar bursitis

    B   Gout

    C   A haemarthrosis

    D   Posterior dislocation of the hip

10.   The capsule of the knee joint:

    A   May form extensions posteriorly called Baker's cysts

    B   Extends upwards about 2 cm above the patella

    C   Contains fat pads below the patella

    D   Contains the menisci

Answers are available at the end of the book. For an explanation of these answers and further resources visit the companion website at:

www.wiley.com/go/bradley/musculoskeletal

The ankle and foot

Aim

To develop an in-depth understanding of the anatomy and physiology, history, examination and early management of minor musculoskeletal injuries and conditions of and around the ankle and foot.

Outcomes

That, by the end of this study, and all the associated activities and clinical experiences, you will be able to:

- demonstrate an in-depth knowledge of the anatomy and physiology of musculoskeletal structures of the ankle and foot
- take an effective history and examine patients presenting with ankle or foot problems, forming a differential diagnosis
- demonstrate an in-depth knowledge of minor musculoskeletal injuries and conditions of the ankle and foot
- apply these skills to the early management of patients, recognising any need for referral.

Section 1
Applied anatomy and physiology

In this final chapter, you are in for a mixture. The ankle is fairly straightforward to appreciate, whereas the foot is a complex '3D' collection of bones and soft tissues. It is very difficult to appreciate the inter-relationships of the foot bones without models in front of you.

Bones

The major parts of the bones that you need to learn now are:

Managing Minor Musculoskeletal Injuries and Conditions, First Edition. David Bradley.
© 2014 John Wiley & Sons, Ltd. Published 2014 by John Wiley & Sons, Ltd.
Companion website: www.wiley.com/go/bradley/musculoskeletal

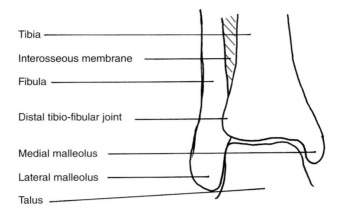

Tibia
Interosseous membrane
Fibula
Distal tibio-fibular joint
Medial malleolus
Lateral malleolus
Talus

Figure 11.1 The bones of the ankle, AP view.

The ankle

- Tibia:
  - Medial malleolus.
  - Articular surface for fibula.
  - Articular surface for talus.
- Fibula:
  - Lateral malleolus.
  - Articular surface for tibia.
  - Articular surface for talus.
- Talus:
  - Articular surface for tibia.
  - Neck.
  - Head.
  - Articular surface for fibula.
  - Articular surface for navicular (*see* Figure 11.1).

The foot

The complexities of the foot are next for you to consider. You need to learn the names of all the bones now; the intricacies of their relationships can come a little later (*see* Figure 11.2).

- Talus.
- Calcaneus.
- Navicular.
- Cuboid.
- Cuneiform:
  - Medial.
  - Intermediate.
  - Lateral.
- Metatarsals (MTs).
- Phalanges.

Activity 11.1   **Time: 15 minutes**

X-rays of the foot and ankle often cause confusion because of three additions that are quite often seen:

1. Sesamoid bones.
2. Accessory bones.
3. Epiphyseal lines.

Do you know of any of these? If so, write a brief note in your book and then continue.

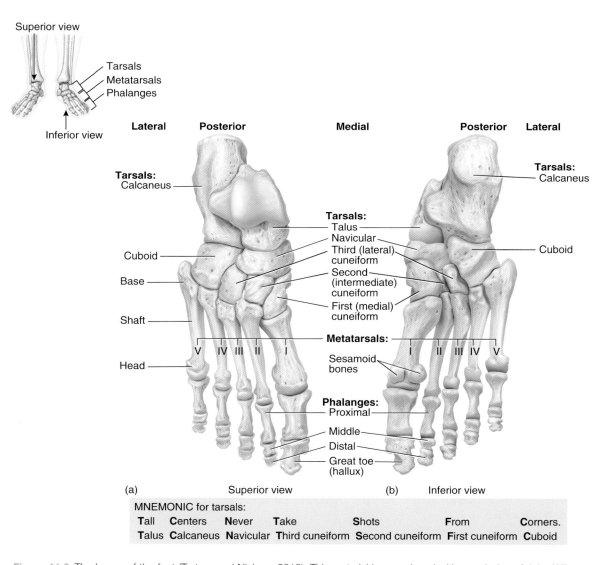

Figure 11.2 The bones of the foot (Tortora and Nielsen, 2012). This material is reproduced with permission of John Wiley & Sons, Inc.

Observations on Activity 11.1

Sesamoid bones

Two sesamoid bones are found in the tendons of flexor hallucis longus (FHL) at the level of the first MTP joint.

Accessory bones

These are quite common in the foot and near to the ankle joint; some are at:

- the base of the fifth MT, **os vasalaneum**
- the posterior talus, **os trigonum**
- the medial border of the navicular, **os tibiale externum**.

Epiphyses

These are at:

- the fifth MT base
- the posterior of the calcaneus
- the distal fibula
- the distal tibia.

Put these names into a search engine now to see several X-rays of them. Examples of some can be seen in the X-ray section of the website associated with this book; use it as a break from just reading. Variation in study methods aids retention.

Joints

The ankle

The ankle is the joint to consider first. It is a mortise formed by the articulation of the talus with the tibia and fibula. Carrying tremendous weight and requiring both stability and flexibility, it is a common site for both minor and major injury.

The surface of the talus that articulates with the tibia is **wider anteriorly than posteriorly**. This has the effect of **tightening and stabilising the mortise when** the foot is **dorsiflexed**, in part explaining why injuries like the sprain occur more commonly when the ankle is in plantar flexion and more lax. (*see* Figure 11.3).

Tibio-fibular syndesmosis

This is the rather grand name given to the slightly moving joint at the lower end of the tibia and fibula, where they are held firmly together by two strong ligaments and the **interosseous membrane**, making the ankle mortise (*see* Figure 11.4).

The ligaments are called:

- anterior inferior tibiofibular
- posterior inferior tibiofibular.

Depending on the exact angle of an anterior-posterior (AP) X-ray, the bones can look just overlapped or the actual joint space can be seen.

Ankle ligaments

The lateral ankle ligament complex must be understood completely, because injuries to it will form a major part of your work (*see* Figures 11.5a and 11.5b).

There are three distinct bands of ligament, listed anterior to posterior:

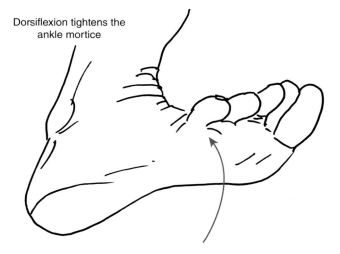

Dorsiflexion tightens the
ankle mortice

Because of the shape of the
articular surface of the talus

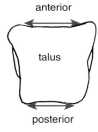

anterior

talus

posterior

Figure 11.3 The ankle mortise, wedge shape and tightening.

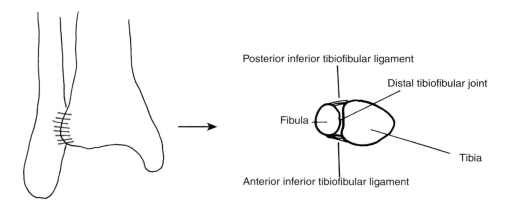

Posterior inferior tibiofibular ligament

Distal tibiofibular joint

Fibula

Tibia

Anterior inferior tibiofibular ligament

Figure 11.4 Tibiofibular syndesmosis.

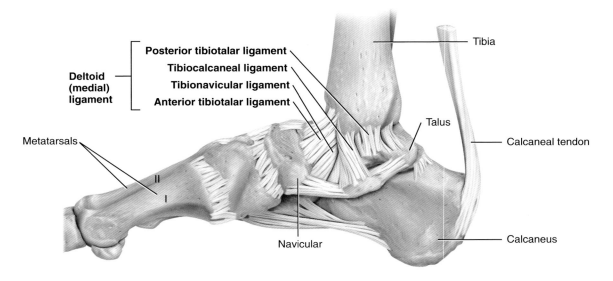

Figure 11.5a Ankle ligaments complex: medial view (Tortora and Nielsen, 2012). This material is reproduced with permission of John Wiley & Sons, Inc.

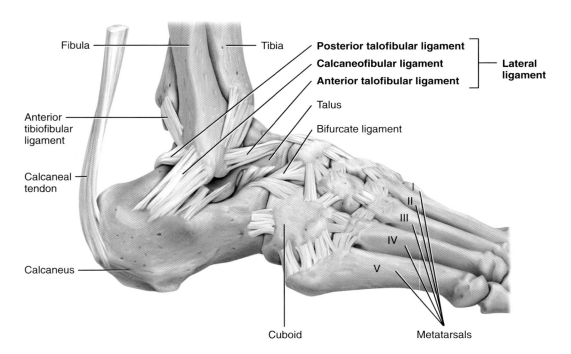

Figure 11.5b Ankle ligaments complex: lateral view (Tortora and Nielsen, 2012). This material is reproduced with permission of John Wiley & Sons, Inc.

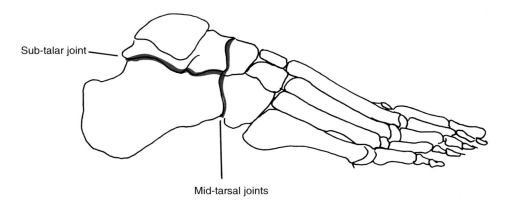

Sub-talar joint

Mid-tarsal joints

Figure 11.6 A lateral view of the right foot, to show the sub-talar and mid-tarsal joints.

1. Anterior talo-fibular (ATFL).
2. Calcaneo-fibular (CFL).
3. Posterior talo-fibular (PTFL).

These ligaments are **quite weak structures** compared with those on the medial side of the joint – a design fault if you wish!

Medially is the deltoid ligament, rarely damaged because of its **superior strength**.

Below the ankle joint, the synovial joints of the tarsal bones are many, some with intricate connections, all supported by ligaments that may be damaged. Tarsal joints are **roughly** grouped as follows:

Sub-talar joint

As the name suggests, this joint is basically between the articular surfaces of the inferior of the talus and the superior surface of the calcaneus. Few even know of its existence, let alone understand anything about it (*see* Figure 11.6).

It is a plane synovial joint allowing some movements of inversion and eversion.

Mid-tarsal joints

These are basically between the talus and navicular medially and between the calcaneus and the cuboid laterally (the talocalcaneonavicular joint and the calcaneocuboid joint) (*see* Figure 11.6).

All the remaining tarsal joints interconnect, so as a whole can be thought of as one joint. There are degrees and mixtures of many movements to be made here:

- Plantar flexion with adduction.
- Dorsiflexion, with abduction.
- Supination and pronation.

The movements of the ankle sub-talar and mid-tarsal joints mentioned earlier can interact considerably with one another.

 Activity 11.2   Time: **60 minutes**

An excellent method of increasing your familiarity with the bones of the foot, if you do not have access to actual bone models, is to draw them. If you are hopeless at drawing, this can be done reasonably simply with the method I showed you with simple shapes in the previous chapter (activity 10.1). Figure 11.7 shows you a rough example, and I would like you to try now.

You can omit this activity, but, if so, don't expect to be able to understand more than the basics about the foot.

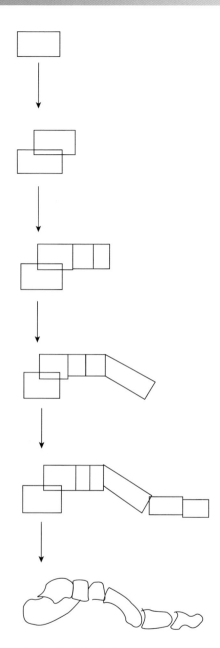

Figure 11.7 An easy way to make a simple sketch of the foot.

Retinaculae

These are found throughout the foot and ankle and are fibrous bands, similar to the retinaculum making the carpal tunnel in the wrist. They hold soft tissues, especially tendons that run through the foot and ankle.

A large and very strong sheet of fibrous tissue, the **plantar fascia (plantar aponeurosis)** supports the longitudinal arch of the foot. Its origin is the anterior surface of the calcaneus (*see* Figure 11.8).

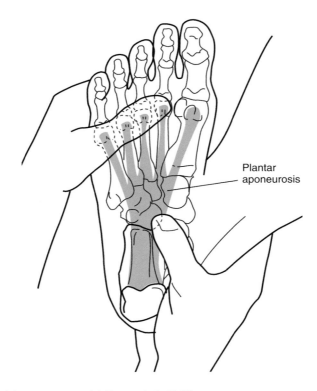

Plantar
aponeurosis

Figure 11.8 Plantar fascia (plantar aponeurosis) (Gross *et al.*, 2009).

Muscles and their tendons

You are not required to learn detail of all the muscles and the positioning of their tendons at this stage of your career
–just those that are most commonly affected. However, as you progress and slowly build on your experience, a working
knowledge of the vast majority will become second nature to you.

Below are the essentials:

Calf

- Gastrocnemius, soleus.
- A thin 'strap-like' muscle, the plantaris.

Lateral foot and ankle

- Peroneus longus.
- Peroneus brevis.

Medial foot and ankle

- Tibialis anterior.
- Tibialis posterior.

Dorsal

- Extensor hallucis longus and brevis (EHL and EHB).
- Extensor digitorum (ED).

Plantar

- Flexor hallucis longus and brevis (FHL and FHB).
- Flexor digitorum longus (FDL).

Section 2
History and mechanism of injury

An ankle sprain

Of all of the mechanisms that you must study and understand in this region, those causing a sprained ankle are the most important for you to have clear in your mind.

There are two forces involved: **inversion of the ankle** and **plantar flexion of the foot**.

With these two features, first the ATFL is placed under stress, followed by the CFL and finally the PTFL (*see* Figure 11.9).

As the weight of the foot comes to be placed on the ground, the toes and metatarsal (MT) heads are the first to come into contact because of plantar flexion. Fractions of a second later, if there is no support for the lateral aspect of the foot coming to the ground (because of an uneven surface), the ankle inverts. This places a tremendous strain initially on the ATFL. Depending on the amount of the force involved, the damage may either stop there or continue sequentially through the CFL and PTFL.

Activities causing this combination of inversion and plantar flexion are almost too numerous to mention, but include the majority of sports and literally anywhere where the foot takes the body weight on an uneven surface (*see* Figure 11.10). The **heavier the patient** is, sadly the **more force** is involved and **more damage** can be expected.

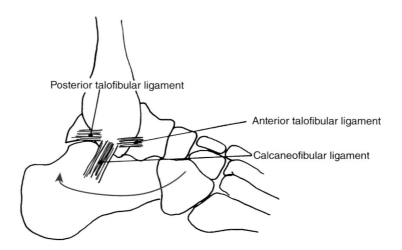

Posterior talofibular ligament

Anterior talofibular ligament

Calcaneofibular ligament

Figure 11.9 The three lateral ankle ligaments failing sequentially. Depending on the force, the ligaments are damaged sequentially from anterior to posterior.

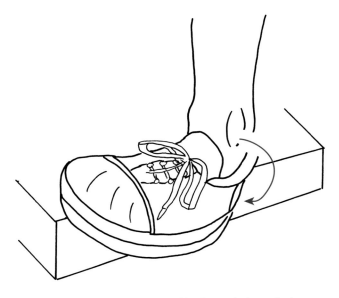

Figure 11.10 The classical mechanism for a sprained ankle: adduction and plantar flexion.

The lateral joint ligaments are almost exclusively affected because they are comparatively flimsy. Sprains of the medial side do occur (following a different mechanism) but, if the force causing the wrench is of any significance, the **ligament is stronger than the bone** and the medial malleolus usually fractures.

A **previous history** of an ankle sprain makes a **subsequent sprain more likely**, so this is an important part of your questioning.

Fractures of the ankle joint **may be fairly trivial**, in effect little more than a sprain. Alternatively, they may have a rather **complex mechanism** of injury, forming **complex patterns** of fracture and, finally, requiring rather **complex management**.

Where does the minor injuries professional fit in with this? Well, because it is pure luck whether twist causes a serious fracture or a trivial sprain, you must understand the basics of various mechanisms and the resulting injuries.

When gathering a history from a patient, there are four points to note about **the force** involved.

 Activity 11.3　　　　　　　　　　　　　　　　　　Time: **10 minutes**

Cover up my observations on this activity.

What are these four major groupings? You have had a similar question earlier in the book, so this should be fairly easy for you.

I want you to write them down in your book before continuing.

Observations on Activity 11.3

1. Strength
   - Is the patient heavy?
   - Was their body weight on one limb?
   - Did the force come from a height?

2. Direction
   - Which way did the ankle twist?
     - Adduction inversion (supination).
     - Abduction eversion (pronation).
     - External (lateral) rotation.
     - Vertical compression, plus plantar or dorsiflexion.
   - Where did the force come from?
3. Strength of the patient's bones and soft tissues
   - Are they young and fit?
   - Or elderly and frail?
   - Has there been a previous injury?
4. Surroundings
   - What surface did they land on?
   - What footwear were they wearing?
   - Was the ground soft or hard?

Effects of forces on the tissues

Vertical compression

This force is from below – for instance, in jumping or pressure through a foot pedal in an RTC. The forces may push the talus into the ankle mortice in one of two ways (see A & B in Figure 11.11) each would damage different parts of the joint.

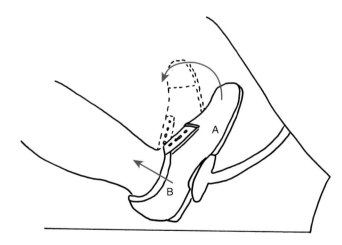

Figure 11.11 Mechanism for a vertical compression force to the ankle in an RTC.

Avulsion

A force that pulls away from a bone is called an **avulsion**. Figure 11.12 is a diagram of the fibula with the following possible effects:

1. No damage.
2. Ligament tears.
3. Flake of bone is avulsed.
4a. A larger horizontal fracture occurs, but remains in position.
4b. Fragment becomes separated.

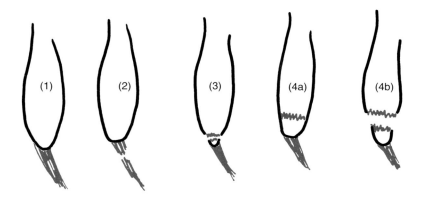

Figure 11.12 Forms of damage caused by an avulsion force – for instance to the lateral malleolus.

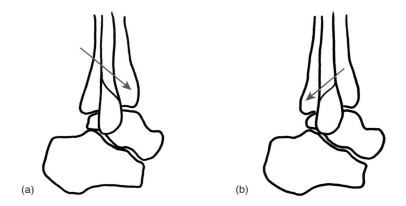

Figure 11.13 Spiral patterns of a fractured fibula: (a) downwards and forwards (b) downwards and backwards.

As well as the fibula, avulsions may also occur at the inferior tibiofibular joint. Rotational or abduction forces applied to this joint may cause the anterior and posterior tibiofibular ligaments to either tear or form an avulsion fracture.

Rotation

This twisting causes oblique or spiral fractures. The direction of the fracture line also shows the direction of the force. For instance, in Figure 11.13a, the fracture line of the fibula **spirals downwards and forwards**. This is **the most common pattern** of ankle fracture and is caused by a supination (inverted)/lateral (external) rotation injury.

In Figure 11.13b the spiral pattern is **downwards and backwards**. This is **far less common** and caused by a lateral (external) rotation injury, with the foot in pronation. You should be able to accurately describe both these patterns to a colleague over the phone.

Shearing

One example is illustrated in Figure 11.14a, where you see the talus pushing against the medial malleolus causing it to be sheared off at an oblique or upright fracture of varying angles. This is contrasted with an avulsion pattern (see Figure 11.14b).

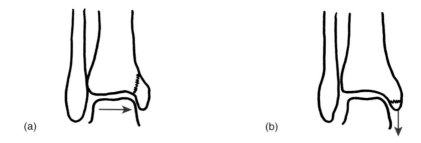

Figure 11.14 Fracture patterns of the medial malleolus: (a) shearing (b) avulsion

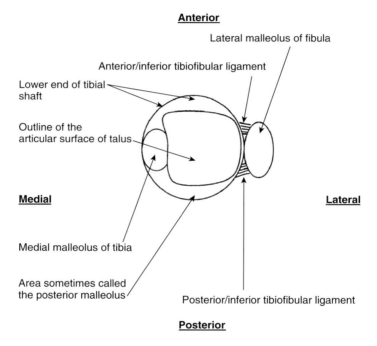

Anterior

Lateral malleolus of fibula

Anterior/inferior tibiofibular ligament

Lower end of tibial shaft

Outline of the articular surface of talus

Medial

Lateral

Medial malleolus of tibia

Area sometimes called the posterior malleolus

Posterior/inferior tibiofibular ligament

Posterior

Figure 11.15a Cross section of the right ankle to show the structures injured with a particular mechanism of injury: for more detailed labelling, see Figures 11.15b, c, d and e.

Eversion/external rotation force

This is the causative mechanism for 'high ankle' sprains.

The recognition of X-ray patterns

There follow details of how common forces cause particular patterns on X-ray.

The associated drawings are based on **cross sections of the right ankle**, at joint level, **viewed from above looking downwards**. The outline of the **articular surface of the talus is superimposed** (*see* Figure 11.15a).

1. External rotation with the foot supinated

This is **by far the most common mechanism**, causing the majority of fractures of the ankle. Like sprains, the structures are damaged in a set sequence as the force reaches them. How far this sequence progresses depends on the very variable factors you have just studied (*see* Figure 11.15b).

2. Abduction with the foot in pronation

Look at the pattern that occurs with abduction (*see* Figure 11.15c).

3. External rotation with the foot pronated

This variation is not very often seen (*see* Figure 11.15d).

4. Adduction with the foot supinated and some internal rotation

You should notice that this is the mechanism for a common sprain of the lateral ligament. However, here the force has been greater and the fibula that the ligament attaches to fractures instead (*see* Figure 11.15e).

All this is quite complex and you should feel no shame if a thorough understanding of the mechanisms and resulting injuries **takes you many weeks**. However, especially if you blend it in with actual patients whom you see, it will soon become clear. Patience, practice and consolidation study will win the day.

 Activity 11.4 **Time: A few minutes**

Before we leave this aspect, do you fully understand what supination and pronation mean when referring to the foot? Think about it briefly before reading the observations.

Observations on Activity 11.4

Pronation and supination of the foot are movements mostly of the sub-talar joint. They can be difficult to appreciate at first, so let me explain a simple way of understanding them that works for me (I presume that you are completely familiar with their use for the forearm).

Place your hands palm downwards (pronated) on a table in front of you. Think of them now as your feet, with you looking down at them. The palms are your soles, the thumbs represent your big toes medially and the little fingers represent your little toes laterally.

Now, just start to turn your palms uppermost (supination). The first few degrees is about the amount of supination that occurs in your feet. They lift up slightly on the insides, the big toe sides.

Similarly, once again with your palms flat on the table (pronated), move them into further pronation by lifting the little finger borders upwards, this corresponds to the pronation seen in the feet.

Both occur only to a tiny degree compared with the forearm, but are still quite noticeable and important.

Fractures of the base of the fifth metatarsal

A very common minor injury and this mechanism should be thoroughly understood. The tendon of the **peroneus brevis** travels posteriorly to the lateral malleolus and then curves anteriorly, inserting into the base of the fifth MT. Any movement that forces the foot into inversion will place a tremendous strain onto the tendon. However, it is very thick and strong, even compared with the bone, and it is usually the bone that fractures instead (*see* Figure 11.16).

 Activity 11.5 **Time: A quick question for you**

Cover up the observations on this activity before you read further.
Where else have you been told of a soft tissue structure that is usually stronger than the nearby bone?

Observations on Activity 11.5

The medial ligament of the ankle usually stays intact, a fracture occurring through the medial malleolus.

External rotation with the foot supinated

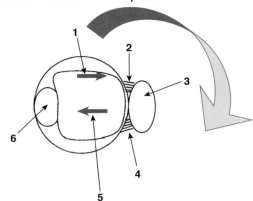

1. The talus externally rotates, pressing against the lateral malleolus.
2. This causes a force to be applied to the anterior tibiofibular ligament which tears, sometimes avulsing some tibial bone with it.
3. As the ATFL gives way, the full force presses onto the fibula itself, causing a spiral or oblique fracture near to the joint (the fracture line runs downwards & forwards).
4. Then if the force is large enough, the posterior TF ligament can either tear, or remain intact and pull off part of the posterior malleolus.
5. If the force continues, the talus may rotate further, pressing against the medial malleolus.
6. Finally, either the medial ligament tears, or the medial malleolus fractures.

Figure 11.15b Mechanism of external rotation with the foot in supination.

Abduction with foot pronated

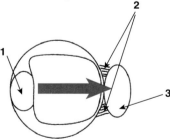

1. The talus is pushed laterally into abduction; this first stresses the medial ligament of the ankle, either tearing it or more commonly avulsing the end of the medial malleolus.
2. With the medial side now free, the talus pushes against the fibula, ripping through both the anterior and posterior tibiofibula ligaments. There is no twisting force here, so the ligaments take the force together. The posterior malleolus is sometimes fractured instead of the PTFL tearing.
3. Finally the fibula itself fractures (horizontally) at the level of the joint.

Figure 11.15c Mechanism of an abduction force with the foot in pronation.

External rotation with the foot pronated

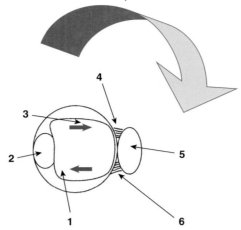

1. The first force is the back of the talus pressing against the medial malleolus as it twists in the mortice.
2. This either tears the medial ligament or causes an oblique fracture of the medial malleolus.
3. Next the talus pushes on the fibula.
4. This either tears the anterior tibiofibular ligament, or avulses bone at its insertion into the tibia (Tillaux fracture).
5. The force continues, producing an oblique or spiral fracture of the fibula above the tibiofibular ligaments (but this time the fracture line is downwards and backwards when viewed from the side).
6. With yet more force, the posterior tibiofibular ligament then tears or avulses some of the posterior malleolus. Because of the site of the fibula fracture, the interosseous membrane is then torn, allowing the fibula to come free from the tibia (diastasis).

Figure 11.15d Mechanism of an external rotation force with the foot pronated.

Adduction with foot supinated and some internal rotation

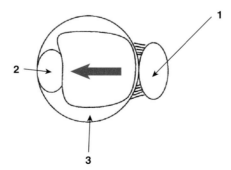

1. The lateral ligament of the ankle joint may be torn, or the lateral malleolus itself may fracture.
2. If the force continues, the talus pushes against the side of the medial malleolus causing an oblique or vertical fracture, quite different from those we have mentioned previously; whereas if it was pulled off (avulsed), it would be horizontal. The deltoid ligament is intact, the malleolus gives way first.
3. A final force to consider here is the associated internal rotation. If this continues it may cause fracture of the posterior malleolus.

Figure 11.15e Mechanism of an adduction force with the foot supinated.

Fall from a height onto the heels

When jumping, we are designed to land first on the toes and distal MT area and then the force is slowly transferred through our arches towards the heel. To land directly on the heels results in there being no chance for 'give'. The force is applied directly to the calcaneus, which may shatter if the forces are powerful enough.

Most people land on two feet at once, so, if you have one suspected calcaneal fracture, examination of the other heel is essential.

Activity 11.6   Time: 15 minutes

Consider a patient jumping and landing heavily on both heels. The calcanei may or may not be fractured, but where else could the forces continue to cause fractures? Write your comments for possible fracture sites.

Observations on Activity 11.6

This is sometimes famously called the '**Don Juan syndrome'**, named after the rogue who seduced the wives of others and escaped by jumping out of the bedroom window as the husbands returned!

Of course everything depends on the exact angles of the forces involved, the type of ground landed on and the strength of the bones and other tissues involved. But as a rule the force travels up either or both **tibiae** and the **vertebral column**. Once landed, people obviously fall over, putting one or both hands out to save themselves. From that they may get either a single or bilateral Colles fracture. Quite a list isn't it? But it illustrates how important a knowledge of the mechanism of injury can be (*see* Figure 11.17). What at first sight may seem to be a comparatively minor fracture of the heel may be one of multiple injuries; always get the detail.

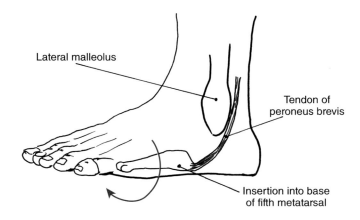

Figure 11.16 Mechanism of injury for a fractured fifth MT.

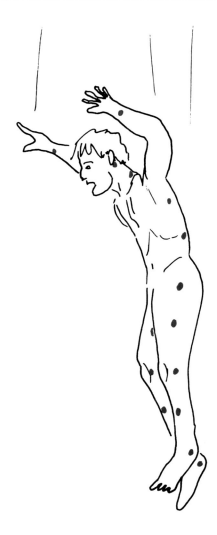

The force of landing on the heels
may carry straight up the body fracturing:

Heels
Tibiae
Knees
Femurs
Acetabulum
Vertebrae
Base of skull
Wrists

Figure 11.17 Don Juan syndrome.

Foot on car pedal

If your patient has been involved in a traffic collision, there is one situation that I would like you to remember. Drivers usually have their feet, or at least the right foot, on a pedal at the time of impact. Depending on the amount of force involved, it is common to have a significant force travel up the pedal into the foot. This could cause considerable bruising and minor fractures, through to severe injuries such as a comminuted fracture of the calcaneus, or the talus could be forced into the lower surface of the tibia causing a fracture running upwards. A great deal depends on how the force is distributed by the exact position of the foot on the pedal.

March fracture

The neck of the second or third MTs are common places to get stress fractures, with the patient presenting with a sudden pain at the site, of unknown cause.

Sesamoid fracture

Yes! Even these tiny bones can fracture. It should be considered following a direct impact, possibly jumping with some hyperextension.

Direct blow to toes

Perhaps the most common fractures of the feet are caused by objects dropping on the toes, or toes getting 'stubbed'. These are common mechanisms in both work, DIY and play. At work, the majority of instances are minimised or completely avoided by 'health and safety' use of footwear with reinforced toecaps, but DIY and play give your departments ample opportunity to practise their skills.

With the above in mind, take every opportunity to pass on gems of accident prevention to your patients and their relatives. It is simply not good enough for us to manage what has occurred. We must constantly analyse the accidents, or start of the condition, and advise our patients to minimise the chances of a repetition.

Common conditions

Pain in the sole of the foot

Listen to this classical presentation. Your patient tells you that when getting out of bed in the morning, as they put weight on their foot they get a severe pain and this pain is always worse first thing. As they start walking about for a while, the acute pain settles a little, but as the day progresses the pain worsens again and they are glad to get their weight off it at bedtime.

Remember this presentation: it is characteristic of **plantar fasciitis**, a very common condition of the sole of the foot that is discussed later.

Women's shoes

Sadly, from their youth, many women have forced their feet into the most amazing shoes. In many instances, the result is crippling deformity with the following:

- Hallux valgus.
- Painful bunions.
- Hammer toes.
- Crossed toes.
- Calluses.

In reality it is their choice, but fashion and peer pressure 'push' them in that direction. This is an area where your health education skills could be exercised. There is no time like a painful time to attempt to get a message over that may save the patient so much pain and discomfort in the future.

Gout

I would like you to consider this condition with any instance of sudden onset of severe joint pain and swelling; sometimes there is a previous history.

Swelling

Anything that causes swelling of the foot and/or ankle area – for instance:

- Tendinitis.
- Causes of inflammation.
- Localised swelling following an injury (bleeding and oedema).
- Scar tissue formation.
- Generalised or gravitational oedema.
- Bony deformity.
- Swellings such as cysts, ganglia, etc.

All have the possibility to increase the pressure and/or cause friction inside the tarsal tunnel, causing **tarsal tunnel syndrome**. Well worth your consideration.

Peroneal tendons

The tendons of the peroneus longus and brevis pass around the lateral malleolus of the ankle. They are held in place by some of the **retinacular fibres**, seen in many places in the foot, holding such structures.

Forced dorsiflexion and eversion of the foot and ankle may tear the retinaculum allowing the tendons to partially or completely slip out of the small **peroneal groove** in the fibula, resulting in pain and discomfort at the site.

 Activity 11.7 **Time: A quick question**

First, cover up the observations on this activity.
 What may the patient come to you saying?

Observations on Activity 11.7

The patient may just come to you saying that they have sprained their ankle, or even a colleague thinking that it is a recurrent 'sprain', the true diagnosis having been missed.

Section 3
Patient examination

Don't approach an examination of the ankle with tunnel vision, just looking for an ankle injury or condition. If you do, you may find an ankle condition, but **nothing else**.

Approach your patient from the MOI/history angle; then injuries or conditions are unlikely to be missed. Classical examples here are an ankle injury also causing a fracture at the **proximal** end of the fibula, and fractures of the heel associated with vertebral and other fractures distant to the site. Now on with the routine.

Observation

Compare both sides for swellings. Subtle swellings are most easily seen as the filling in of hollows in the tissues –for instance, around the malleoli – or not being able to see the extensor tendons on the dorsum of the foot. Ensure that it isn't oedema of both ankles from a 'general' cause.

Look for:

- a firm bony prominence that can sometimes develop over time (an **exostosis**)
- a tense cystic swelling near tendons (a **ganglion**)
- **callus** formation on the sole, at areas of excessive pressure
- fungal infections of the nails or athlete's foot
- bruising
- the pad of fat under the heels, which can hide bleeding – the bruising showing only more distally.

Also notice gait – how your patient walks from the waiting room.

 Activity 11.8   **Time: A few minutes**

Before you complete this small section, don't miss a final revision of the general observation list after Activity 3.7 in Chapter 3; it should be second nature to you now.

Movements

First, see the range of active movements that the patient can make. If in a lot of pain, they may be too apprehensive to move without assistance from you.

If necessary, the following may then be attempted:

- Plantarflexion.
- Dorsiflexion.
- Inversion.
- Eversion.
- Adduction.
- Abduction.
- Circumduction.
- Finally, flexion and extension of all the toes, but especially the big toe.

Forced dorsiflexion of the foot, Homan's sign (*see* Figure 11.18), should be gently attempted with any of your patients who complain of calf pain, tenderness or swelling. It will cause severe pain if a DVT is present. Never centre just on the foot or ankle: a DVT may mimic a lower leg injury or other musculoskeletal condition.

Palpation

As in previous chapters, once you have completed palpation of your own feet, you are advised to initially choose a thin friend or family member to palpate. This allows you to recognise many of the soft tissues against the bony skeleton and will give you confidence before attempting more difficult builds or those with swelling.

 Activity 11.9   **Time: Many hours of practice**

I am not going to individually go through instructions for palpation of major structures in the foot and ankle. But in the observations I list those that I want you to become familiar with initially. Take each in turn and practise until you feel sure and, if not, revert to a mentor.

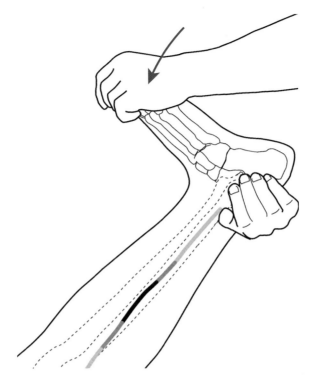

Figure 11.18 Homan's sign, stretching the deep veins of the calf (Gross *et al*., 2009).

Observations on Activity 11.9

The following should be found:

- Medial malleolus.
- Lateral malleolus.
- Body of calcaneum.
- Sustentaculum tali.
- Achilles tendon.
- Soft heel pad.
- Base of fifth MT. This is a good starting place to determine the other tarsal bones.
- Heads of MTs.
- Extensor tendons and shafts of MTs.
- All phalanges.
- Origins and insertions of all three lateral ligaments.
- Medial ligament.
- Laterally: peroneus longus (posterior), peroneus brevis (more anterior).
- Medially: tibialis anterior (in front of tibia) and posterior (behind medial malleolus).

Specifically with children and adolescents, it is important to palpate over the position of the epiphyseal plates of the lower tibia and fibula. These are relatively weak areas that often fail before an associated distal ligament, giving **Salter-Harris** type injuries (*see* Figure 11.19).

On dorsum of foot

Feel for the pulse of the **dorsalis pedis** artery.

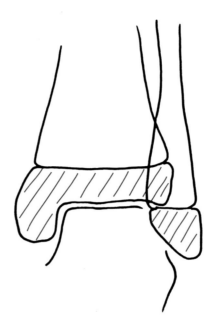

Figure 11.19 Epiphyseal plates at the ankle.

Seemingly minor injuries associated with high sprains and **Maisonneuve** fractures can sometimes have severe tearing of the **interosseous membrane** associated with a great deal of bleeding. Compartmentalisation of the lower leg sometimes means that compartment syndrome may occur, so this test of the pulse and the circulation to the foot in general is an essential routine for you to cultivate.

Palpate for the tendons of:

- extensor hallucis longus
- extensor digitorum longus.

Ottawa ankle rules

This is a set of very useful rules to help you make a decision as to the need for your patient to have an ankle or foot X-ray to exclude a fracture. They have widespread acceptance throughout the world (Stiell *et.al.*, 1992).

However, there is little completely 'black and white' in this world and I'm sure some practitioners still have their own very adequate local rules that you must accept.

In the past, many hundreds of thousands of pounds was spent on unnecessary ankle X-rays, without any research behind the decision.

 Activity 11.10   Time: **A few minutes**

Write in your notebook, or on the line below, what you think the cost of an AP and lateral X-ray view of an ankle will cost the NHS.

£ _____

Now, the next time you pass an X-ray department, ask them for an estimate; you will get a shock. It was costly in my clinical days, so must be worse now.

That is the financial story, but it is not all. The inconvenience and time involved is another aspect for discussion.

Now for the rules themselves. They do not apply to all patients; groups excluded are:

- pregnant women (dangers of radiation)
- those unable to understand the questioning (drunk, head injuries, the very young, confused and elderly).

Activity 11.11   **Time: About 30 minutes**

I would like you to have a change of scene now and go back to your computer. Go onto your search engine, find YouTube and type in 'Ottawa ankle rules'. There are many quite short, good videos for you to watch with excellent illustrations of the examination process.

As you read further, I have listed the basics for you.

Ankle X-rays are required if, following injury, there is any pain in the malleolar zone plus any **one** of the following:

- Bone tenderness, in the posterior, distal 6 cm, or tip of the medial malleolus.
- Bone tenderness, in the posterior, distal 6 cm, or tip of the lateral malleolus.
- The patient cannot weight bear for four steps, immediately following the injury, or in the A&E.

Foot X-rays are required if, following injury, there is pain in the midfoot zone plus any **one** of the following:

- Bone tenderness at the base of fifth MT.
- Bone tenderness over the navicular bone.
- The patient cannot weight bear for four steps, immediately following the injury or in the A&E.

Activity 11.12   **Time: 15 minutes**

Here is one final search for you that may point to the future. I want you to look up in your search engine 'Tuning fork ankle fractures'. Very interesting!

Squeeze test

Something very different: let us look at the '**high ankle sprain**'. This is a very simple and useful test to perform. The patient sits with the knee bent and the lower leg hanging. The leg just at the lower calf is grasped with two hands encircling and gently but firmly squeezed. This will stress the **tibiofibular syndesmosis** causing pain if the ligaments have been injured –the so-called 'high sprain'.

Examination of the Achilles tendon

Have your patient face down on a couch with their feet free over the edge. In this position any gap in the tendon may be palpated, although swelling frequently hides this by the time they seek your help, making palpation difficult for the less experienced.

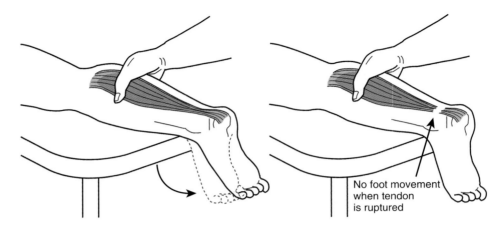

Figure 11.20 Thompson/Simmonds test (Gross *et al.*, 2009).

The position most vulnerable to a tear is approximately 4 cm proximal to the insertion into the calcaneum.

There is one specific test to decide if the tendon is completely torn, but it is confusing because it has two names: the **Thompson** or **Simmonds test**. What should happen with an intact tendon is that, if you squeeze the calf firmly, the tendon pulls on the calcaneum and the foot plantarflexes slightly. If the tendon is torn, the foot remains motionless (*see* Figure 11.20).

With this test and the others you have covered in this chapter, be sure to sign them off in the listing of examination points in Checklist 11.1.

Section 4
Minor musculoskeletal injuries

The ankle sprain

There are three groupings of sprains of the ankle:

1. Lateral.
2. Medial.
3. High ankle sprain of the tibiofibular syndesmosis.

The sprain considered here is of the commonly injured **lateral** ligament complex of the ankle. In previous sections, the anatomy, MOI and examination have already been considered. Much of the advice also applies to the far less commonly seen medial ankle sprains.

There is a fair amount of detail here, but much of it will be applicable to other foot and ankle injuries, so it is not wasted. I will start with a useful practical activity for any new practitioner.

 Activity 11.13   **Time: 15 minutes only**

Cover up my observations and then read on.
    You decide that your patient has a sprained ankle. What words would you choose to tell them the diagnosis? Write them down now.

Checklist 11.1 Record of progress
Physical examination of the ankle and foot

Examination	On self	Friend practice	Friend practice	Patient practice
Patient history, a variety				
Observation:				
Palpation:				
Medial malleolus				
Lateral malleolus				
Base 5th metatarsal				
Lateral ligament				
Medial ligament				
Achilles				
Body of calcaneum				
Sustentaculum				
Metatarsal heads and shafts				
All tarsals				
Range of movement:				
Plantarflexion				
Dorsiflexion				
Inversion				
Eversion				
Adduction				
Abduction				
Circumduction				
Toes flexion and extension				
Sensations:				
Foot- dermatomes				
Circulation:				
Dorsalis pedis				
Specific tests:				
Ottawa rules				
Thompson				
Other:				
Squeeze test				

Observations on Activity 11.13

You need to take care with your terminology, especially when talking to your patient. Most will understand what a fracture is. However, the same cannot be said with regard to a sprain. This means very different things to different people and certainly leads to confusion. Consider the following:

- Sprain.
- Torn ligament.
- Rupture (complete or partial).
- Strain.

If you use any of these, go on to explain in simple terms what you mean. For instance, 'You have sprained your ankle; some of the ligament fibres that hold the joint together on the outside have been torn through. . .'

A golden rule for this could be:

> **GOLDEN RULE**
>
> Informing the patient, so that they clearly understand what is going on, is just as important as other aspects of their management.

This is never more so than when **not** X-raying the limb. This clarity can also have an effect on the your esteem of and that of your Trust.

Let me explain: the tiny word 'only' can upset some patients. Picture this scenario: a patient with a sprained ankle, limping and in quite a lot of pain. In an attempt to reassure them, you say something like, 'Don't worry, it may be painful, but it's **only** a sprain. . .' Their interpretation of this comment may be that you are trivialising their condition, so later on they go elsewhere. At the next department they say, 'They never even X-rayed it, just said it was a sprain, so I thought it best to come to you.'

To most members of the public, it is logical and straightforward to expect an X-ray following a painful ankle injury. They know nothing of Ottawa rules, tuning forks and runaway film costs (Welling, 2011). So, it is a vital part of your management to explain your reasoning clearly. You will not 'win' with everyone, but the practitioner who takes time to get a patient's trust by good explanation is indeed clever.

Paediatric considerations

The medial and lateral ligaments of the ankle are distal to the epiphyseal plates of the distal tibia and fibula. These plates are fairly weak structures and are increasingly likely to be damaged instead of the ligaments, making sprains less common in young children and teenagers.

Classification systems

Grade 1

This is the most common form of ankle sprain, consisting of a complete or partial tear of the ATF ligament, the joint remaining stable. Revise your anatomy now for a few minutes to be sure that the positioning of the parts of the lateral ligament are clear in your mind (*see* Figure 11.21a).

Grade 2

A less common form of sprain. This is a more extensive version of Grade 1, with damage to both the ATF and the CF ligaments, usually with some later joint instability (*see* Figure 11.21b).

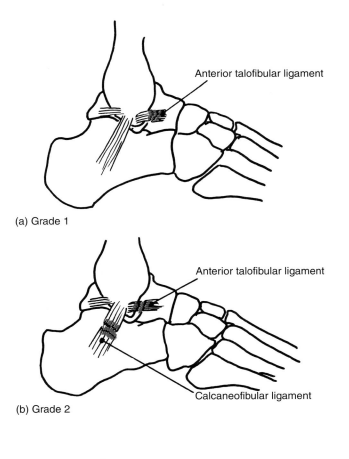

(a) Grade 1

(b) Grade 2

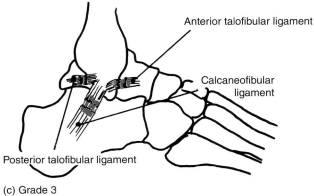

(c) Grade 3

Figure 11.21 A grading system for lateral sprains of the ankle: (a) Grade 1, damage to the ATFL (b) Grade 2, damage to the ATFL and CFL (c) Grade 3, damage to the ATFL, CFL and PTFL

Grade 3

The uncommon complete tear of all three ligaments (ATFL, CFL and PTFL); the joint will therefore be unstable (*see* Figure 11.21c).

Management

Because a sprained ankle can have such variable features, ranging from the patient with minor swelling and scarcely a limp, through to the person with a 'ballooned' ankle in intense pain, so the management will vary. Here I will take the 'middle road', the patient with a painful, swollen but stable ankle, unable to weight bear.

The long-tried and tested acronym RICE:

* **Rest.**
* **Ice.**
* **Compression.**
* **Elevation.**

These are still the basis for patient management in the acute stage. However, other things that are not part of the acronym –**analgesia** and later **exercise** – are also essentials. Let us go through each of these now and add a little detail.

Rest and support

It is not enough to simply say, 'You must rest the joint.' Rest means different things to different patients. Rest is fine and sensible in the early stages of the injury. Helping the micro-circulation to clot prevents further tearing of the delicate injured tissues and eases pain.

Exactly how a patient rests varies tremendously with their **role** in life, their form of **work**, their **support network**, what is **important to them** at the time and, importantly, the degree of physical **support you have applied to their injured ankle**.

For example, oh the joy for a husband office worker, who gets paid when sick, has a wife at home and nothing socially urgent! He can manage resting at home, sitting on a settee watching TV for a couple of days and having everything done for him.

Contrast that with a single mum, bringing up a toddler on her own and shopping daily for basic foods. Rest to her could be hobbling around in pain doing the same as usual.

Note how the patient's circumstances will sometimes dictate the form of support you apply. Even for a grade 1 injury, the first example may be only requiring some form of elasticated support, whereas the single mum may need a form of brace or boot just to survive.

The question of weight bearing also comes under this title of rest. With minor sprains, full weight bearing for essentials can be allowed from the start, whereas, as the grading worsens, partial or supported weight bearing will be necessary. A grade 3 injury is too severe to be detailed in a book like this, but initial management would be non-weight bearing until assessed by orthopaedics.

Ice

Cooling the injured area is next to consider. The vaso-constriction will minimise bleeding and help modify the inflammatory process, but patients will vary with regard to the amount of cold discomfort they will tolerate. Chemical cold packs are freely available for a patient's home use, but are rather costly. More readily available are bags of frozen vegetables, left on the part (over the top of bandages or other supports, not directly against the skin) for approximately half an hour, then replaced to cool again in the freezer.

By the way, I am no food expert, but common sense will tell you that food out of the freezer, thawed and refrozen a few times will not be suitable for eating (worth a mention)!

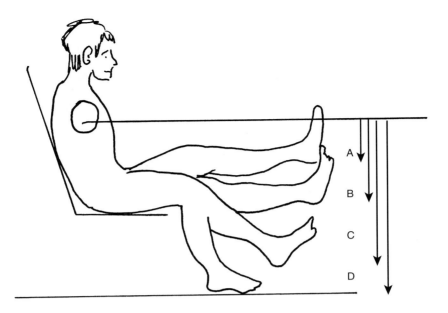

Figure 11.22 Foot elevation.

Compression

The hydrostatic pressure of the tissue fluid in the injured part will be increased by some form of compression support. This will minimise the production of swelling and hasten its removal.

Elevation

With elevation, both blood and lymphatic fluid drain easily from the areas of higher to lower pressure. Elevation is such a simple but effective way of easing both pain and swelling. However, it is often done half-heartedly; if elevation is substantial, it can often eliminate the need for analgesia completely by the following day (*see* Figure 11.22).

Analgesia

Sometimes patients only think of using analgesics like paracetamol for a headache, and may need reminding of their use for this and other musculoskeletal pains. Always ask carefully regarding possible intolerances to suggested NSAIDs; gastric problems alone are common.

Exercise

Elevation good, compression good, but you also have to spell out to most patients that the foot should not just lie there for 24 to 48 hours like a lump of lead. That is a sure way to start the muscles wasting. These are the same muscles that will be essential for a fast return to normal function in the coming weeks.

So to start with, every time the adverts come on the TV, ask the patient to wriggle their toes as a very minimum. Depending on the form of support given to the ankle and the limits of comfort, they should also try putting the whole of the foot and ankle through a gentle range of movements. Exercise will help to prevent muscle wasting and go a long way to 'pump' the venous return, easing swelling and therefore pain. It is quite satisfactory for the patient to mobilise themselves, if you feel that they will go about it properly and without additional physiotherapy (Higgins, 2001; Shaw, 2005).

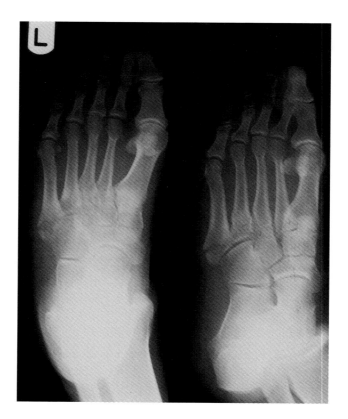

Figure 11.23 Fifth MT fracture.

Fractured base of fifth metatarsal

This is a very common fracture indeed and often talked of by the patient as a 'sprained ankle'. Because of this, it is important that you get into the routine of always palpating the fifth base with any ankle or foot injury.

The most common is a transverse **avulsion fracture**, pulled off by the **peroneus brevis** during pronation (*see* Figure 11.16). Near the proximal tip of the base, the fracture line will pass through the joint with the cuboid (*see* Figure 11.23), but if the fracture is more distally situated it will enter the joint with the base of the fourth MT. Further views and pointers may be seen on the book's website.

Another variation is the so-called '**Jones fracture**', which is even more distal at the metaphysis/diaphysis junction.

When looking at X-rays, take care not to mistake the longitudinal epiphyseal line or the tiny accessory bone sometimes found nearby (**os vesalianum**).

Because there is usually no displacement of note, the initial management of a simple avulsion fracture varies from gentle support bandaging to a brace or plaster (Martin, 2001). Much depends on the patient's pain and requirements. The amount of weight bearing will also vary.

Stress fracture of metatarsals

This fracture is usually caused by the bone being stressed over time. Most of the body weight initially transfers down the medial side of the foot. Because of this, the first MT is very strong, but the next in line, **the second and third, are**

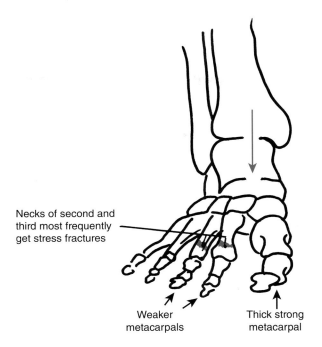

Necks of second and third most frequently get stress fractures

Weaker metacarpals

Thick strong metacarpal

Figure 11.24 Stress fractures of the MTs.

often frail in comparison and sometimes give way under frequently repeated weight bearing, especially if the person is not used to it. Another name for the condition, '**march fracture**', gained popularity in World War II when many conscripts suddenly had to spend their days marching, running and jumping (*see* Figure 11.24).

The third MT is the most commonly affected. There is no direct history of an injury, just recent overuse. It presents with pain and tenderness at the fracture site in the sole of the foot, made worse by weight bearing.

Initially the diagnosis should be clinical, because there may be nothing to see on X-ray until callus starts to form. Explain this to your patient, so that they don't consider you negligent, and manage and advise them from the start as though a fracture were there.

Fractures and dislocations of the toes

When talking about toes, don't confuse minor injuries with small bones. Certainly none of your patients will die with a toe injury, but, small as the bones may be, these fractures can be very painful and often result in loss of earnings.

Despite the difficulty because of size, thoroughly examine the digits, palpating the toes and assessing joint movements. X-ray will not always be necessary if the fracture is considered to be simple and with no or minimal displacement.

Clinical features are obvious and not to be repeated here. But there is one observation that I would pass on to you. If you find that your patient has an **ecchymosis** of the toe, a **blood blister** or **subungual haematoma**, a fracture is often present.

If the fracture is **simple and undisplaced**, a standard management is to use the neighbouring digit as a support by padding between and using a form of strapping. Care has to be taken with several points here. First, especially if an ecchymosis or blistering is present, the skin will be very fragile. Try to avoid placing any adhesive directly onto the injured skin; all will be fine as the patient leaves you, but the skin can rapidly break down. Second, if they have come to you quite rapidly following the injury, there will be much more swelling to be expected, whereas if the visit is the following day the swelling will probably be at its maximum already.

With more than minimal **displacement**, a ring block and manipulation will probably be required. Traction alone, sometimes with a helping manipulation from a finger or thumb, will usually result in an acceptable position.

A subungual haematoma associated with an underlying fracture should be drained if the skin and nail are intact. This is because of the severe pain that will otherwise last for days. Local protocols may ask for antibiotics afterwards because the fracture is effectively being made compound. Similarly, all effort should be made to save a nail overlying a fracture, because it acts as protection.

Finally, stress the additional points that assist a trouble-free recovery. Elevate the whole limb at every opportunity, cut the toe area out of an old slipper to ease pressure, advise walking mostly on the opposite side of the foot to the injury, spreading the weight load with a stick if necessary. Advise the fairly free use of some simple analgesics in the first 24 hours.

Achilles tendon injuries

A rupture of the Achilles tendon is common and usually caused by a pure overloading injury; but there are also degenerative, overuse and pharmacological mechanisms that can cause rupture as well. The site of the damage is usually a few centimetres above the insertion into the calcaneus, and may be partial or complete.

 Activity 11.14   Time: **A quick question for clarity**

Can you remember which muscles use the Achilles to insert into the calcaneum?

Observations on Activity 11.14

The soleus and the gastrocnemius use the Achilles. The tendon of the **plantaris** (a thin weak strap-like muscle) usually remains intact because it inserts separately, deep to the Achilles.

Achilles rupture occurs, as with so many musculoskeletal conditions, in either a sports context where frequent extreme exertion is required by a younger age group, or, at the other extreme, with older people whose soft tissues are often degenerating. Danger factors are:

- sports people
- older people
- a previous tear or tendinitis of the Achilles
- the patient taking long-term **steroids** or
- the patient on the **quinolone group of antibiotics** (ciprofloxacin).

Having said all that, it could easily be you or I, just walking down the street and not on any drugs. Much in life is a lottery.

The pain is so sudden and unexpected that the patient sometimes feels that someone has kicked them in the back of the leg. Often a 'pop' is heard, as with an ACL rupture. Specific examination has been detailed previously in section 3.

Management may be operative. However, with partial ruptures and those who are more (shall we say?) 'sedentary', the ankle is held in a brace, initially in equinus, for many weeks. Some feel that re-rupture rates are minimised by initial operative repair (Gilpin, 2003).

Lisfranc fracture

This term refers to an important group of serious fracture dislocations at the **tarso-metatarsal joints** (the joint itself is called the '**lisfranc joint**' by some). The injuries range from those with fairly minimal displacement, difficult to notice on X-ray, to widespread disruption.

Because of the ligament structure, any fracture near the base of the second MT should alert you to the possibility of this Lisfranc injury.

These are major injuries and frequently misdiagnosed. They are mentioned here so that you are aware and can quickly refer any patients you are not 100% sure of.

Get into a routine of checking the alignment of the bones in this area on foot X-rays; details are provided for you on the book's website.

Compartment syndrome

Here, yet another very major condition, mentioned to you because it may sometimes present as something minor – a patient walking in with a tense swollen leg.

All the soft tissues in the calf are sectioned off, **subdivided into compartments** (*see* Figure 11.25a). This is all very well until a blunt injury occurs, bursting several small blood vessels. Over time, sometimes hours or occasionally days, **a haematoma develops inside one of the compartments**. If the compartments have remained intact, the **pressure of this blood steadily rises** until it equals the pressure of the blood in the arteries of the leg. Obviously, when this occurs, **blood flow stops** (*see* Figure 11.25b).

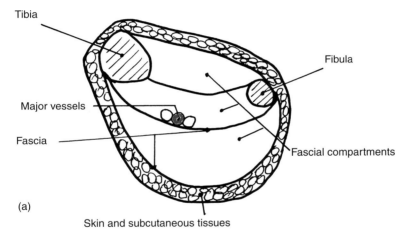

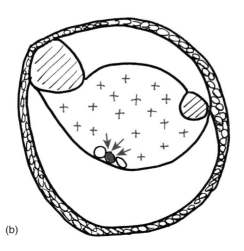

Figure 11.25 Cross section of the mid-calf: (a) the normal and (b) in compartment syndrome.

What you have to do is recognise the possibility of this happening and treat the patient as an **orthopaedic emergency** the moment you see them. If you have never seen this condition before and are in doubt, just refer immediately: take no risk.

Management is by opening the leg up in theatre, cutting through the fascia forming the compartment and releasing the pressure. The first time I saw this done in theatre, I was staggered at the amount of blood clot released.

Section 5
Minor musculoskeletal conditions

Footballer's ankle

In this overuse condition, there is pain, tenderness and inflammation of the tissues in the front of the ankle. The tendons and ligaments become impinged, trapped between the tibia and the talus (*see* Figure 11.26a). Sometimes a **bony spur** occurs accelerating the problem.

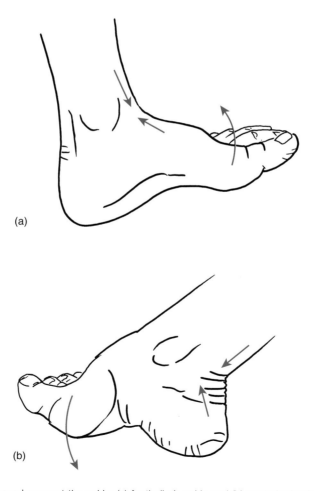

(a)

(b)

Figure 11.26 Impingement syndromes at the ankle: (a) footballer's ankle and (b) posterior impingement.

Although commonly called 'footballer's ankle', this impingement is not confined to this sport: it can occur in any cases of frequent and extreme dorsiflexion.

A similar type of impingement syndrome can occur in the posterior of the ankle (*see* Figure 11.26b).

Gout

This is a disorder of **purine metabolism**. It results in the formation of **uric acid crystals inside joints** causing severe inflammation. This form of arthritis, which commonly starts in the first MTP joint, is possible in any joint.

Rumour has it that it occurs most commonly in those who overindulge alcohol and 'the high life', but this is not the truth. The reality is that sugar-enriched drinks, excessive beer and red meat do predispose to the condition, but no more. It is more frequent in males and those aged over 60.

Flat-foot deformity (Pes planus)

This is a series of conditions in which there is loss, or non-appearance, of the medial arches of the foot (*see* Figure 11.27).

These arches only form throughout early childhood. If worrying a patient or their parents at any age, referral is best. Although reassurance is all that is needed in many instances, the causes and associated conditions are many and sometimes complex.

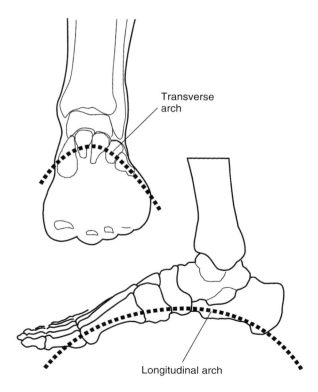

Figure 11.27 The arches of the foot (Gross *et al.*, 2009).

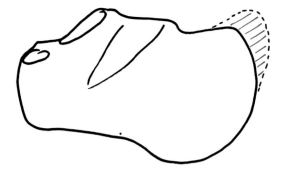

Figure 11.28 Haglund's deformity of the heel. The black outline of the calcaneum is the normal; the shaded area is what occurs with a Haglund deformity.

Haglund's deformity

In this condition, the posterior of the calcaneum is enlarged and prominent, causing discomfort at the back of the heel and making it very difficult to get well-fitting shoes. It can lead to irritation and inflammation of the local bursae, tendinitis of the Achilles and excessive production of hard and thickened callous (*see* Figure 11.28).

Shin splints (medial tibial stress syndrome)

Not quite the ankle, but low down in the leg! 'Shin splints' is a rather poor but common term used for pains in the anterior medial aspect of the lower legs near the tibiae.

It has an insidious onset of activity-related leg pain.

It is the **most common cause of chronic leg pain in runners**, but can occur in other activities in the general population.

There is a 'tibial periostitis' due to stress at the junction between muscle and bone. Figure 11.29 shows where tibialis anterior and posterior attach to the tibia in the anterior compartments.

Symptoms decrease as runners warm up. It is worse in the morning and after exercise.

Intermittent claudication

This is very different from the medial tibial stress syndrome, but something that should be considered especially in **smokers**. Classically, the middle-aged to elderly patient develops pain as they walk in one or both calves, and this eases rapidly as they rest.

A careful history is vitally important for a correct diagnosis.

Sever's disease

This is an apophysitis of the posterior epiphysis of the calcaneum. In effect, the continued pull on the epiphysis causes inflammation and fragmentation (which sometimes shows on X-ray). It affects pre-teenagers, especially those who are more athletic in their pursuits. It is to be considered if you see a painful tender posterior heel, not following an injury.

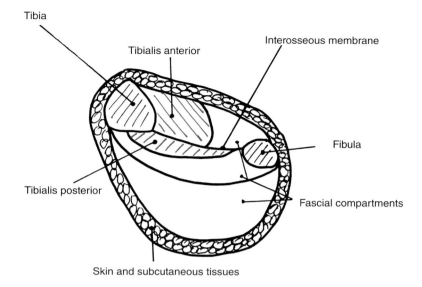

Figure 11.29 The muscles mostly affected by 'shin splints'.

Kohler's disease (navicular osteochondritis/osis)

This is a condition seen mostly with boys, in early school years. It starts with pain and tenderness over the area of the navicular, and limping develops. An X-ray of this condition can be seen on the book's website.

Plantar fasciitis

This very common chronic condition, affecting the origin of the strong plantar fascia to the calcaneum, is often associated with a **calcaneal spur**. Learn more about this on the book's website. However, it is not quite as clear-cut as the spur causing the irritation. Rather it is what comes first, the chicken or the egg? Damage to the periosteum causes the formation of the spur, which may worsen the situation, although the spur can be found in asymptomatic individuals.

This fasciitis can occur in two groups; first, the **young athlete** overdoing things, and, second, the **older person whose tissues start to degenerate** and easily become inflamed with little more than normal wear and tear.

The pain of fasciitis centres around the heel while weight bearing and can be severe. It is not uncommon for both heels to be involved.

The condition usually responds to some of the following:

- Analgesics and anti-inflammatory drugs.
- Rest.
- Physio treatments.
- Pads to minimise weight bearing to the area of a spur.
- Orthotics.
- Exercises.

Hallux rigidus

This is simply a rather grand name for OA of the first MTP joint; say no more.

Hallux valgus; metatarsus primus varus; bunions; hammer toes; crossed toes

All these conditions are very common and related to one another. Although with some feet there is more to consider regarding the anatomy, a simple sequence of events is set out here. All the conditions are far more common in women, but men are also affected.

Women's feet are frequently, and for prolonged periods, forced into wedge-shaped shoes and high heels. Over the years, increasing bony deformities develop. The first MT starts to point medially (**metatarsus primus varus**). The great toe angles away from the midline (called **hallux valgus**), overlapping the second and other toes. The first MTP joint develops OA (called '**hallux rigidus**'), a bursa and thickened inflamed bony (**exostosis**), and soft tissues develop over the medial aspect of the first MTP joint (**a bunion**).

These deformities are rare in cultures that do not use footwear. So it would be wrong to say that poor shoes are the direct cause, but they certainly are a very major precipitating factor to someone who is susceptible.

Sesamoiditis

These are tiny, insignificant bones at the first MTP joints, but they are **easily inflamed by overuse** and the use of high heels, which concentrate pressure in places not designed to take such stress (*see* Figure 11.30).

The patient has tenderness on deep palpation over the position of the sesamoids, near the MT head.

Ingrowing toe nail

An ingrowing toe nail (IGTN) is very painful, very common and often ignored in the early stages, until only surgical management can offer relief.

The cause is excessive pressure on the nail fold, usually of the great toe. The soft tissues of one or both sides are pushed against the nail. This irritates, inflames and infects the tissues with a degree of **granuloma formation**.

Primary causes range from the poor cutting of the nails to nail deformities. However, an overriding factor in the majority of instances is tight-fitting socks and shoes actively pushing the tissues together.

Morton's metatarsalgia or neuroma

If there is slowly increasing pressure on a nerve, it may sometimes become irritated and start to swell. In this condition, usually the **small nerve between the third and fourth MT shaft** becomes compressed and a fusiform swelling occurs (*see* Figure 11.31). This is called a 'Morton's neuroma' or 'Morton's metatarsalgia'. It is considerably more common in women, leading to the belief that the abnormal position of the structures following the use of high-heeled shoes is a factor in its development.

Clinical features include severe pain and parasthesiae in the sole of the foot centred around the area. The symptoms are worsened by weight bearing, compression of the MTs and tight-fitting shoes, but eased with rest.

Freiberg's disease

This condition usually affects the **second MT head**. It is a form of **osteochondrosis** and the precise cause is unknown. Pain, swelling and tenderness occur locally in teenage athletes and should alert the professional to the possibility of referral.

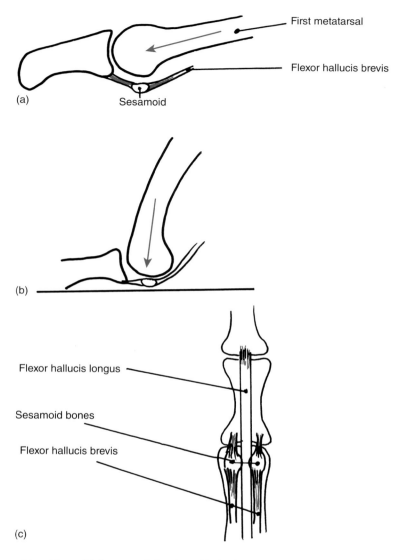

First metatarsal

Flexor hallucis brevis

(a)

Sesamoid

(b)

Flexor hallucis longus

Sesamoid bones

Flexor hallucis brevis

(c)

Figure 11.30 Sesamoid problems: (a) the normal situation with the foot on the flat (b) concentrated pressure with high heels (c) the inferior view showing the tendon system, with the sesamoids in FHB.

Bursitis

There are two bursae that cause problems in the foot: one superficial (calcaneal bursa [*see* Figure 11.32]) and one deep (retrocalcaneal bursa) to the Achilles tendon at the heel.

The superficial (posterior calcaneal) is the more frequently affected, being easily rubbed by ill-fitting shoes. Careful palpation should discriminate between the two.

Initial simple management is based around rest, anti-inflammatory drugs, elevation and attention to footwear.

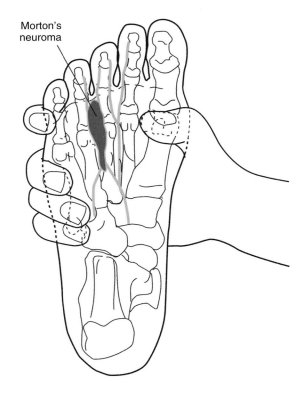

Figure 11.31 Morton's metatarsalgia (Gross *et al.*, (2009).

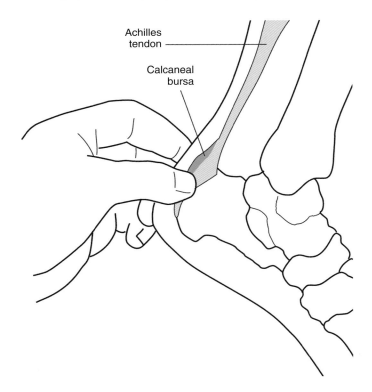

Figure 11.32 Calcaneal bursa (Gross *et al.*, 2009).

Exostosis

There are several places throughout the foot where outgrowths of bone occur called 'exostoses'. These also **occur throughout the body**, but are often hardly noticed. However, feet carry tremendous weight and are enclosed, so outgrowths are quickly noticeable. They may cause pain and sometimes need removal.

Osteochondritis dissecans of talus

This is typically associated with a history of a previous acute sprain or repetitive twisting trauma.

The condition is thought to initially occur because of a tiny chip fracture to the lateral border of the articular surface of the talus. This damages the blood supply to the fragment and a small part of surface of talus softens and breaks off through cartilage and bone underneath.

Tarsal tunnel syndrome

The main problem with any tunnel system (tarsal and carpal) is that any **swelling inside can cause acute compression** of structures passing through. The main structure in this instance is the **posterior tibial nerve**, which travels through the tunnel, behind the medial malleolus on its journey to the sole (*see* Figure 11.33).

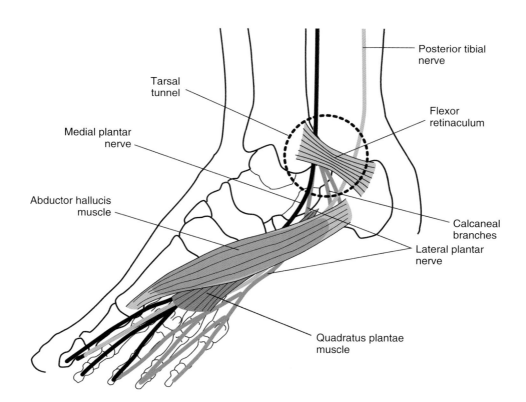

Figure 11.33 The tarsal tunnel (Gross *et al.*, 2009).

If you are still unsure of the anatomy, re-read the first section of this chapter; there is no shame in doing this. Until you see a person with this condition, it is very difficult to tie in the theory.

Clinical features include pain, pins and needles or numbness in the distribution of the nerve in the sole of the foot.

Possible causes have been mentioned in the section 1 of this chapter, but in many instances the cause is obscure. If you are suspicious, your patient will need advice and referral.

Diabetes and the foot

This chapter would not be complete if a special mention was not made of diabetes. With known diabetic patients, **the foot is a danger zone**. Simple conditions that would be trivial to you or me, such as traumatic wounds, ulcers, ingrowing toenails, sores, pressure from shoes, corns, etc. all need to be **carefully monitored in the diabetic** patient with frequent podiatry visits.

Not only are lesions **far more likely to become infected**, but diabetic neuropathy means that the **patient can easily be unaware** that they are developing problems.

Of even more importance are patients with undiagnosed diabetes. Here it is vital that you remain suspicious of lesions that are acting out of character; **vigilance could mean that you are the first to make the connection that leads to the diagnosis**.

 Activity 11.15　　　　　　　　　　　　　　　**Time: A couple of hours**

Here is a list of ankle and foot conditions that need studying at some time in the future, for completeness. However, for the time being, concentrate on the conditions detailed in this book.

- Septic arthritis.
- Osteomyelitis.
- Tumours.
- Bone cysts.
- Club foot.
- Plantar warts.
- Athlete's foot.

REFERENCES AND SUGGESTED READING

Gilpin, T. (2003) Operative Repair is best for an Acutely Ruptured Achilles Tendon, www.bestbets.org (accessed 24 May 2013).

Gross, J.M., Fetto, J. and Rosen, E. (2009) *Musculoskeletal Examination*, 3rd edn, Wiley Blackwell, Oxford.

Higgins, G. (2001) Lateral Ligament Ankle Sprains should be Mobilised Early, www.bestbets.org (accessed 24 May 2013).

Martin, B. (2001) Support Bandage is Best for an Avulsion Fracture of the Base of the Fifth Metatarsal, www.bestbets.org (accessed 24 May 2013).

Shaw, J. (2005) Physiotherapy in Acute Lateral Ligament Sprains of the Ankle, www.bestbets.org (accessed 24 May 2013).

Stiell, I.G., Greenberg, G.H., McKnight, R.D., *et al.* (1992) A study to develop clinical decision rules for the use of radiography in acute ankle injuries. *Annals of Emergency Medicine*, 21 (4), 384–390.

Stiell, I.G., Greenberg, G.H., McKnight, R.D., *et al.* (1993) Decision rules for the use of radiography in acute ankle injuries. *Journal of the American Medical Association*, 269 (9), 1127–1132.

Stiell, I.G., McKnight, R.D., Greenberg, G.H., *et al.* (1994) Implementation of the Ottawa ankle rules. *Journal of the American Medical Association*, 271 (11), 827–832.

Tortora, G.J. and Nielsen, M.T. (2012) *Principles of Human Anatomy*, 12th edn, Wiley Blackwell, Oxford.

Welling, A. (2011) 006 Tuning fork testing on ankle injuries: does it improve the accuracy of the Ottawa ankle rules. *Emergency Medicine Journal*, 28, A2–A3.

Multiple choice questions

Before you start, take in the reasoning behind these MCQs, how to answer them and how to interpret the results, from the section at the end of Chapter 1.

1. **The tarsal tunnel consists of:**

    A A sheet of retinaculum on the lateral border of the foot

    B A hollow above the sustentaculum tali

    C A sheet of fibrous tissue above the posterior tibial nerve

    D A sheet of flexor retinaculum between the tibia and the calcaneum

2. **The peroneal tendons:**

    A Lie in a groove in the fibula

    B Insert into the base of the fifth MT

    C Sometimes slip from behind the fibula, if the holding retinaculum is torn

    D Help to invert the foot

3. **Impingement can occur to the soft tissues of the ankle, but:**

    A It only occurs in the anterior of the joint

    B It may be associated with synovitis of the joint capsule

    C It can be worse if an os trigonum is present

    D Ballet dancers may get it because of extreme plantar flexion

4. **In the commonly seen sprained ankle:**

    A The MOI is pronation and inversion

    B The posterior tibiofibular ligament is the first to tear

    C The anterior tibiofibular ligament is not affected

    D The Ottawa ankle rules should always be applied

5. **Plantar fasciitis:**

    A Is caused by a spur of bone developing on the calcaneum

    B Causes tenderness centred around the first and second MT heads

    C Can occur in both heels simultaneously

    D Affects the origin of the palmar apponeurosis at the calcaneum

6. **A rupture of the Achilles tendon:**

    A Usually occurs 1 cm above its insertion into the calcaneum

    B Is sometimes associated with taking steroids and/or ciprofloxacin

    C Always requires operative repair

    D May be suspected by the patient's inability to stand on their toes

7. **The very common fracture at the base of the fifth MT is:**

    A Usually caused by an avulsion mechanism

    B Called a Jones fracture

    C Horizontal and involves one of two joint surfaces

    D Sometimes confused with an epiphysis.

8. **The second MT bone:**

    A   Is a common site for a stress fracture
    B   Is the site of Freiberg's disease
    C   Could be involved in a lisfranc injury
    D   Articulates with the medial cuneiform

9. **A fracture of the medial malleolus:**

    A   Will usually occur before the deltoid ligament ruptures
    B   Often requires open reduction because of soft tissue interposition
    C   Is a common site for osteomyelitis
    D   Has its own epiphysis

10. **The condition commonly called 'shin splints' is:**

    A   Most commonly seen in athletes, rather than the general population
    B   Also termed 'fibular stress syndrome'
    C   May be anterior or posterior
    D   Basically an overuse condition

Answers are available at the end of the book. For an explanation of these answers and further resources visit the companion website at:

www.wiley.com/go/bradley/musculoskeletal

Answers to multiple choice questions

Detailed explanation of these answers can be found on the website for this book.

Chapter 1

1. BD
2. AB
3. ABCD
4. ABCD
5. BCD
6. ACD

Chapter 2

1. ABC
2. BC
3. B
4. ACD
5. ABCD
6. None
7. BC
8. C
9. ABCD
10. AB

Chapter 3

1. B
2. ABD
3. CD
4. C
5. D
6. A
7. B

Managing Minor Musculoskeletal Injuries and Conditions, First Edition. David Bradley.
© 2014 John Wiley & Sons, Ltd. Published 2014 by John Wiley & Sons, Ltd.
Companion website: www.wiley.com/go/bradley/musculoskeletal

8. ABC
9. AB
10. BCD

Chapter 4

1. ACD
2. ABCD
3. C
4. BCD
5. C
6. B
7. B
8. D
9. B
10. C

Chapter 5

1. ABD
2. BD
3. ABD
4. BC
5. C
6. CD
7. ABCD
8. BC
9. ABCD
10. B

Chapter 6

1. ABC
2. D
3. B
4. C
5. BC
6. CD
7. BD
8. CD
9. ACD
10. ABCD

Chapter 7

1. B, C
2. CD
3. BD
4. ABCD

5. AC
6. B
7. ABC
8. AB
9. D
10. AC

Chapter 8

1. ABC
2. BC
3. B
4. BC
5. ABD
6. AD
7. CD
8. None
9. BC
10. AD

Chapter 9

1. AC
2. CD
3. ACD
4. B
5. None
6. ABC
7. BD
8. D
9. A
10. CD

Chapter 10

1. None
2. BD
3. BC
4. BD
5. ABCD
6. A
7. C
8. ABCD
9. CD
10. ABD

Chapter 11

1. CD
2. AC

3. BCD
4. C
5. C
6. BD
7. ACD
8. ABC
9. AB
10. ACD

 Full explanation of the answers can be found on the Wiley companion website at:

www.wiley.com/go/bradley/musculoskeletal

Index

Key

Bold: most likely place to start your search.
'*see website*': refers to the official Wiley Blackwell website associated with this book: www.wiley.com/go/bradley/musculoskeletal.
The particular resource on the website that should be looked at follows in roman, e.g.: '*see website* X-rays' refers to the PowerPoint slides of X-rays hosted on the companion website.